W9-BBD-896

The Heath Handbook

Langdon Elsbree
Claremont McKenna College

Gerald P. Mulderig
Newcomb College, Tulane University

The

Heath

Handbook

Eleventh Edition

D.C. Heath and Company
Lexington, Massachusetts   Toronto

Acknowledgments

Emily Dickinson, "This quiet Dust was Gentlemen and Ladies." From *The Complete Poems of Emily Dickinson,* edited by Thomas H. Johnson. Copyright 1914, 1942 by Martha Dickinson Bianchi. By permission of Little, Brown and Company. Excerpt from "Tell all the Truth but tell it slant," reprinted by permission of the publisher from *The Poems of Emily Dickinson,* Thomas H. Johnson, editor. Cambridge: Harvard University Press © 1951, 1955, 1979, 1983 by the President and Fellows of Harvard College.

Ogden Nash, "Reflections on Ice-Breaking." From *Verses From 1929 On* by Ogden Nash. Copyright 1930 by Ogden Nash. First appeared in *The New Yorker.* By permission of Little, Brown and Company.

Wallace Stevens, excerpt from "Thirteen Ways of Looking at a Blackbird." From *The Collected Poems of Wallace Stevens.* Copyright 1923 and renewed 1951 by Wallace Stevens. Reprinted by permission of Alfred A. Knopf, Inc.

Acquisitions Editor: Paul Smith

Developmental Editor: Holt Johnson

Production Editor: Holt Johnson

Designer: Victor A. Curran

Production Coordinator: Michael O'Dea

Text Permissions Editor: Margaret Roll

Preface

This eleventh edition of *The Heath Handbook* is a comprehensive guide to writing, combining all the contents of a traditional handbook with a modern rhetorical perspective and an organization that regards writing as a *process*. In the long history of *The Heath Handbook,* reaching back to 1907, this edition has been one of the most completely rethought and revised. During revision, the collaboration between the authors and the editors has been particularly close, from the initial planning through the various stages of the text's preparation. And the assistance from colleagues and reviewers has been especially helpful, whether the questions involved minor details or guiding principles. While working with the contributions of so many others, we have retained the proven materials from previous editions and added new material to make this the most complete edition of the *Handbook.* Like earlier editions, this one presupposes that writing is a craft based on knowable principles and conventions. Our aim throughout has been the traditional one for this text—its usefulness for students and teachers.

Additions to the eleventh edition include the following:

1. A new introductory section on discovery ("prewriting"), featuring new chapters on analyzing one's audience of readers, developing one's voice as a writer, and understanding the four forms of discourse (description, narration, exposition, argumentation). The result, we believe, is a more rhetorically oriented text that reflects contemporary developments in the teaching of writing.
2. A new section on revising, including individual chapters on revising diction, sentences, paragraphs, and the essay as a whole. This section stresses the major challenges in revision—the reworking of phrasing, organization, and logic for greater clarity, economy, and depth.
3. A largely new chapter on sentence style, concentrating on some basic strategies by which writers can make their sentences more fluent and powerful.
4. A new chapter on writing about literature, including an analysis of the assumptions students often make about literature that inhibit full response and clear thinking, some key questions and techniques students can employ

to discover meaning and form, and an illustrative essay on the patterns of imagery in poems.

5. A new section on special writing tasks, including fresh chapters on writing business letters, applications, and résumés, and an expanded section on writing essay examinations.

In addition to these new features, this edition of the *Handbook* has been significantly rearranged and expanded. These changes include the following:

1. A complete reorganization of the book's contents, to reflect the three major phases of the composing process—discovery, writing, and revising.
2. A completely revised chapter on exploring ideas for writing, including extensive illustration of three methods of discovery—brainstorming, free writing, and systematic questioning.
3. Complete revised chapters on paragraph structure and development, featuring new samples of student writing.
4. Expansion of the treatment of sound reasoning into two chapters for greater clarity. The first chapter covers premises, key assumptions, and the distinction between fact and judgment, and includes a new section on believability and tone. The second chapter discusses basic errors in reasoning and incorporates new material and illustrations.
5. A completely revised section on the research paper, including greatly expanded coverage of periodical indexes; material on computerized database searches; a new, clearly illustrated section on plagiarism and acceptable paraphrase; and a thorough explanation of ways to incorporate quotation and paraphrase into one's own writing. The section also presents a complete review of the new Modern Language Association system of documentation and features two sample student research papers—the first on a general topic, "Recovery from the Florence Flood: A Masterpiece of Restoration," and the second on a literary subject, "Anne Bradstreet's Homespun Cloth: The First American Poems"—each with extensive commentary.
6. Revisions and additions in the Glossary of Usage to delete outdated entries and to include new items and in the listing of Grammatical Terms to be more comprehensive.

While making these substantial additions and changes, we have also preserved the time-tested strengths of earlier editions which users have found especially helpful. These include, among other features, the frequent and varied use of student essays, paragraphs, and sentences; the separate chapters on spelling, punctuation, and mechanics for easy reference; and the exercises within and at the end of chapters for further practice.

Whether major or minor, revision usually depends on the assistance and criticism of others. We continue to be grateful to colleagues, students, and reviewers who helped with earlier editions. We are deeply indebted to our editors, Holt Johnson and Paul Smith of D. C. Heath, for their contributions during all stages of writing. We wish to thank Robert Fossum, Michael Riley, and Nicholas Warner of Claremont McKenna College for their valuable suggestions for and criticisms of Chapter 18, "Writing About Literature," and James V. Catano of Tulane University for his careful reading of Section I, "Discovery." We are especially pleased to acknowledge the detailed, precise, and very full critiques we received from the following readers:

Paul G. Bator, California State University, Chico
Barbara Carson, University of Georgia
Charles R. Duke, Utah State University
Theresa Enos, Southern Methodist University
Thomas L. Franke, Lansing Community College
Ernest C. Giordani, Broome Community College
Philip Keith, St. Cloud State University
Edward A. Kline, University of Notre Dame
Paul Mitchell, Pan American University
Samuel D. Watson, Jr., University of North Carolina at Charlotte

Finally, we wish to thank Ron Butters of Duke University, not only for his comments on the entire manuscript but also for his significant contributions to Chapter 11.

L.E.
G.P.M.

Contents

Part IV   *Critical Reading and Thinking*

Part VIII **Punctuation, Spelling, Mechanics**

Part I

Discovery

1 Reasons for Writing

It may surprise you to know, as you begin this book on writing, that no less a person than Plato had serious doubts about the value of learning to write. More than 2400 years ago, the Greek philosopher argued in one of his works on rhetoric that a person's education is better served by oral discussion and debate than by writing. Unlike a speaker or teacher, a printed book cannot answer its readers' questions, nor can it in turn pose questions to make sure that the readers have correctly understood what they have read. Those who become dependent on the written word, according to Plato, will gradually lose their powers of memory and the ability to think on their own. Believing their knowledge greater than it actually is, they will become conceited and complacent, a burden rather than an asset to their society.

Plato's attack on writing and reading reflects his belief that a better way of arriving at truth was through the process of careful and precise questioning, a process that he learned from his own famous teacher, Socrates. Still, we cannot overlook the fact that while Plato may have doubted writing's value, he nonetheless chose to express those doubts in writing. If he had not, his ideas would probably be unknown today. Plato's written attack on writing suggests in a paradoxical way the inevitability of written communication in the exchange and transmission of ideas. Even today, the telephone, the broadcast media, and sophisticated computer networks have not eliminated the need for clear and effective writing; on the contrary, our world would be unimaginable without the written word. People write, quite simply, because they must. At home, in school, at work, we live in a world of writing tasks ranging from the note casually jotted in a friend's birthday card to the job application letter painstakingly revised and meticulously typed.

1a Why write?

For the moment, though, let us suppose that writing was not an inevitable part of our daily lives, that it was instead an activity which we could choose to engage in or not, as we wished. What value could we assign to writing under these circumstances?

In the first place, writing brings us into contact with language in a special way, demanding that we examine the words we use in communicating with others, observe the effects of those words, and make choices among them. Consider, for example, the different implications of the following alternative ways of expressing similar ideas:

The office was left unlocked because of an oversight on my part.	I forgot to lock the office.
Jim is a devoted supporter of the President.	Jim is a fanatical supporter of the President.
The socialization process of post-pubescent youth may be inhibited by excessive solitary interaction with computers.	Teenagers who spend most of their time with computers may have trouble getting along with people.

The patterns of our language are inevitable reflections of our patterns of thought and our perspectives on the world; with our linguistic choices, therefore, we define a place for ourselves in our society. No wonder that skill with language has been the cornerstone of Western education for 2500 years. When we write, we not only participate in one of the world's oldest intellectual traditions, but also develop our linguistic and cultural awareness.

Writing offers us opportunities to increase our intellectual awareness as well. It brings us to a fuller understanding of our ideas by forcing us to give those ideas concrete form. As an activity that is at the same time deliberate and intuitive, the writing process necessarily involves both reflection and inspiration. It naturally leads us into a kind of internal dialogue with ourselves as we search for the words and sentences that will best capture our elusive thoughts. Unlike an impromptu debate over a late-night pizza, a written argument focuses attention on the quality of our ideas and the reasonableness of our arguments; the logical leaps that pass unnoticed in conversation show up in writing as glaring fallacies. Because it demands such precision, the very act of writing is a means of discovering and refining our ideas about any subject.

Writing not only leads us to the discovery of new ideas, but also offers opportunities for discovery of the self. When we commit ourselves in writing to an idea, a perspective, a belief, or an argument, we also come to understand ourselves better. Bound up with the intellectual growth that always accompanies serious writing is the personal growth that comes from taking a firm position on an issue, from choosing to see the world in one way rather than another. The commitment that is part of every important writing act forces us to come to terms with what we really believe, with who we really are.

1b The communication triangle

Beyond these general reasons for writing, every individual writing act naturally has an immediate purpose as well. We write out directions across town in order to be helpful to a visitor. We write a letter to a distant friend in order to reaffirm and preserve our friendship. We write a research paper to acquire knowledge about a subject and at the same time, no doubt, to satisfy the requirements of a course.

But the concept of "purpose" in writing involves something more complex than these examples suggest. When we speak of purpose in this other sense, we mean writing as an act that occurs in relation to a set of elements often called the **communication triangle**:

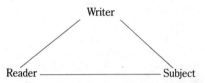

It would be difficult to imagine any act of writing that did not involve these three components. In the first place, virtually all writing is addressed to an audience of some sort; even a private journal has at least a single reader, for what writer of a journal does not go back and read entries written weeks, months, or even years before? Obviously, every act of writing also involves a subject, simple or complex, familiar or unfamiliar. And linking writer, reader, and subject is the written text itself, whether in the form of a letter, an essay, a memo, a novel, or a poem.

These elements, the set of circumstances that surround us in any writing situation, vary endlessly and thus demand endless adaptability from us as writers. When our audience changes, so must the style and content of our writing; no one would use the same language to address an intimate friend and a senior business colleague. Our approach to writing also changes when our subject or our closeness to the subject changes. The familiar tone of an autobiographical essay differs from the more formal tone of a research paper partly because of a writer's different relationship with the material in each case. Finally, our writing changes as the form in which we write changes. Letters of application, for example, require that we follow conventions different from those that govern the writing of sonnets or of term papers. Purpose in writing, then, means awareness of the ways in which changes in the communication triangle call for corresponding changes in the content, style, tone, and form of what we write.

Much of this book is based on the elements of the communication triangle. The remainder of this first section will be devoted to the concept of audience and its relation to the writing process, to the nature of a writer's "voice," and to a consideration of some methods of exploring a subject before you begin to write. Later chapters will examine many of the forms that good writing takes—clear paragraphs, well-organized essays, substantial research papers, and effective business letters, to name just a few. Throughout the book, however, you should remember that subject, audience, form, and purpose are interrelated, inseparable elements. Experienced writers keep all these considerations in mind whenever they write.

Exercise 1

Make a list of the last five writing tasks you completed, including everything from casual notes to formal papers. Who was the audience in each case? What was your primary purpose in writing?

Exercise 2

Imagine each of the five pieces of writing listed in Exercise 1 addressed to a different audience. How might you have changed your handling of the subject? How might you have altered your writing style?

2 Considering Your Audience

The term **rhetoric** has long been associated with the concept of persuasion. The politician seeking the votes of his constituents is practicing rhetoric, as is the courtroom attorney arguing for her client's innocence. But rhetoric may also refer more broadly to the use of language in order to produce any effect—pity, anger, euphoria, contempt—in an audience of hearers or readers. If we think of rhetoric in this larger sense, we can see that virtually every act of human communication contains a rhetorical element. We may not spend our days asking for votes or pleading for the lives of clients, but at the very least we usually want the people around us to believe that we are worth listening to. Inspiring that belief in our friends and associates is itself a rhetorical act, no matter what our topic of conversation may be.

2a The rhetorical situation

The relationship between your audience and yourself—whether in conversation or in writing—is called the **rhetorical situation.** In spoken dialogue, you can see whether or not other people understand what you are saying, whether they approve, when they object. The case is much different when you write. Alone with your thoughts and your typewriter, you can only imagine how readers will react to what you write. Whenever you pause to think about the best arguments to use or to consider how a sentence will sound to your readers, you are demonstrating your sensitivity to the rhetorical situation in which you find yourself.

Good writers are able to alter their writing to suit widely different audiences and rhetorical situations. All of us, in fact, make similar adjustments of tone and style every day. If you are explaining a bridge to a small child, you don't use the vocabulary of a structural engineer. If you are showing a visitor through the research labs on your campus, you don't use the familiar tone that is suitable with close friends or family members. If you are embroiled in a heated debate, you don't use arguments that you know will only antagonize your opponent. The person who is sincerely trying to communicate, rather than merely to impress or confound, makes every effort to find language appropriate to the audience.

In a writing course, students are often directed to consider others in the class as their audience. In most business and professional writing, however, your readers will not be as familiar to you as your fellow students are. Being able to cope with writing tasks in the real world—with application letters and office reports, for example—will demand that you be able to adapt to the specific rhetorical situations involved. And such adaptation will require that you know how to analyze your audiences and how to approach them in writing.

2b Analyzing audiences

Many beginning writers like to think that they are writing for the "general reader." In fact, such a person doesn't actually exist. No subject, after all, can realistically be said to interest all people, or even most people. If you think carefully about any paper you have written, you will realize that no matter how broad its appeal, you can imagine readers for whom it would be inappropriate or simply uninteresting. Even the members of your composition class—the audience you may consider most like yourself—come from differing geographical areas, ethnic and religious backgrounds, and family situations, and those differences may profoundly affect their reactions to what you write.

Once you recognize that your audience is never people in general, but always a particular selection from humanity, you must consider ways of identifying and understanding that audience, for only if you understand the disposition of your readers can you write effectively for them. Every complex argument has several sides, and no single approach will satisfy all possible audiences. Do your readers already understand your subject, or must you provide background information? Do they already share your beliefs, or must you persuade them to see your subject as you do? The answers to such basic questions will necessarily affect the content and tone of your writing.

Some writers try to visualize an individual member of the audience they are addressing. But this strategy will not be of much value if you lack specific knowledge about your audience. Instead, you might try posing a series of specific questions about your readers. Such questions, like those below, take some of the guesswork out of understanding your audience.

Audience's background

What do I know about my audience's

1. age?
2. social status?
3. level of education?
4. political positions?
5. moral beliefs?

Audience's relation to subject and writer

1. What does my audience already know about this subject?
2. What else do I want my audience to know?

3. What do I want this audience to think of me as a person?
4. What evidence/arguments will be convincing to this audience?

Not all of these questions will be relevant in every case. Their purpose is simply to provide a systematic way of examining audiences and rhetorical situations, a checklist of key items to consider whenever you approach a writing task. Of course, as you answer these questions, you must decide how your answers will affect the writing you are about to do.

In the audience analysis below, note how one student's use of these questions leads him to a fuller understanding both of his audience and of his purpose. In this case, the student has decided to write a letter to be published in his college newspaper about damage to furnishings in the college library. Should such a letter be directed to the students responsible for the damage, or to the rest of the students on campus, the indirect victims of the vandalism? The writer's analysis of these two audiences helps him decide which one to address.

Audience's background

1. Age
   All students on campus approximately my age—vandals act younger than they are—socially immature?
2. Social status
   Most students from middle-class backgrounds—about a third have part-time jobs—some paying entire college tuition without help from parents.
3. Level of education
   Academically speaking, same as mine—but what about social education, i.e., respecting other people's property and rights?
4. Political positions
   Not relevant.
5. Moral beliefs
   Wrecking furniture a kind of stealing: steals from college, which must pay to replace damaged items—steals from other students, who are deprived of good study conditions—do vandals see matter this way, as a moral issue?—probably not—if they do, then little apparent sense of guilt.

Audience's relation to subject and writer

1. *What does my audience already know about this subject?*
   Students who use the library to study know about extent of damage to chairs, couches, and study carrels—other students may not know about issue at all—vandals know what has been done *and* who's responsible.
2. *What else do I want my audience to know?*

If audience is student body at large, I want them to know the seriousness of the problem, and to know that there are students like me who are angry, who feel that something should be done to stop vandalism—if audience is vandals, I want them to know that there are students who oppose their actions—which approach will be more effective in stopping vandalism?—which audience should I address?

3. *What do I want this audience to think of me as a person?*
   Reasonable?—or outraged?—is it possible to be sympathetic to vandals?—or should I appear angry?—is *any* approach going to matter if my audience is the vandals themselves?—do they care what I think?—probably not.

4. *What evidence/arguments will be convincing to this audience?*
   If audience is vandals, could try to appeal to their respect for others' rights—but do they have any respect?—can I expect to change such people's actions by a single letter?—better possibility: try to persuade other students that vandalism can be stopped if students mobilize against it—examples from other campuses available?—also, present vandalism as an attack on their rights—their tuition pays for damage—vandals are stealing from them—no one is more directly concerned than students themselves—their responsibility to take action.

By systematically examining his two possible audiences—the vandals and their victims—this writer was able to define both his audience and his purpose more clearly. The vandals, he gradually realized, represented an audience whose actions he could not possibly hope to affect with a single letter to the college newspaper. On the other hand, such a letter might be able to mobilize the majority of the student body against the few who were guilty of the destruction.

As this example suggests, you must understand your readers before you have completely defined your subject, since the audience you choose to address inevitably affects the content of your writing. The more complete the notes you can make about your audience, the better prepared you will be for the next stages of the writing process: deciding on an appropriate tone and exploring the subject of your writing.

Exercise 1

Using the questions on pages 8–9, write out an analysis of the next audience for whom you intend to write. Underline what you consider to be the most important points in your analysis. How will these points influence what you write?

Exercise 2

Examine the letters to the editor in a recent edition of your local newspaper. Who is the intended audience of each? Who is *outside* the audience that the writer is addressing? How well does the writer demonstrate his or her knowledge of the audience? How does the writer fail to do so?

3 Choosing a Voice

Writing begins as dialogue; it is one person speaking to another about something important to both. We write because we wish to extend this one-to-one relationship to a larger number of persons. One of the pleasures of writing is discovering that as writers we do not have to give up the sense of self that enlivens conversation. The many different voices we use in speaking with others can be created in our writing as well.

3a A writer's voice

In spoken dialogue, your facial expression, gestures, and tone of voice determine to a great extent the way your audience responds to what you say. The pitch, volume, and pace of your speech tell your listeners whether you are serious or mocking, decisive or doubtful—in short, how you feel about your subject matter. In writing, you must translate these physical and auditory signals into visual symbols so that the eyes of your readers will hear the tone of your voice. The more proficient you become as a stylist, the more voices you will have at your disposal. Your written voice—like your speaking voice—can vary in tone from ironic to passionate, from annoyed to outraged, from humorous to grim.

Of course, developing a personal voice in writing is complicated by the fact that our language comes from a public stock. We cannot each invent a new language; no one would understand us. Yet the linguistic symbols that limit us also enable us to be who we are. We assert our identity by choosing from the language we find around us the words and styles that best suit our personalities and our purposes.

The first step in developing your writer's voice, therefore, is recognizing that you can make choices. If you carefully examine the voice in your past writing, you may be surprised by how often you have surrendered your power of choice and unconsciously borrowed the phrasing and tone of people around you. The language of parents and friends, of the media and the bureaucratic world, inevitably creeps into the writing that most of us do. In some situations, though, you have no doubt found yourself writing with genuine feeling and power. The composition of a letter to someone you care for or the assertion of a value you believe in can move you to choose your words carefully, to rewrite sentences again and again until you feel certain that what you have written will move your reader. In such a creative act you can almost hear your voice in the words on your page and see the look of recognition on the face of the person you are addressing. Making this experience a part of every writing act is the goal of all serious writers.

To a large extent, the voice in our writing—what we might also call the tone of our writing—depends on two relationships: our attitude toward our subject, and our attitude toward our reader. We will consider both of these relationships in the sections that follow.

3b Voice and subject

Before you can write with any distinguishable voice, you must first decide for yourself how you feel about your subject. In the broadest terms, writers might be said to regard their subjects either positively or negatively. But the range of possible attitudes within each of these large categories is enormous, limited only by each writer's range of emotional responses. The city council's plan to curtail public transportation may *concern* one citizen, *disturb* another, *anger* a third, *outrage* a fourth. An act of kindness between acquaintances may inspire appreciation, affection, admiration, or devotion, depending on the people involved.

To convey our attitude toward our subject in writing, we must rely on carefully chosen words and details. In the passage below, for example, the writer does not explicitly state his attitude toward nurses, but his admiration and respect are nonetheless clear because the details he includes emphasize efficiency, sensitivity, and personal concern.

> The nurses, the good ones anyway (and all the ones on my floor were good), make it their business to know everything that is going on. They spot errors before errors can be launched. They know everything written on the chart. Most important of all, they know their patients as unique human beings, and they soon get to know the close relatives and friends. Because of this knowledge, they are quick to sense apprehensions and act on them. The average sick person in a large hospital feels at risk of getting lost, with no identity left beyond a name and a string of numbers on a plastic wristband, in danger always of being whisked off on a litter to the wrong place to have the wrong procedure done, or worse still, *not* being whisked off at the right time. The attending physician or the house officer, on rounds and usually in a hurry, can murmur a few reassuring words on his way out the door, but it takes a confident, competent, and cheerful nurse, there all day long and in and out of the room on one chore or another through the night, to bolster one's confidence that the situation is indeed manageable and not about to get out of hand.
>
> —Lewis Thomas

In the same way, May Sarton helps us to understand her feelings about the life she lives by presenting details from her daily routine:

> For me the most interesting thing about a solitary life, and mine has been that for the last twenty years, is that it becomes increasingly rewarding. When I can wake up and watch the sun rise over the ocean, as I do most days, and know that I have an entire day ahead, uninterrupted, in which to write a few pages, take a walk with my dog, lie down in the afternoon for a long think (why does one think better in a horizontal position?), read and listen to music, I am flooded with happiness.
>
> —May Sarton

Sarton's paragraph might perhaps be reduced to the assertion, "My solitary life is satisfying." But without the details with which she has described her day, we would not fully understand her sense of satisfaction. As writers, we must remember that merely asserting our attitude toward our subject is insufficient. If we want our readers to understand our feelings, and perhaps even to share them, we must rely on carefully chosen diction and details that will show our readers why we feel as we do.

All of this is not to suggest that every writer's attitude toward his or her subject can be precisely labeled, or even that every piece of writing will always reveal its writer's attitude. Many writing situations call for the objective reporting of information, such as we find in the following passage.

> If low-income and working-class nonvoters suddenly appeared at the polls, would they change American politics? According to careful studies of the question, the answer is no. Pollsters find that the political views of nonvoters—at least on matters that appear on the ballot—are not terribly different from those held by voters. Careful analysis by political scientists suggests that if nonvoters were to vote, they would shift the electorate slightly to the left on economic issues, such as jobs, government spending, public works, and the like, but slightly to the right on social issues, such as busing, abortion, and other life-style questions.
>
> —David Osborne

Of course, we should remember that apparent objectivity in writing is also the result of a writer's choice—the decision *not* to reveal one's attitude toward the subject.

3c Voice and audience

If we have clearly defined our attitude toward our subject, we have laid the groundwork for writing with an honest voice. But equally important to a writer's tone is the relationship that the writer seeks to establish with his or her readers. Just as we easily shift our spoken language to suit the many different people whom we address throughout the day, from family members to strangers, we must be ready to adapt our written language to each rhetorical situation that we confront as writers.

Some writing situations naturally require that we use language that suggests a personal relationship with our readers. In letters to close friends, for example, we tend to use the simplified sentence structure of conversation, the diction of colloquial speech (including contractions and slang), and the first-person and second-person pronouns *I, we,* and *you.* If we did not, our writing would seem stilted and artificial. For other writing tasks, however, such as the writing of a research paper, distance between writer and reader is more suitable than intimacy. In such writing, we strive to create polished sentences that will suggest our careful thinking; we adopt a more formal diction (including, perhaps, specialized words appropriate to the discipline in which we are writing); and we tend to avoid the first-person and second-person pronouns.

It is important to realize, however, that no absolute rules will help us in determining how to approach our readers when we write. "Never use *I*" might be an acceptable guideline for formal academic writing, but in other writing situations it would be as absurd as a rule like "Always use slang." Instead, we must think carefully about the kind of relationship with our audience that is appropriate to our rhetorical situation, and about the means available to us for creating this relationship in our writing.

The examples of a letter to a friend and a formal research paper are just two points on a vast continuum of potential writer/reader relationships. Along the continuum are an infinite number of degrees of closeness between writer and reader, ranging from the greatest distance to the greatest intimacy. At one end, for example, is the writing found in many professional journals, which uses distance between writer and reader as one means of suggesting the writer's authority:

Great distance between writer and reader

> This paper has shown that a direct generalization of assumptions that Davis and Hinich have shown to be sufficient for multidimensional median voter results in *deterministic* voting models is sufficient for multidimensional median outcomes in *probabilistic* voting models. Among other things, this is an indication of just how strong the assumptions that they originally studied are. The generalization that was studied here is similar in spirit to the original assumptions of Davis and Hinich—both in its explicit use of pseudo-norms and scaling functions and in its retention of symmetry for the distribution of the voters' ideal points in the society. As a consequence, it should be recognized that this generalization itself is also highly restrictive—and could easily fail to hold in a specific economy that is of interest.
>
> —Peter J. Coughlin

The distance between writer and reader in this passage results partly from the writer's highly technical vocabulary—"multidimensional median voter results," "probabilistic voting models," "pseudo-norms and scaling functions"—which places the passage outside the realm of ordinary conversation between two individuals. This distance is reinforced by the writer's deliberate avoidance of personal pronouns. In the first sentence, for example, he has chosen to write "This paper has shown . . ." rather than "I have shown. . . ." Similarly, he later uses the passive voice to remove both himself and his reader from the text:

> "The generalization that was studied here. . . ."
> [rather than, "The generalization that *I studied* here. . . ."]
>
> "As a consequence, it should be recognized that. . . ."
> [rather than, "As a consequence, *you should recognize* that. . . ."]

In this case, as in much writing intended primarily to report or inform, the writer's main interest is his subject rather than his reader. The formal voice of a scholar is more appropriate to such a writing situation than the familiar voice of a friend.

Informative writing need not be impersonal, however, even when the subject is a grand one. In the following passage, for example, Kenneth Clark compares two major artists of the Middle Ages, the painter Giotto and the poet Dante, yet his tone borders on the informal.

Moderate distance between writer and reader

> Although I think that Giotto was one of the greatest of painters, he has equals. But in almost the same year that he was born, and in the same part of Italy, was born a man who is unequalled—the greatest philosophic poet that has ever lived, Dante. Since they were contemporaries and compatriots, one feels that it should be possible to illustrate Dante by Giotto. They seem to have known each other and Giotto may have painted Dante's portrait. But in fact their imaginations moved on very different planes. Giotto was, above all, interested in humanity: he sympathised with human beings and his figures, by their very solidity, remain on earth. Of course there is humanity in Dante—there's everything in Dante. But he also had certain qualities that Giotto lacked: philosophic power, a grasp of abstract ideas, moral indignation, that heroic contempt for baseness that was to come again in Michelangelo; and, above all, a sense of the *un*earthly, a vision of heavenly radiance.
>
> —Kenneth Clark

On the whole, Clark's diction here is as lofty as his subject. Phrases like "philosophic power" and "heroic contempt for baseness" are not part of most people's everyday conversation. But Clark pulls the tone of this passage toward the informal by interjecting himself in its first sentence ("I think"), by using a contraction ("there's everything in Dante"), and by starting several sentences with the conjunction "but," often regarded as a somewhat colloquial sentence opener.

These features, sparingly used in Clark's passage, are among the characteristics that we usually expect to dominate less formal writing. In the student paragraph below, for example, written as an introduction to a personal essay, the writer combines the personal pronouns "I" and "you" with generally informal diction to draw the reader into the world of his experience.

3c

Moderate intimacy between writer and reader

The solid vibration that goes through your arms and body when you perfectly connect a wooden bat with a leather-covered baseball is a feeling of pure exhilaration. My love affair with hitting baseballs began with stickball games on my street, continued through Little League, junior high, and high school, and persists even now when I go to the Revere batting cages, where occasionally some Boston Red Sox players hit. I've consistently been a good hitter through the years, with the exception of a period of steady decline from the end of my sophomore year in high school through half of my junior year. During this batting slump, I wondered whether I had completely lost the ability to hit a baseball well. What was I doing wrong? Was I striding too soon? Were my hands coming around too fast? Was I rotating my hips improperly? I consulted every book on hitting to check the mechanics of my swing. I changed my stance a hundred times. But still my batting slump hung on.

—David A. Miller

The attempt to establish a close bond with the reader is characteristic of the language of much advertising and popular journalism. Notice the direct appeal to the reader in the following magazine advertisement, soliciting suggestions for new articles. Here the writer liberally uses personal pronouns, contractions, colloquial diction, and even slang to create an extremely informal tone.

Great intimacy between writer and reader

Our Eyes and Ears

"Frontlines" needs you, the legions of *MJ* faithful and faithless, the fifth column in the war for irreverence and investigation. Send us your troubling and bubbling items, yearning to breathe free.

Although we can't acknowledge every item sent in, we do acknowledge those we use. What's more, if we use something you tip us off to, we'll rush you $15 and a *Mother Jones* T-shirt.

—Mother Jones

The tone of all writing results from choice. Effective writers are so conscious of their writing voice that they bring a distinctive touch even to routine writing situations. If you resolve to be personally committed to any act of writing, to care about what you say and how you say it, such involvement will compel you to write vigorous prose. Writing becomes a mechanical task only when we fail to listen to our voice and to the imagined response of our reader.

Exercise 1

Analyze the writer's voice in each of the passages below. What is the writer's subject? In which cases do details or diction reveal the writer's attitude toward that subject? Does the writer's relationship with the reader tend toward distance or intimacy? How does the writer create this relationship?

1. It is time for the baby's birthday: a white cake, strawberry-marshmallow ice cream, a bottle of champagne saved from another party. In the evening, after she has gone to sleep, I kneel beside the crib and touch her face, where it is pressed against the slats, with mine. She is an open and trusting child, unprepared for and unaccustomed to the ambushes of family life, and perhaps it is just as well that I can offer her little of that life. I would like to give her more. I would like to promise her that she will grow up with a sense of her cousins and of rivers and of her great-grandmother's teacups, would like to pledge her a picnic on a river with fried chicken and her hair uncombed, would like to give her *home* for her birthday, but we live differently now and I can promise her nothing like that. I give her a xylophone and a sundress from Madeira, and promise to tell her a funny story.

—Joan Didion

2. In England, until the end of the fourteenth century, the government, the business community, the courts, the towns, kept their records in French or Latin; lords and knights conducted their correspondence in French, when they corresponded at all. Then with amazing suddenness, in a span of less than fifty years during the first decades of the fifteenth century, French well nigh disappeared and Latin faded. The rolls of Parliament, chronicles, letters, town records, were cast in the vernacular. The Englishness of England had arrived. At this same time there developed the impulse not only to enjoy with keener awareness the flavor of living, the drama of character, but also to record these manifestations.

—Paul Murray Kendall

3. I think the observable reluctance of the majority of Americans to assert themselves in minor matters is related to our increased sense of helplessness in an age of technology and centralized political and economic power. For generations, Americans who were too hot, or too cold, got up and did something about it. Now we call the plumber, or the electrician, or the furnace man. The habit of looking after our own needs obviously had something to do with the assertiveness that characterized the American family familiar to readers of American literature. With the technification of life goes our direct responsibility for our material environment, and we are conditioned to adopt a position of helplessness not only as regards the broken air conditioner, but as regards the overheated train. It takes an expert to fix the former, but not the latter; yet these distinctions, as we withdraw into helplessness, tend to fade away.

—William F. Buckley, Jr.

4. If you have never attempted to trace your lineage, and would enjoy an interesting and fascinating adventure that may well develop into a family project, and lead to a lifetime avocation, I heartily recommend that you inaugurate a search for your very own family tree which is located somewhere in the great forest of humanity. I can almost hear you ask: "Where do I start?" Start right in your own home where you will find evidences of family history all about you.

There is no magic formula to follow in tracing family history because each search presents different problems, and the solution of one problem usually leads to several new and unsolved ones. You simply take a logical approach, as in any

3c

other field of research, and work from the known facts to the unknown. *Time* and *place* are the basic factors in the solution of all genealogical problems.

—Ethel W. Williams

5. For the Northern Plains, it was a year plagued by disasters. First came the drought, the result of sparse rainfall in the spring and summer. Then came the grasshoppers, great brown clouds that descended on crops of wheat, barley, oats, and finally the grasslands. What the grasshoppers left behind, the hailstorms battered to the ground. In August, lightning from a dry thunderstorm struck randomly across the state, igniting rotten logs, brush, and needles in Montana's forests. As strong winds fanned the tiny flames, the fire rose like an angry dragon, sucking in air, heating it, and blasting it through the trees at speeds of up to sixty miles an hour. Herds of elk and deer raced ahead of the wall of fire. Coyotes scampered on singed feet into nearby canyons. For days, the flames crowned the tops of Ponderosa pine and Douglas fir, leaping from ridge to ridge in a brilliant nighttime spectacle of soaring embers that could be seen thirty miles away.

—Carol Ann Bassett

4 *Exploring Ideas*

The process of writing would be enormously simplified if we could always be assured of having good ideas to write about. In reality, though, even important subjects don't always yield successful essays. Why is one writer able to create a substantial, convincing paper, while another, working with a similar subject, produces writing that is stale and flat? The difference often has less to do with the intellectual abilities of the two writers than with the ways in which they have thought about their subjects. Good ideas for writing don't come to most of us spontaneously; instead, we have to take deliberate action to get our minds working. This chapter will examine several different ways of stimulating thinking in order to generate ideas for writing.

The methods of discovery described here can work regardless of the kind of paper you are writing. If your assignment is an autobiographical paper or personal experience essay, these approaches to discovery should yield material from your life that you can use as the substance of your paper. If you are writing in an academic discipline such as art or political science or psychology, these procedures may raise the kinds of questions that you will want to pursue with library research. In either case, you will have discovered lines of thought that can be valuable to you later in the writing process.

4a Unstructured methods of discovery

We might define an unstructured approach to discovering ideas for writing as one in which you let your mind go in whatever direction it chooses. The important thing, though, is that you focus your attention on your mind's activity, noting all the ideas it turns up. Only at the end of the discovery process, as you begin to shape your paper, should you go back over your list of ideas to decide which ones to use and which to discard (for suggestions about organizing your raw material, see **6a, 6b, 6c,** and **6g**).

1. Brainstorming

Brainstorming is the free and uncontrolled play of the mind with any idea. When we engage in brainstorming, we let our mind's natural powers of association shape the discovery process. The difference between brainstorming and mere random thought is that in a brainstorming session we *write down* all

4a

of the ideas that come to us; the very act of noting each idea often prompts the mind to generate still more related ideas.

You may jot down the ideas that occur to you through brainstorming in an ordinary list like the one below. In this case, a student began to consider writing about some aspect of the subject "gymnastics":

Gymnastics

—many people think gymnastics is boring
—they're right
—practice boring, especially stretching, warm-up exercises, setting up and breaking down equipment
—leg lifts are very boring
—very painful
—how you do them
—flat on your back
—if you do them wrong you get extras
—leg lifts for punishment as well as exercise
—gymnastics is good for you, though
—getting a high score is worth the effort
—one of the top sports
—becoming increasingly popular thanks to the Olympics
—more people beginning training . . .

When you brainstorm, you should not "edit" your thoughts in order to produce a neat, orderly list of ideas. Brainstorming, as its name suggests, is a wild and furious activity; its initial results are supposed to be chaotic and disorganized. The time to edit, to look over the ideas you have generated and select those that seem most promising, will come later, as you plan the structure and development of your paper.

Some writers like to use a "mapping" diagram like that on page 21, rather than a straight list, in the brainstorming process. At the center they place the main idea that they wish to explore. Then, as new ideas come to mind, they write them down on connecting lines drawn out from the center of the page, grouping related ideas together and extending the subgroups as far as possible. One advantage of mapping is that it links related ideas. Like a straight list, though, the mapping diagram is also tentative and exploratory, and like any method of discovery, it should be expected to generate much more material than you can use in a single well-focused essay. Only when you have extended your ideas as far as possible should you go back to decide which ones might work in your paper.

Brainstorming also works when your writing is based on printed sources rather than personal experience, although the notes you make in such cases will

4a

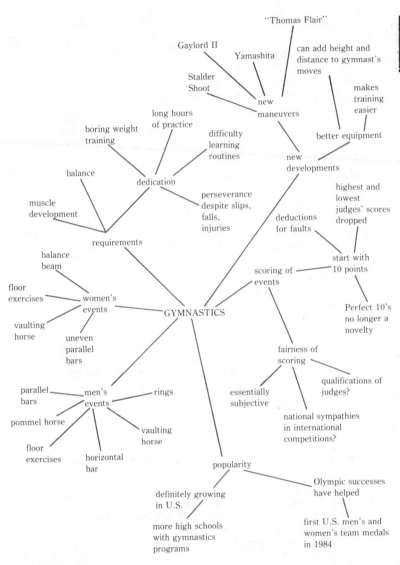

Mapping diagram

naturally be less spontaneous and more reflective. When you are writing a paper based on a reading assignment, you may expect your brainstorming notes to fall into two categories: ideas *from* the readings that strike you as important, and ideas *about* the readings that occur to you as you read. With such notes, you can often discover the focus and basic content for your paper.

Consider this assignment from an introductory sociology course:

> Compare the structure and the functions of the family and the values surrounding children and community in modern China and the Israeli kibbutz. Refer to assigned readings by Melford E. Spiro ("Is the Family Universal?") and Bruce Dollar ("Child Care in China"). Length: 2–4 pages, typed.

After reading the two articles, one student made these preliminary notes:

"Is the Family Universal?"
  Murdock: four functions of nuclear family
      1. sexual
      2. economic
      3. reproductive
      4. educational
  Kibbutz one such group
      —an agricultural collective in Israel: communal living, collective ownership of all property, communal rearing of children
  Education + socialization function of "nurses" and teachers, not parents
  Parents are important to psychological development of child

"Child Care in China"
  Several major ideas about childrearing
      —subordination of personal to social needs, respect for productive labor, altruism, cooperation, integration of physical w/intellectual labor—tend to develop kind of citizen China wants—values
  Importance placed on group activities
  Toys too heavy for one child
  "Multiple mothering" of Chinese tradition

She then sketched out the following thoughts about the two articles:

Likenesses
  both value children
  both emphasize group rather than individual
  both separate economic and educational function from others
  cooperation preferred over individual action
  both provide psychological security for the child
  family life strong
  both altruistic

Why important?
  family is institution that guarantees future of society
  I see this now better than before—all values are focused on children
  society's way of life and values are impressed in the way children are treated—
      socialization isn't just education; it's the whole atmosphere of the society in its attitude toward children

The notes taken on her readings led the student to a perspective on the material and to a possible focus for her paper—the similar ways in which cultural values are impressed on children in Israel and China. Formal research, of course, requires much more thoroughness in note taking and documentation. But this student's work illustrates that brainstorming can offer a valuable approach to thinking about the ideas we encounter in our reading.

2. Free writing

When you brainstorm, you write down bits and pieces, fragments of ideas that occur to you as you let your mind roam freely. Another way of capturing your thoughts in flight is free writing. Free writing differs from brainstorming in that you attempt to catch the flow of your thoughts by writing them not as a list of fragmentary ideas, but as a continuous thread of sentences.

Free writing often begins with an idea or question that sparks your thought. Your opening question may be as vague as "What can I say that's worth reading?" or as specific as "What does Ruth Benedict mean by 'cultural integration'?" Once you have written your question down, follow it by writing quickly whatever comes to mind as you think about your reply to it. Remember that, since your question is merely a starting point, you do not need to attempt to answer it in your free writing. Try not to pause at all as you write, particularly not to consider such matters as correct punctuation or spelling. If you think you have run out of things to write or are not able to think of words for what you want to say, try rewriting your last five words again and again until something new comes to mind. Your object is to fill your pages with writing, not to compose a perfect essay on the spot.

Some writers actually time themselves when they engage in free writing, trying to get as many words as possible on the page in ten- or fifteen-minute intervals. The idea behind free writing is that our minds will come up with many good ideas if we simply give our thought processes free rein. As in brainstorming, though, it is important that you write down all your ideas as they come to you. It's the written record of your thoughts that distinguishes free writing from daydreaming and that provides concrete material for writing later on.

Here is a brief sample of one student's free writing on the topic of television hospitals:

> How are TV hospitals different from real ones? TV hospitals are very unreal. When a patient arrives at an emergency room everyone stops what they're doing and their attention goes to the patient—That's on TV. In real life it's different. When I had a bad accident, no one at the hospital was concerned, and it took an hour for the Dr. to arrive. This one lady was yelling and crying desperately that her baby needed help and treatment but no one came to help as they do on TV.—A clerk told her to wait because there were others waiting and she had to fill out forms before the Dr. could examine the baby.
>
> What is an emergency room like? On TV it is antiseptic, well-lit, focus on one patient, a very dramatic place with music to underline the drama. Only one patient

sick at a time. The one I was in was darker. And busier. Two-tone walls green and white—not dirty but not sparkling white either. Hadn't been painted in a while, a noisy place, full of sick people, no drama, basically it was boring. Sickness in real life is basically boring.

In this free writing sample, the student has correctly been more concerned with getting her ideas down on the page than with structuring her sentences precisely. The details in this passage, combined with the writer's insights into some differences between television hospitals and real ones, could become the basis of a successful paper. As in this case, free writing will almost always lead you in interesting directions if you give it the opportunity.

Like brainstorming, free writing also works with writing based on reading assignments. You may find it particularly useful to begin with notes taken from your sources. With your notes before you, simply let your mind and your pen take over. Below, for example, is some of the free writing done by the student who had assembled notes on child rearing in China and on the Israeli kibbutz.

Emphasizes group rather than individual. What does this mean? The community values of the society are focused on communal success not on the individual. Best illustrated by the way children are brought up—most activities occur in groups not in individuals—examples of the building blocks that are too heavy for children to pick up. This forces (Chinese teachers said) group cooperation. More than one child was needed to pick up blocks—whole Chinese society is focused on group effort. Thus we see that children are taught values they will live by for the rest of their lives, thus maintaining the society's values (maybe this should be part of the introduction). Well, it's not really teaching—the blocks are designed to force students to learn to cooperate. It's the whole atmosphere that is intended to reinforce the values.

How is this related to the family? Family is institution that guarantees the future of a society. In China the family has three of the four functions which what's his name mentions (look it up): economic, sexual, reproductive, not education, also one that Spiro mentions, affection. This means that the family is not fully part of educational system because the family would tend to individualize—in a society that emphasizes group identity you would have to take children away from the family, but even the substitute family is very loving. Do not punish, only correct.

Note that in the second paragraph the writer did not permit her forgetting one source's name to interfere with the flow of her thinking.

Neither of the two "paragraphs" above is perfectly coherent, nor should we expect them to be. More important is the fact that both contain ideas that can be developed further in other, more deliberately planned, paragraphs. After she has produced several more pages of free writing, the writer can begin to reflect on the best way of organizing her ideas. She may underline sentences that seem especially important; she may copy out key sentences onto another sheet of paper; she may even group ideas together in a rough sort of outline. With pages of written notes before her, she is in a good position to think about the content and structure of her essay.

Exercise 1

Using either listing or mapping, explore one of the general subjects below, or another subject of your choice. Generate as many ideas as you can in one sitting. Wait at least a few hours and then come back to the same subject. Can you add some new ideas to those you wrote down earlier? Repeat this procedure several times, and then review all the ideas you have jotted down. Which ones interest you? Which do you think you could make interesting to someone else?

1. Fitness	6. Solitude
2. Personal computers	7. Jealousy
3. Learning to drive	8. The environment
4. Television commercials	9. Music
5. Children	10. City life

Exercise 2

Select a chapter from one of your textbooks, and use the brainstorming method described on pages 19–23 to explore its contents. What key ideas in the chapter did you identify? What ideas of your own were you able to generate in response to the chapter you read?

Exercise 3

Write steadily for ten minutes on one of the topics below, or on another subject of your choice. At the end of ten minutes, select what you consider to be the most important idea in your free writing, copy it over at the top of a clean page, and write again for ten minutes without stopping. When you have finished, underline the best ideas from your two sessions of free writing and try to rewrite them into a single coherent paragraph.

1. My greatest accomplishment so far in life has been _____.
2. The most important person in my life is _____.
3. Television would be much better if _____.
4. I always feel good when _____.
5. The most important decision I will have to make this year is _____.

4b Structured methods of discovery

We called the approaches to discovery above "unstructured" because they follow no predetermined pattern. The results of brainstorming and free writing depend solely on the unpredictable way in which ideas surface in your mind. In contrast, structured approaches to discovery follow a prescribed pattern, usually a fixed set of questions to answer or a checklist of topics to consider. Like the methods of discovery described above, structured methods demand mental alertness and concentration. For some writers, though, structured methods of discovery are easier to use than brainstorming or free writing, since they depend less on the random workings of the mind.

One of the simplest—and most effective—structured approaches to discovery is the set of questions learned by every novice journalist:

Who?
What?
When?
Where?
Why?
How?

Armed with these questions, a journalist should be able to assemble the essential information about any subject that he or she is investigating. By expanding this formula with additional questions under each of these main headings, we can create a useful structured approach for examining any subject for writing.

Before we do that, however, a few words are in order about the most effective way of using such a set of questions. Many students trying such a discovery procedure for the first time mistakenly believe that their task is to come up with a single answer for each of the questions involved. Two things are wrong with that conception of structured discovery procedures. First, if this approach is to be successful, your goal must be to produce *as many responses as possible* to each question. You should not treat these questions like examination questions for which there is only one correct answer; instead, reflect on each one carefully, using it to squeeze out of your mind as much information about your subject as you can. Second, you must recognize that not every question will be relevant to every topic. Don't feel that this approach is not working if you don't have answers for all the questions.

Remember, too, that the answers you get from asking these questions are not themselves topics for a variety of different papers. Instead, as with brainstorming and free writing, your goal is to accumulate as much diverse information about your subject as possible. Later, as you begin to organize your paper (see Chapter **6**), you will be able to pull out the best ideas from your notes and consider how they can be most effectively organized, and whether they can be further developed. Like brainstorming and free writing, therefore, structured methods of discovery are useful only if you work through them with pen in hand, jotting down all the ideas that occur to you and assembling pages of working notes on your subject.

Now let's look at an expanded version of the journalist's set of questions. In the questions below, X represents the subject you are thinking or writing about.

Who?

Who is involved in X?
Who benefited from X?
Who suffered?

What?

How is X defined?

How would you describe X?

What is X similar to?

What parts make up X? How are they related to each other?

When?

When did X occur?

How long did X take?

What happened before X?

What happened after X?

Where?

In what setting did X occur? What were the physical surroundings?

What other circumstances made X possible?

How would X have been different if the circumstances were different?

Why?

What are the causes of X?

What are the consequences of X?

How?

How did X come to be? Who made X?

How does X work?

To see the versatility of these questions, consider the way in which one student used them to generate ideas about her hobby, photography. Reflecting on the questions above yielded several pages of notes, among which she was gradually able to find a controlling idea for an essay on the subject. Here is just a portion of the student's notes, those in response to the second set of questions, under the heading "What?"

What?

How is photography defined?

A chemical process involving light, an image, and a light-sensitive material.

How would you describe photography?

As a knack or gift. As a hobby—but photography requires more equipment than most hobbies—can be expensive (film, developing)—takes time to become really skilled. As a talent. As a profession. As an art form—photography is more

4b

highly technical than most art forms—artist also restricted by many conditions beyond her control. As a form of personal expression.

What is photography similar to?
Painting—but the photographer's imagination is limited by lighting, setting, subjects, equipment. Writing—photographs can tell a story—either a single picture, or a series of photographs—images and setting establish mood—subjects' faces can convey emotion.

What parts make up photography? How are they related to each other?
Photographer herself. Equipment: camera (more than one?), lenses (normal, telephoto, zoom, wide-angle—necessary for maximum creativity); filters (UV, skylight, polarizing, star-effect, colored—for effective color reproduction and special effects); tripod; flash; camera case and equipment bag. Subjects: human (posed, candid), landscapes, animals (hard to control). Experts for developing, printing, enlarging (without first-rate processing, all the photographer's efforts are futile). Purchasers of photographs: magazines, newspapers, friends.

These and the other notes that the student made led her to recognize clearly for the first time the conflict that existed between her instinctive creativity and the elements of photography beyond her control—equipment limitations, unpredictable conditions for work, unreliable processing, and the like. In the contradiction that she discovered beteween her natural abilities and the inescapable restrictions imposed on those abilities she was able to find a focus for a paper that balanced the rewards of photography with its intrinsic frustrations.

Thinking about a subject in this systematic way is not easy; it takes concentration, imagination, and persistence. But such thorough exploration of a topic can help to make us more critical thinkers and more careful writers.

Exercise 4

In Exercise 1 (page 25) you used brainstorming to explore a possible subject for writing. Now examine the same subject using the set of questions on pages 26–27 above. Are you able to generate new information?

Exercise 5

Choose another subject and explore it first with free writing (follow the directions in Exercise 3, page 25) and, a day later, with the set of questions presented in this section. Which approach to discovery—unstructured or structured—seems to work better for you?

5 Understanding the Modes of Discourse

At the end of the last century, composition teachers became fond of classifying writing as either description, narration, exposition, or argumentation—a breakdown known as the four modes (or forms) of discourse. This classification system is admittedly less perfect than some nineteenth-century teachers wanted to believe, since it largely ignores the possibility of overlap among the four categories. Much effective narration, for example, is based on vivid description; similarly, a convincing argument almost always involves clear exposition.

Still, the modes of discourse have remained popular for more than a hundred years, and despite their roughness as categories, they continue to provide a convenient way of thinking about one's primary purpose in writing. Whether your writing falls squarely within one mode or encompasses several, you should be familiar with the basic strategies of description, narration, exposition, and argumentation. The examples below offer an introduction to these strategies, which will be discussed at greater length in chapters to come.

5a Description

When we describe, we attempt to make the reader see our subject exactly as we do. One of the most basic of language skills, description is part of our everyday communication with those around us. In writing, effective description almost always depends on precise diction and the careful selection of details. Skilled writers often use such exact language not only to appeal to a reader's senses, but also to suggest their feelings about a subject. In the following passage, for example, notice how the writer's vivid images of a boyhood cabin by a Maine lake convey his fondness for the place.

> I guess I remembered clearest of all the early mornings, when the lake was cool and motionless, remembered how the bedroom smelled of the lumber it was made of and of the wet woods whose scent entered through the screen. The partitions in the camp were thin and did not extend clear to the top of the rooms, and as I was always the first up I would dress softly so as not to wake the others, and sneak out into the sweet outdoors and start out in the canoe, keeping close along the shore in the long

shadows of the pines. I remember being very careful never to rub my paddle against the gunwale for fear of disturbing the stillness of the cathedral.

—E. B. White

Smells, sounds, and sights are fused in this remarkable passage, which suggests with its final image of the cathedral White's deep respect for the lake.

Descriptive writing does not have to be so intensely personal to be effective, however. Many writing situations call for more objective detailing of a subject, as in this account of the sensations that accompany falling asleep:

> A number of curious experiences occur at the onset of sleep. A person just about to go to sleep may experience an electric shock, a flash of light, or a crash of thunder—but the most common sensation is that of floating or falling, which is why "falling asleep" is a scientifically valid description. A nearly universal occurrence at the beginning of sleep (although not everyone recalls it) is a sudden, uncoordinated jerk of the head, the limbs, or even the entire body. Most people tend to think of going to sleep as a slow slippage into oblivion, but the onset of sleep is not gradual at all. It happens in an instant. One moment the individual is awake, the next moment not.
>
> —Peter Farb

Although the almost clinical tone of Farb's passage is far different from White's hushed veneration, these two writers share a regard for the precision of language that makes description work. (For further discussion of specific detail in description, see **8a** and **13a**.)

5b Narration

Narration tells us what happened. Like description, the reporting of events is part of our daily interaction with other people. Like description, too, narration often depends on the exact selection of details, arranged in such a way that the reader can clearly follow the sequence of events in question.

When the writer of narration is a figure in the narrative, we call the work a first-person narrative:

> In fourth grade I embarked upon a grandiose reading program. "Give me the names of important books," I would say to startled teachers. They soon found out that I had in mind "adult books." I ignored their suggestion of anything I suspected was written for children. (Not until I was in college, as a result, did I read *Huckleberry Finn* or *Alice's Adventures in Wonderland*.) Instead, I read *The Scarlet Letter* and Franklin's *Autobiography*. And whatever I read I read for extra credit. Each time I finished a book, I reported the achievement to a teacher and basked in the praise my effort earned. Despite my best efforts, however, there seemed to be more and more books I needed to read. At the library I would literally tremble as I came upon whole shelves of books I hadn't read.
>
> —Richard Rodriguez

In a third-person narrative, in contrast, the writer reports events of which he or she is not a part:

> In 1904, Abbot Kinney, who had made a fortune on Sweet Caporal cigarettes, traveled to Europe and so loved what he saw that he conceived of building a replica of Venice in southern California. Kinney raised the money to build canals, lagoons, roller coasters, bathhouses and bridges of fake Italian design, and cottages with docks so people could visit one another by gondola. The idea caught on: "Venice of America" became a fashionable resort. Douglas Fairbanks and Mary Pickford, Charlie Chaplin and Paulette Goddard, kept hideaways on the canals or beach front.
>
> In time, the novelty wore off and the resort went to seed. The canals turned stagnant, and the unheated cottages became substandard housing for the poor. In the Sixties, Venice became one of the few places in Los Angeles where numbers of hippies and radicals lived. It was an outlaw gulch—a haven for draft resisters, artists, and drug addicts. At the same time, a real estate development was under way that threatened to alter permanently the character of Venice.
>
> —Sara Davidson

This narration of Venice's rise and fall illustrates the difficulty of separating narration from the other modes of discourse. The framework of Davidson's paragraphs, clearly, is a chronological series of events, but without the carefully chosen descriptive details that she has woven into the narration, we would have little concrete sense of the place that Venice was.

<u>5c</u> Exposition

Perhaps the broadest of the modes of discourse, exposition is writing that explains. Expository prose takes many forms; it may define a subject, or give examples of it, or discuss its causes, or compare it to another subject (see **8b–8g**). This passage of expository prose, for example, is structured around a comparison between the climates of Plymouth, England and Plymouth, Massachusetts:

> It is still not generally recognized that if the Pilgrims had landed on a nearby planet instead of the New England coast, they could scarcely have made a more abrupt switch in thermal environments. In Plymouth, England, they left a moderate climate, with a very stable temperature, without extremely cold winters or very hot summers; snows and droughts were rare; tornadoes and cyclones unknown. In Plymouth, Massachusetts, they found a thermal environment whose annual cycle was far more severe, with a temperature spread from July to December more than twice as great as in Plymouth, England. They also found heavy snowfalls, long freezes, enormous gales.
>
> —James Marston Fritch

In the passage below, the writer explains her main idea with a definition and examples.

5d

If I could have one wish for my own sons, it is that they should have the courage of women. I mean by this something very concrete and precise: the courage I have seen in women who, in their private and public lives, both in the interior world of their dreaming, thinking, and creating, and the outer world of partriarchy, are taking greater and greater risks, both psychic and physical, in the evolution of a new vision. Sometimes this involves tiny acts of immense courage; sometimes public acts which can cost a woman her job or her life; often it involves moments, or long periods, of thinking the unthinkable, being labeled, or feeling, crazy; always a loss of traditional securities. Every woman who takes her life into her own hands does so knowing that she must expect enormous pain, inflicted both from within and without. I would like my sons not to shrink from this kind of pain, not to settle for the old male defenses, including that of a fatalistic self-hatred. And I would wish them to do this not for me, or for other women, but for themselves, and for the sake of life on the planet Earth.

—Adrienne Rich

Expository writing need not follow such firm patterns of development. In the passage that follows, notice how the writer explains his opening assertion with careful analysis rather than with any of the specific methods of organization mentioned above.

There is a popular conviction that war and battle are the sphere of ugliness, and, since aesthetic delight is associated with the beautiful, it may be concluded that war is the natural enemy of the aesthetic. I fear that this is in large part an illusion. It is, first of all, wrong to believe that only beauty can give us aesthetic delight; the ugly can please us too, as every artist knows. And furthermore, beauty in various guises is hardly foreign to scenes of battle. While it is undeniable that the disorder and distortion and the violation of nature that conflict brings are ugly beyond compare, there are also color and movement, variety, panoramic sweep, and sometimes even momentary proportion and harmony. If we think of beauty and ugliness without their usual moral overtones, there is often a weird but genuine beauty in the sight of massed men and weapons in combat.

—J. Glenn Gray

5d Argumentation

When we argue, we seek to win our reader's acceptance of our ideas about a subject. Sometimes argumentative writing is based on strict logic, sometimes on emotional appeals to the reader, most often on some combination of the two. Usually, the writer of argumentation also wants to be regarded as a thoughtful and reasonable person, a person whose ideas are deserving of the reader's serious consideration. (For a detailed discussion of principles of argumentation, see Chapters **16** and **17**.)

One familiar kind of argument is the argument that something ought to be done. In the following passage, for example, John Holt proposes and then begins to argue for a change in the prevailing conception of children's education.

Young people should have the right to control and direct their own learning, that is, to decide what they want to learn, and when, where, how, how much, how fast, and with what help they want to learn it. To be still more specific, I want them to have the right to decide, if, when, how much, and by whom they want to be *taught* and the right to decide whether they want to learn in a school and if so which one and for how much of the time.

No human right, except the right to life itself, is more fundamental than this. A person's freedom of learning is part of his freedom of thought, even more basic than his freedom of speech. If we take from someone his right to decide what he will be curious about, we destroy his freedom of thought. We say, in effect, you must think not about what interests and concerns *you*, but about what interests and concerns *us*.

—John Holt

Another common type of argument is an evaluation, a judgment about the good or bad features of a subject:

In our time it is broadly true that political writing is bad writing. Where it is not true, it will generally be found that the writer is some kind of rebel, expressing his private opinions, and not a "party line." Orthodoxy, of whatever colour, seems to demand a lifeless, imitative style. The political dialects to be found in pamphlets, leading articles, manifestos, White Papers and the speeches of Under-Secretaries do, of course, vary from party to party, but they are all alike in that one almost never finds in them a fresh, vivid, home-made turn of speech. When one watches some tired hack on the platform mechanically repeating the familiar phrases—*bestial atrocities, iron heel, bloodstained tyranny, free peoples of the world, stand shoulder to shoulder*—one often has a curious feeling that one is not watching a live human being but some kind of dummy: a feeling which suddenly becomes stronger at moments when the light catches the speaker's spectacles and turns them into blank discs which seem to have no eyes behind them.

—George Orwell

In a real sense, of course, all writing involves a degree of argumentation. Whenever we write, we seek to interest our readers in our subject, to gain their respect, to encourage them to think as we do. If we were not concerned about our readers' reactions, there would be little reason for writing in the first place.

Exercise 1

Read each of the following passages and identify the primary writing mode being used by the author—description, narration, exposition, or argumentation. Do any of the other modes also contribute to some of these passages? Explain.

1. Bobby and I were pals. Seven years old was plenty old enough to be partners, and we were inseparable—I with my blond crew cut and bitten fingernails, he with his curly, cowlicked brown hair and toothless grin. Each summer day we made our long, barefoot way down to our secret glimmering valley. Each evening, knowing that young adventurers are oblivious of time, the sun would tilt in the sky, reminding us to tote our discoveries back through the

5d

cavern, across the oily, rocky road to our place beneath the poplar tree in Bobby's side yard. We talked of plans for the next day as the sun's orange light played on our secret handshake. Bobby had invented it, and each night his eyes glowed with pride as we sealed the day with the clumsy sequence of grips and gestures. Back under the curl in the fence I would go, home just in time to escape a switching for being gone past dark.

—Scott Ourth [student]

2.   It is not my contention that chemical insecticides must never be used. I do contend that we have put poisonous and biologically potent chemicals indiscriminately into the hands of persons largely or wholly ignorant of their potentials for harm. We have subjected enormous numbers of people to contact with these poisons, without their consent and often without their knowledge. If the Bill of Rights contains no guarantee that a citizen shall be secure against lethal poisons distributed either by private individuals or by public officials, it is surely only because our forefathers, despite their considerable wisdom and foresight, could conceive of no such problem. . . .

There is still very limited awareness of the nature of the threat. This is an era of specialists, each of whom sees his own problem and is unaware of or intolerant of the larger frame into which it fits. It is also an era dominated by industry, in which the right to make a dollar at whatever cost is seldom challenged. When the public protests, confronted with some obvious evidence of damaging results of pesticide applications, it is fed little tranquilizing pills of half truth. We urgently need an end to these false assurances, to the sugar coating of unpalatable facts. It is the public that is being asked to assume the risks that the insect controllers calculate. The public must decide whether it wishes to continue on the present road, and it can do so only when in full possession of the facts.

—Rachel Carson

3.   Assuming for the moment that the Earth is round, the first person who measured its circumference accurately was another Greek, Eratosthenes (276–195 B.C.). Eratosthenes noted that on the first day of summer, sunlight struck the bottom of a vertical well in Syene, Egypt, indicating the sun was directly overhead. At the same time in Alexandria, 5,000 stadia distant, the sun made an angle with the vertical equal to 1/50 of a circle. (A stadium equaled about a tenth of a mile.) Since the sun is so far away, its rays arrive almost in parallel. If you draw a circle with two radii extending from the center outward through the perimeter (where they become local verticals), you'll see that a sun ray coming in parallel to one of the radii (at Syene) makes an angle with the other (at Alexandria) equal to the angle between the two radii. Therefore Eratosthenes concluded that the full circumference of the Earth is 50 x 5,000 stadia, or about 25,000 miles. This calculation is within one percent of the best modern value.

—Alan Lightman

4.   Now, if I, as a black man, profoundly believe that I deserve my history and deserve to be treated as I am, then I must also, fatally, believe that white people deserve their history and deserve the power and the glory which their testimony and the evidence of my own senses assure me that they have. And if black people fall into this trap, the trap of believing that they deserve their fate, white people fall into the yet more stunning and intricate trap of believing that they deserve *their* fate, and their comparative safety; and that black people, therefore, need only do as white people have done to rise to where white people now are. But this simply cannot be said, not only for reasons of politeness or charity, but also because white people carry in them a carefully muffled fear that black people long to do to others what has been done to them. Moreover, the history of white people has led them to a fearful, baffling place where they have begun to lose touch with reality—to lose touch, that is, with themselves—and where they certainly are not happy. They do not know how this came about; they do not dare examine how this came about. On the one hand, they can scarcely dare to open a dialogue which must, if it is honest, become a personal confession—a cry for help and healing, which is really, I think, the basis of all dialogues—and, on the other hand, the black man can scarcely dare to open a dialogue which must, if it is honest, become a personal confession which, fatally, contains an accusation. And yet, if we cannot do this, each of us will perish in those traps in which we have been struggling for so long.

—James Baldwin

5.   I invented a plan to test my theory that males feel no pain; males don't feel. At school, I stood under the trees where the girls play house and watched a strip of cement near the gate. There were two places where boys and girls mixed; one was the kindergarten playground, where we didn't go any more, and the other was this bit of sidewalk. I had a list of boys to kick: the boy who burned spiders, the boy who grabbed me by my coat lapels like in a gangster movie, the boy who told dirty pregnancy jokes. I would get them one at a time with my heavy shoes, on which I had nailed top taps and horseshoe taps. I saw my boy, a friendly one for a start. I ran fast, crunching gravel. He was kneeling; I grabbed him by the arm and kicked him sprawling into the circle of marbles. I ran through the girls' playground and playroom to our lavatory, where I looked out the window. Sure enough, he was not crying. "See?" I told the girls. "Boys have no feelings. It's some kind of immunity." It was the same with Chinese boys, black boys, white boys, and Mexican and Filipino boys. Girls and women of all races cried and had feelings. We had to toughen up. We had to be as tough as boys, tougher because we only pretended not to feel pain.

—Maxine Hong Kingston

Part II

Writing

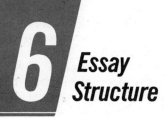

6 Essay Structure

We have seen that the first step in the writing process is accumulating as much information as possible about your subject and audience. All of this information will help to give your writing the kind of authority that only depth of knowledge can bring, even though only some of it will find a place in your final paper. This chapter and the five that follow deal with the process of shaping your rough material into a unified, well-developed, readable whole.

6a A limited subject

Effective writing often depends on the writer's ability to limit the scope of a subject appropriately. We are never able to write everything that could be said about a topic, simply because all writing tasks have length limits of some kind. In the case of college writing, this limit is usually imposed by the instructor to whom the paper is submitted. Your instructor is probably not going to count the number of words in your paper, but he or she may not be pleased by a paper that is several pages longer than what was assigned. When you write an essay exam in class, the limits are even more absolute. Once class time is up, you will be expected to have isolated the important points in the questions you answered and discussed them completely, but without including extraneous detail.

One of the purposes of college writing in all disciplines is to provide you with such practice in deciding what is really important about your subject. You practice limiting a subject in college writing because the writing situations you will confront in the world after graduation impose similar strict limits. Business reports, advertising copy, magazine articles, dissertations, books—all of these force writers to limit their subjects according to the time and interests of their readers. A business report must be thorough and complete, but it must also get to the point; its readers cannot be expected to wade through pages of tangential background material and piles of preliminary observations. A book in any field, similarly, interests its intended readers by appealing to their desire to know something new about the subject at hand. No one wants to find a new book padded with information that is readily available elsewhere.

As these examples suggest, limiting a subject is principally a writer's response to fundamental questions of purpose and audience, the inevitable

39

constraints in every writing situation. Consequently, there are no easy procedures for limiting a subject that will work in all situations. But recognizing the
role of purpose and audience in this process makes it possible to construct some
useful questions to pose as we approach any writing task.

Suppose, for example, that you have been concerned about the importance
of conserving the world's natural resources. When you begin to consider this
large subject, you may be tempted to throw up your hands in despair over the
number of important topics that you could write about: the threats to natural
wilderness areas; the diminishing amount of agricultural land available to grow
food for the world's population; the limited supplies of oil and natural gas; the use
of other sources of energy (solar, geothermal, nuclear) and their potential
advantages and hazards; the pollution of the air by exhaust gases from factories
and cars; the pollution of rivers and lakes by industrial wastes, sewage, and acid
rain; the production of pure drinking water in urban areas; the necessity of
controlling population growth. All of these are certainly important subjects, yet
they could not all be treated adequately even in a book-length study.

How do you start? You might try using the three questions below, or any
one of them, to narrow your view of the subject.

1. *What aspect of your subject is most interesting or important to you? Why?*

If you have lived in America's farming belt, then you are probably concerned
about such issues as the increasing urbanization of rural land, the erosion of
topsoil, the declining number of family farms, and the financial burdens faced by
many farmers. If you live in a large urban area, then you have no doubt
experienced the effects of smog and read about sewage treatment and waste
disposal. You may have grown up near one of the nation's massive nuclear power
plants; in that case, you have certainly formed opinions, favorable or unfavorable, about the use of nuclear reactions to produce electricity. If you enjoy
outdoor activities like boating or backpacking, then you have probably been
grateful for the existence of clean lakes and unspoiled mountain trails. There's a
simple point here: choose an angle on your subject that genuinely interests you.
All successful writers care about their subjects; they use their backgrounds and
natural inclinations to steer them toward the kinds of subjects that they will be
able to write about with genuine interest and concern. You should too.

2. *If you could tell your reader only one thing about your subject, what would
it be? Why?*

As we suggested in the first section of this book, thinking about a subject
without considering a reader is usually frustrating. If you have thought carefully
about your readers, then you can use that conception of your audience to help
limit your subject. Suppose, for example, that your essay is to be duplicated and
distributed for comments to the members of your English class. In what ways
are their interests similar to yours, or different? For what points will they
demand convincing evidence? You can narrow a paper on any subject by

regarding it as an argument directed to specific readers, an essay with a point that you want your readers to carry away with them.

    3. *What aspect of your subject could you develop best with the material you have at hand?*

    Behind this question is the simple fact that you can't write effectively without something to say; thus, you should not limit your subject to an area in which you have only scanty knowledge. For some topics, you will be able to use the discovery methods discussed in Chapter **4** to generate information from your own personal experience; on other occasions, you will think of potentially interesting approaches to your subject that can be researched in a library. But don't try to take on a narrow subject without adequate information about it; doing so will invariably make the writing process exasperating and will result in a finished essay that is thin and unconvincing. Always select from among the many possible aspects of your subject the ones about which you have substantial and important knowledge.

6b The thesis statement

    Like all stages of the writing process, the process of limiting a subject cannot be described by rigid rules or formulas. Sometimes, the questions above may immediately lead you to see how your subject should be focused; at other times, you may fully understand what you want to say only after you have begun to draft a paper. Regardless of your method, as your understanding of your precise subject evolves, you should try to formulate your controlling idea in a single sentence or two known as a **thesis statement.**

    A thesis statement may begin as a tentative expression of your paper's main point, subject to change as your ideas work themselves out on your page. In its final form, however, the thesis must be specific and unambiguous, for it establishes a kind of contract between writer and reader, a promise about the content of the paper that is to follow. Typically, a thesis contains two elements: the precise subject of the essay, and a word or phrase that even further limits this subject. The importance of that restricting word or phrase is illustrated in the following sample thesis statements, which show how a single subject may be limited in different ways:

a. The pollution of underground water supplies threatens the existence of many cities in the American West.
b. The pollution of underground water supplies is difficult to detect.
c. The pollution of underground water supplies has reached serious proportions in the American West only within the last twenty years.

A clear thesis often implies a method of development. Though the subject in each of these thesis statements is the same, the different ways in which it is restricted will produce three quite different essays. The first thesis will lead to a

6b

paper that explores the threat that underground water pollution poses to human life, examining its effect on the health and livelihood of Americans in western states. The paper that develops from the second thesis statement will be much more technical in nature; we might expect it to deal with such matters as the engineering difficulties involved in reaching underground water supplies and the scientific process of testing them for pollution. In the third case, we might anticipate a paper that takes a historical perspective, examining the causes of underground water pollution and explaining why this phenomenon is a relatively recent one.

Much of a thesis statement's potential usefulness is lost if either its subject or focus is vaguely stated. Sometimes a writer may believe that he or she has composed a thesis with a clear subject, when in fact the thesis contains only a generalized topic, not the actual subject that the writer intends to develop:

> **Vague subject** Many experiences help a person develop a respect for the rights of others.

This general statement may perhaps provide a kind of background for a paper, but notice that it does not contain a specific subject. What experiences does the writer intend to describe? Compare the thesis statement above with this one, which substitutes a specific subject:

> **Precise subject** *Sharing a college dorm suite with five other students* helps a person develop a respect for the rights of others.

Sometimes the problem with a thesis is not that its subject is too vague, but that the thesis does not limit the subject adequately. In each of these thesis statements, for example, the writer begins with a sufficiently specific subject but fails to restrict it in a way that makes the paper's point clear:

> **Vague restriction** Climbing Long's Peak as a teenager was a very important experience for me.
>
> **Vague restriction** The Vietnam War years had a great impact on this country.

In what ways was climbing Long's Peak "important"? What effects of the war in Vietnam have endured in America today? Without such information, these thesis statements merely announce a subject; they do not commit the writers to anything specific, nor do they help the reader to anticipate what will follow. In contrast, the thesis statements below add to the same subjects a more precise restriction:

> **Precise restriction** Climbing Long's Peak as a teenager *restored my faith in my abililty to set and accomplish goals.*
>
> **Precise restriction** The Vietnam War years *created divisions in American society that have lasted into the 1980s.*

In both of these thesis statements, the subject is focused in a way that provides the writer with direction and that arouses expectations in the reader about the paper's development.

Typically, a thesis statement is placed near the beginning of an essay, often in the opening paragraph. In that position, it serves both the reader and the writer in several important ways. For the reader, it provides a way of focusing attention that will make the task of reading easier. Some beginning writers mistakenly feel that a precise thesis near the beginning of a paper gives away too much of the paper's point and may therefore cause readers to lose interest in an essay from the very start. What such writers forget is that readers need to know where a paper is leading if they are to follow its development and evaluate its arguments. Your readers, after all, do not have the same familiarity with your subject that you do. They do not begin to read with an understanding of the connections between points that you have worked out for yourself, nor will they necessarily grasp the logic of your organization immediately. A clear, specific thesis gives the reader a helpful context in which to place the ideas and details that follow.

6c

A well-formulated thesis is of as much value to the writer as to the reader. For the writer, it serves as a constant reminder of the direction that the paper should be taking. Every new argument, each specific detail, should in some way advance the focus of the thesis statement. Once a draft of the paper is complete, you can check its development against the idea stated in the thesis. Does the paper stick to the subject and focus that you established in the thesis? Does it develop these ideas completely and specifically? A good thesis provides an important standard for evaluating a paper's development and logic.

Theoretically, a thesis may be placed anywhere in an essay, as long as it is prominent enough to be recognized as the thesis by the reader. In an inductive argument (see **17a**), for example, the thesis—the main idea being argued—is often held until the end, after all the relevant evidence has been presented. A thesis placed in the concluding paragraph may also provide a dramatic turn to an essay and give the reader a sense of discovery. But no matter where the thesis occurs, it should offer your readers a clear and precise statement of your paper's focus.

6c Organizing ideas

Sometimes, the subject of a paper will itself determine the best arrangement of the ideas to be used in developing a thesis. A student explaining how to install a new tile floor, for example, might naturally organize her paper around the steps involved in the process:

1. Tools and materials
2. Removal of old flooring
3. Preparation of surface
4. Laying new tile

Most topics for writing, however, are more complicated than this example suggests. Moreover, writers who have used methods of discovery like those described in Chapter **4** will usually have more material at hand than they can fit into a single paper and will need to select from among the ideas they have noted. When your material doesn't clearly determine the organization of your paper, begin by formulating as precise a thesis statement as you can, and then experiment with several ways of arranging your supporting ideas, each based on a different approach. Sketch out your ideas on paper, so that you will be able to spot opportunities for adding, deleting, and rearranging your material. A writer who wishes to argue the thesis "Grades in college are an obstacle to education" might start by selecting from his notes all the arguments that fit logically under the heading of grades and students:

Effects of grades on some students

> Become an end in themselves
> Lead students to select easy courses
> Sometimes provoke cheating or plagiarizing
> Limit students' attention to material for tests
> Cause anxiety

Among the remaining notes he might find some that address the subject from the standpoint of teachers:

Effects of grades on teachers

> Sometimes force teachers to make difficult distinctions between students
> Change teacher's role from instructor to judge
> Force teacher to develop distance from students

With both lists before him, the writer might see that his thesis could be developed by presenting the effects that grades have on students' attitudes toward teachers and courses:

Students' attitude toward teacher

> See teacher primarily as judge rather than instructor
> Develop reluctance to consult teacher outside class

Students' attitude toward course

> Avoid challenging courses to protect average
> Concentrate only on what is required for tests
> Ultimately develop narrow intellectual range

Remember, of course, that such preliminary organizing is temporary and can be changed as the paper begins to take shape. Don't take your headings so seriously that they become a straitjacket instead of a support. The actual process of writing may suggest new material, or reveal a lack of material, and may thus lead you to modify your original thesis and plan of development.

Section **6h** will consider formal outlining as an aid to arranging ideas, and Chapter **8** will examine some basic patterns for arranging ideas within paragraphs. The point to be made here is that you must consciously search for an effective pattern, experimenting with different arrangements until you discover one that makes sense. Look for natural divisions in your subject, and trust your instinctive sense for logic and clarity. As an example of one writer's ability to group details effectively, consider the thesis, preliminary outline, and opening paragraphs from the following student essay.

6c

Thesis: Groucho and Chico Marx relied on verbal comedy, but Harpo played with the language visually; since he was mute, his jokes had to be related to sight.

Preliminary Outline: Harpo's visual style of punning
Harpo's visual use of overcoat
Harpo's visual play with clichés

Harpo and the Marx Brothers

When I read Peter Farb's *Word Play*, I was delighted with his four pages devoted to the Marx Brothers and their attitude toward language. Although I believe that Farb accurately summarized the Marx Brothers' style of comedy (they attacked the rules and conventions of the English language), I don't think he caught Harpo's style as well as he did those of the other brothers. Farb was correct when he described Groucho's puns as those of a shrewd and "fast-talking sharpie" and Chico's speech as a "phony-Italian dialect" that "misconstrues both the meaning and manners of the 'foreign American speech community.'" However, his analysis of Harpo's manner of comedy, as one that throws language "back to the level of the beasts," is incomplete. Whereas Groucho and Chico relied on verbal means, Harpo played with the language visually; since he was mute, almost all of his jokes had to be related to sight.

An excellent example of Harpo's style can be found in *Monkey Business* (1931). Harpo is leaning against a sign on one side of a door appearing to be marked in bold letters, "MEN." Along ambles a well-dressed fellow who opens the door, enters the room, and seconds later is seen by the audience flying out the door and landing on his rear. At this point, Harpo strolls away from the wall, revealing that the sign actually reads "WOMEN." Harpo also leads his brothers in the taking of English homonyms and other words literally. A movie packed full of many of these gems is *Horsefeathers* (1932)—the *Animal House* of the 1930s. For example, when Groucho demands a "seal" to make the contract process valid and binding, his mute brother extracts a live, black, slippery, flipper-clapping sea mammal from his baggy overcoat and dumps it on the desk. In another scene, when Chico and Harpo pose as icemen and enter carrying a large chunk of ice in each other's arms, Groucho questions the practicality of their methods. He demands, "Where's your tongs?" whereupon the other two open their mouths wide and stick out their tongues.

Harpo's magical overcoat is essential to this visual type of comic punning. He always comes up with anything a person demands, as in the episode with the seal and

6d

in the gag where a ragged hobo approaches him with the request, "Say, buddy, I'd like to get a cup of coffee." The man is obviously looking for a handout of money, but Harpo's response is to reach into the inside pocket of his tattered overcoat, pull out a white saucer and a cup of steaming coffee, and hand it to the dumbfounded bum. A witty variation of this style—a put-on—occurs in *Monkey Business* when the brothers are trying to get off a steamship and they cut through a line to the customs table. When they are stopped by officials, a bald, uniformed man demands a "passport" from Harpo. Harpo proceeds to pull everything out of his overcoat that has a somewhat similar sounding name, from a washboard to a cupboard, infuriating the inspector a little more each time.

Harpo even takes clichés and trite phrases literally and vivifies them. In *A Night in Casablanca* (1949), a policeman spots Harpo loitering and leaning against a wall and asks him, "What are you doing? Holding up the building?" Harpo vigorously nods his head affirmatively. As the policeman drags him away, the bricks, glass, and wood of the building rumble to the ground, leaving a rising cloud of dust, a stunned cop, and a grinning Harpo. . . .

Although this passage is only part of the essay and its outline, it illustrates how a precise thesis and a clear plan of development can help a writer achieve the momentum that makes writing satisfying.

6d The introduction

Few rules of writing are binding, but it is ordinarily desirable that an essay's introductory paragraph (1) attract and hold the reader's attention, (2) indicate the subject matter of the paper, and (3) reveal in some way the writer's attitude toward the subject. As these guidelines suggest, you can usually write an effective introduction only *after* you have formulated your thesis statement. In fact, since the success of an introductory paragraph depends on a writer's understanding of the complete essay, many writers work on their introductions after they have written everything else for a paper.

If you remember that any beginning can be changed, or even discarded, you should not be hesitant about starting an introduction. One way of getting started, especially for short papers, is to begin with your thesis statement:

> *The so-called "generation gap" of the 1960s and 1970s has today been replaced by feelings of open, deep indifference.* In the 1960s youth was attacked for its involvement in political and peace movements and its rebellion against sterile education and the war-as-usual. In the 1970s it was criticized for its preoccupation with careers, its apathy about social issues, and its interest in "doing one's own thing." Knowing that earlier generations were denounced for contradictory reasons, many students of the 1980s can see no reason at all why they should listen to adult America.

If your subject is a published work, you might try opening with a key quotation from the text you are going to discuss, as the student writer of the following example did.

It is the "quick, compact imagery of a single statement that forms the basis of Navajo poetry," says Oliver LaFarge. *This remark can well be illustrated in LaFarge's own story of Navajo life,* Laughing Boy, *a novel in which things are perceived and identified through "quick, compact imagery."* The first image of the novel ties the protagonist, Laughing Boy, to his environment: "His new red headband was a bright color among the embers of the sun-struck desert, undulating like a moving graph of the pony's lope"—a simple statement, but a "compact image" of the movement of a man on his horse over flat ground.

6d

In this paragraph, the writer has used a quotation from LaFarge to provide the focusing phrase for the thesis statement: *"Laughing Boy* [is] a novel in which things are perceived and identified through 'quick, compact imagery.'"

Perhaps the most sophisticated introduction, though, is one that gradually builds up to the thesis statement. Placing the thesis at the end of an introduction enables you to begin with background information that establishes a context for your main point. Moreover, a thesis in this position leads smoothly into the first paragraph of the body of the paper. In the following introductory paragraph, for example, notice how the student writer uses a brief historical survey to frame her thesis.

Beginning in the 1960s, the United States saw a growing militancy among native Americans. During this time, these people began to put aside their inter-tribal difficulties and feuds, and to unite and support each other's causes. The American Indian Movement (AIM), with its militancy and activism, soon drew national attention to the oppression and discrimination of Indian peoples. AIM, however, worked outside the established system, battling for Indian rights on the streets. *Now native Americans have gone beyond this strategy and are waging battle from a new front—the courtroom.*

Without the perspective provided by the opening sentences of this introduction, we would not understand the significance of the writer's thesis, which focuses on the new legal action being taken by native Americans.

In the following introductory paragraph, another student writer has used the same strategy to establish a context for his analysis of a short story.

It's often difficult for us to pause and analyze our relationships with other people. Instead, we find it easier to live each day as it comes without forming personal commitments or attachments. Sooner or later, though, everyone realizes that it is impossible to live with a person and not really care whether he or she will be there tomorrow. *The two characters in Dan Jacobson's short story "Led Astray" come to this realization and discover that no relationship can exist without feeling.*

To appreciate the effectiveness of this approach, notice that the thesis statement and the introductory sentences in this paragraph could not simply be flipped around in the reverse order. The thesis is not merely attached to the introductory sentences; rather, it appears to develop out of them.

In the following student paragraph, the writer uses his opening sentences for a different purpose—to create an informal tone and to establish himself as an authority on his subject.

> The Hawaiian Islands are anchored in a position where they receive sea swells the year round. The contour of the ocean floor and the structure of the reefs turn these swells into beautiful breaking waves, which make Hawaii a surfer's paradise. I have been surfing in this paradise every day for the last seven years, and I can tell you that there is probably no more purely natural act than surfing. You are at one with nature's most basic element—the living sea. *But as changing times bring "progress" to the islands, surfing in Hawaii will also be forced to change.*

6e

No matter what form of introduction you use, a few general guidelines apply. First, try to create for your reader the impression of a fresh beginning, even though you may have written and discarded half a dozen versions of your introduction before you were satisfied. Second, be certain that your thesis statement is prominent enough for your reader to have no trouble identifying it among the other sentences of your introduction. Finally, remember that confidence, authority, and solid content characterize the most successful opening paragraphs. Stay clear of any beginnings that sound trite and obvious: "Our modern world is an ever-changing one." "It is obvious to everyone that today's children watch too much television." Avoid formulas like "This essay will discuss . . ." or apologies like "Although I am far from being an expert on this subject. . . ." All such beginnings discourage even the most determined reader.

<u>6e</u> The body

The sections on outlining later in this chapter and the discussion of paragraphing in Chapters **7** and **8** offer the fullest treatment of the material that comes between the introduction and the conclusion—the body of your paper. But this is an appropriate place to mention the principle of **emphasis** and its role in shaping the body of an essay.

The more space you give an idea, the more important it will appear to your reader. As you begin thinking about how to present your ideas in the body of your paper, therefore, plan to develop points that are approximately equal in importance with roughly equal amounts of evidence and discussion, and devote more space to any ideas that you wish to stand out above others. Keep in mind the distinction between what your readers already know about your subject and what else you want them to know (see **2b**). Commonly accepted judgments or matters of fact, for example, can be stated briefly, but your position on a controversial issue may need the support of concrete evidence presented in one or more fully developed paragraphs with tight logical structure.

You can achieve appropriate emphasis in an essay through arrangement as well as balance. Whenever you use several facts, examples, or arguments to establish a point, consider arranging them in order beginning with the weakest argument or the least important fact and moving to the strongest and most important. Evidence organized in this way gives you the chance to convince a skeptical reader through what seems to be the accumulating of solid proof. If you use your best evidence first, the rest of your paper will seem anticlimactic, and the force of your entire argument may be undercut.

6f The conclusion

6f

Not every paper requires a conclusion. A particularly short essay, for example, may not need the added sense of completeness that a conclusion provides. When a conclusion is called for, however, it should be more than a sentence or a paragraph attached to the end of an essay with a mechanical transition like "Therefore . . ." or "In conclusion. . . ." Rather than merely summarizing what has gone before, the best conclusions mark the arrival of the essay at the destination announced in its introductory paragraph. An essay should end with the ease and authority of a musical composition that brings its themes to a unified, harmonious resolution, giving the reader a sure sense of finality. For example, consider this ending to a student's seven-hundred-word essay on Chekhov's play *The Seagull.*

> When the curtain falls on *The Seagull,* one has the feeling that the story is not at all ended, that the action continues behind the curtain. Reflecting on this, one may find that the secret of Chekhov's effect lies in avoiding the overly dramatic, the play in which everything builds to one climax centered in one character. Chekhov has allowed the themes of love and death, of dreams and reality, to unfold in the random, senseless way that they occur in our lives.

Often the feeling of completeness that a well-written conclusion conveys can be created by picking up a word or phrase from the introduction, or by recalling an earlier example. The student surfer whose introduction we quoted above went on to argue that the increasing number of surfers in Hawaii would either have to discipline themselves to share the waves or have to expect state regulation of the sport, and he concluded by emphasizing the concept of the living sea and the inevitability of change—two key ideas from his introduction:

> Unless we treat the sea with the consideration that it deserves as a source of wonder, pleasure, and life, sacrificing our own selfish desire to catch the big wave regardless of who or what is in the way, we can look forward to the regulation of surfing. Police patrolling the beaches, floodlights stuck into the sand for day and night surfing, licenses, permits, tickets—these are not pleasant prospects. But neither are the fights, the racial name-calling, the indifference to another surfer's safety which one encounters all too often in Hawaiian waters. To live in a world of change we must learn to change ourselves.

A writer may also conclude strongly by making connections between ideas explored earlier in the paper. In the following student example, an analysis of Robert Pirsig's *Zen and the Art of Motorcycle Maintenance* and Ralph Ellison's

Invisible Man, note how the writer links Phaedrus and the Invisible Man, the protagonists of the two novels.

> Participation in life and the celebration of its possibilities are what both Phaedrus and the Invisible Man finally affirm. They are able to do so as a result of their personal quests. Yet they both set out in ignorance, not knowing the direction they are actually headed in. At the end, when the Invisible Man says, "Who knows but that, on the lower frequencies, I speak for you?" it is a warning that most of us are still back at the very beginning simply because we think we're not or, worse yet, because we don't even think about it.

No competent writer dashes off a conclusion at the last moment. When we finish reading an essay we should feel that it had to end as it did. Writing that creates this sense of completion is the result of careful thought and painstaking revision, but its effectiveness justifies the effort.

6g The formal outline

For many writers, one of the most effective means of planning and revising papers is outlining, the systematic listing of an essay's main points. Even the most experienced writers usually begin with some kind of informal outline, however much they may modify it or deviate from it as they expand upon their subject. For less experienced writers, outlining can be an essential tool.

Outlines serve several purposes. Perhaps the most important use of the formal outline is to help a writer organize ideas generated during the discovery stage of the writing process (see Chapter **4**). The visual model of an essay's structure that an outline provides can help the writer anticipate the logical divisions of a topic, decide on appropriate supporting evidence and detail, and consider connections between the paper's main points. The more complex the topic and the more elaborate its supporting evidence, the more essential outlining becomes.

A second use of the formal outline is to assist in the revision of a rough draft or an unsatisfactory final version. When a paper seems to lack coherence, balance, or tight logical structure, a formal outline of the paper's contents can help to diagnose its problems. An outline enables you to translate the vague feeling that something is wrong with a paper into specific knowledge about which points need further development and where stronger transitions would improve coherence.

Finally, outlines often provide a fruitful way of examining another writer's plan and structure. Suppose, for example, that you have read three essays on Lincoln's use of power during the Civil War and are to write on the authors' differing assumptions about the presidency. By constructing three accurate outlines and thereby highlighting in visual form the crucial differences among the essays, you can save yourself from skimming over and over the same paragraphs and snatching at random phrases or details. Formal outlining is also useful when you are asked to refute another writer's argument. By outlining his or her essay, you can isolate the key issues and examine the evidence and logic that support them. Outlining your reading, in short, enables you to discover someone else's views as you clarify your own.

Informal outlines may follow any pattern that a particular writer finds helpful, but formal outlines fall into three groups: the paragraph outline, the topic outline, and the sentence outline. Each has its particular uses and limitations.

The first of these, the paragraph outline, is a list of sentences numbered so that sentence one summarizes paragraph one, sentence two summarizes paragraph two, and so on. For example:

6g

1. Outlining is a systematic listing of an essay's most important points.
2. The first use of a formal outline is to help the writer anticipate the main divisions of the topic and connect ideas and evidence.
3. The second use of the formal outline is in the revision of a rough draft. . . .

The paragraph outline helps you review the progression of major ideas in a paper. For that reason, it is often a good starting point in planning an essay. What the paragraph outline does not show clearly, however, are the kinds of evidence used to develop the paragraphs in an essay or the precise logical relationships between them. As you become more certain about your paper's probable organization and development, you may want to rely more heavily on the outline forms that do indicate this material—the topic and sentence outlines.

The topic outline begins with the entire thesis statement, the main idea being developed in the paper. After the thesis, though, its entries are words or brief phrases, numbered and lettered to show the relative importance of the paper's supporting ideas. (The paper written from the topic outline on page 52 may be found on pages 318–33.)

For brief papers in class, tests, and short analyses or reports, the topic outline is useful and usually sufficient. Carelessly used or misunderstood, however, it merely deceives the writer and very often causes vagueness and disorder. Headings like "Introduction," "Main Body," and "Conclusion" and subheadings like "Example," "Reasons," and "Results" delay concrete thinking and reveal nothing. Consider the following example:

Vague topic outline

The Change from School to College

  I. Introduction
      A. High school ideas
      B. Reasons for these ideas

  II. What my first impressions were
      A. Two examples
      B. Results

6g

Anne Bradstreet's Homespun Cloth:
The First American Poems

Thesis: In its combination of revulsion and submission, Anne
Bradstreet's poetry represents an American variation on the "Puritan dilemma."

I. Biographical Introduction
   A. Anne Bradstreet's voyage to Massachusetts Bay
   B. Her reaction to the New World

II. The Puritan Dilemma
   A. Conflict between impulse and dogma
      1. Love of this world
      2. Love of God and submission to His will
   B. Bradstreet's dilemma
      1. Rebellion against the New World
      2. Submission to God's will

III. Handicaps of a woman poet in colonial America
   A. Physical Handicaps
      1. Harsh living conditions
      2. Endless labor raising eight children
   B. Psychological handicaps
      1. Woman's duty to do housework
      2. General distrust of poetry as "Devil's
         Library"
      3. Writing believed dangerous for female minds
         a. Governor's wife
         b. Sister Sarah
         c. Anne Hutchinson

IV. Bradstreet's best poetry produced by tension
   A. Conflict between love of this world and of Heavenly
      Kingdom in her later poems
   B. Increased interest in personal experiences as
      themes
      1. Fear of death in childbirth
      2. Autumnal splendor declaring the glory of God
      3. Adjustment to early death of grandchildren
      4. Destruction of house in fire

V. Conclusion: Final success of Bradstreet's homespun
   muse

III. Conclusions
    A. Why I have changed my mind
    B. Advice to high school seniors

The vague entries here largely undercut the potential value of outlining. Though they suggest the paper's general direction, they do little to help the writer organize his ideas or consider his supporting evidence.

    For long papers, a sentence outline may be even more valuable than a good topic outline. Since each entry in a sentence outline is a complete sentence, this form of outline makes a thorough analysis of a paper's contents possible. Note how a good topic outline can be expanded into a sentence outline:

6g

Topic outline

The Complexity of Experience of Laughter

Thesis: Although there are several theories of laughter, no single one accounts for the quite distinct emotions that cause it.

  I. Single explanation theories of laughter
    A. Social punishment
      1. Mocks differences
      2. Shows feeling of superiority
    B. Defense against social taboos
      1. Relies on dirty jokes
      2. Is relief of tension
    C. Sudden surprise
      1. Stimulated by the unexpected act
      2. Is delight in being startled

  II. Complex experience of laughter
    A. Descriptions of feelings
      1. "To have the last laugh"
      2. "To laugh at"
      3. "To laugh off"
    B. Descriptions of vocal expressions
      1. "To chuckle"
      2. "To giggle and titter"
      3. "To snicker"
      4. "To guffaw"

  III. Inadequacies of theories of laughter to experience of laughter
    A. Failure to account for description of feelings
      1. No sudden pleasurable surprise in social punishment theory
      2. No sense of superiority in social taboo theory
      3. No self-embarrassment in pleasurable surprise theory
    B. Failure to account for sheer joy
      1. No explanation of lovers' spontaneity by any theory
      2. No explanation of delight in success by any theory

Expansion to sentence outline

The Complexity of Experience of Laughter

Thesis: Although there are several theories of laughter, no single one accounts for the quite distinct emotions that cause it.

 I. The theories tend to explain laughter by a single emotion or cause.
   A. Laughter is social punishment inflicted by the majority.
      1. It mocks differences in dress, behavior, and belief.
      2. It is a feeling of superiority and satiric awareness.
   B. Laughter is a defense against social taboos.
      1. It is stimulated by the dirty joke and obscene remark.
      2. It is a safety-valve response relieving tension.
   C. Laughter is the expression of pleasure in the sudden surprise.
      1. It is stimulated by the unexpected physical or verbal act.
         a. The physical is often the sudden fall or thump.
         b. The verbal is usually a witty remark.
      2. It is delight in being startled.

 II. The experience of laughter is not a simple one.
   A. Our feelings while laughing vary.
      1. Vindictively we "have the last laugh."
      2. In amusement we "laugh at" something.
      3. In embarrassment we "laugh it away."
   B. The vocal expressions of laughter vary.
      1. We "chuckle" in a low tone when inwardly satisfied.
      2. We "giggle and titter" in rapid, high-pitched sounds when silly.
      3. We "snicker" in sly, half-suppressed tones at another's plight.
      4. We "guffaw" in loud tones when heartily enjoying ourselves.

III. The theories are inadequate to the experience of laughter.
   A. No theory accounts for the ways we describe our feelings.
      1. The theory of laughter as social punishment neglects the laugh of sudden pleasurable surprise.
      2. The theory of laughter as a defense against social taboos minimizes the laugh of punishment and mockery.
      3. The theory of laughter as pleasurable surprise slights the laugh of self-embarrassment.
   B. All theories omit the laughter of sheer joy of being and doing.
      1. They do not account for the spontaneous laughter of children, lovers, and parents.
      2. They do not account for the triumphant, delighted laugh of the successful artist or athlete.

Notice that the sentence outline contains far more information and reveals a more detailed analysis than the topic outline. The sentence outline has the advantage of compelling you to formulate more explicitly the material you intend to use. For longer papers on complex topics—say, 1,500 words on the effects of automation on the unions or 2,000 words on methods of crime prevention—a sentence outline may be the best help.

<u>6h</u> Conventions of topic and sentence outlines

The following system of alternating numbers and letters is nearly universal in outlines:

Thesis:
  I.
      A.
          1.
          2.
              a.
              b.
      B.
  II.
      A.
      B.
      C.

6h

In topic outlines, capitalize the first letter of the word beginning each heading, but do not punctuate the end of the entry since it is not a sentence. In sentence outlines, start with a capital letter and end with a period or other terminal punctuation.

An outline begins with the thesis statement, the main idea to be developed in the paper. Roman numerals indicate the major *subdivisions* of the idea stated in the thesis. Capital letters, Arabic numbers, and small letters mark further and further subdivisions. The key to the logic of every outline is coordination and subordination. Coordinate points—those of equal importance—are indented the same distance from the left margin; under them, farther from the left margin, come subordinate, or supporting, points. In the outline above, for example, I and II are main points of equal importance, A and B are points of equal importance supporting I, and 1 and 2 are points of equal importance supporting A.

If an outline is to function as a tool for analysis, these conventions must be taken seriously. A writer who divides material like this negates the whole reason for outlining:

Illogical and confusing

    I. Advantages of outboard motors
        A. Relatively inexpensive
        B. Attachable to any small boat
   II. Easily transportable

"Easily transportable" is logically a subtopic under I, "Advantages of outboard motors." It should be made parallel with A and B:

Clear coordination and subordination

    I. Advantages of outboard motors
        A. Relatively inexpensive
        B. Attachable to any small boat
        C. Easily transportable

    II. Disadvantages of outboard motors
        A. Troublesome to repair on the water
        B. Limited fuel capacity

6h

When one subheading includes material covered in other parallel headings, the subdivisions are said to overlap. Overlapping subdivisions show that you have not analyzed your material fully.

Poorly analyzed—overlapping

    I. Organized welfare groups
        A. Early relief organizations
        B. Red Cross
        C. Community Chest
        D. Relief organizations today

Logically, "Relief organizations today" *includes* the Red Cross and Community Chest. If you are subdividing on a chronological basis, stick to it consistently, and make a subdivision for Red Cross and Community Chest:

Clearly subdivided

    I. Organized welfare groups
        A. History of early relief organizations
        B. Relief organizations today
            1. Red Cross
            2. Community Chest

One last word about subdivisions: convention demands that each topic which is subdivided must have at least two headings. The argument runs that dividing something must produce at least two parts. Occasionally, however, a lone subhead is a useful means of *reminding yourself* of an example, illustration, or reference you don't want to forget:

Reminder for full illustration

    I. Extension of Mohammedan power under the early caliphs
        A. Eastward and northward
            1. For example, Persian and Greek lands
        B. Westward
            1. For example, Syria, Egypt, and northern Africa

Though sometimes useful in working outlines, such lone headings should be eliminated from the final version of an outline.

Exercise 1

The questions for narrowing a subject (pages 40–41) will work best *after* you have explored a subject and considered your intended audience (see Chapters **2** and **4**). But to test their effectiveness, try using them to limit one or more of the following broad subjects, or another equally general subject of your choice. Which of the questions seem to be most helpful?

1. Family relationships
2. Music
3. Science
4. Your hometown
5. International relations
6. Religion
7. Transportation
8. Animals
9. Space exploration
10. Peace

6h

Exercise 2

Complete each of the following thesis statements in two *different* ways by adding two different restricting phrases. Make a list of the main points you might use to develop a paper for each of the thesis statements you produce.

Example

The campus radio station . . .

Thesis #1: The campus radio station gives students firsthand experience with sophisticated broadcasting equipment.

Thesis #2: The campus radio station plays a blend of music that fails to attract either students on campus or the public at large.

1. My best friend . . .
2. Extracurricular activities in high school . . .
3. Outstanding teachers . . .
4. College math [or English or biology] courses . . .
5. Having [or not having] a car on campus . . .

Exercise 3

On which of the subjects below do you already have a reasonably firm position? For each such case, formulate a thesis statement that would be the foundation for an essay of between five hundred and seven hundred words. How might you develop your essay?

1. Violence in television
2. The appeal of science fiction
3. Sex education in schools
4. The role of the SAT in the college admissions process
5. The death penalty
6. Defense spending
7. The study of foreign languages
8. The eating habits of American young adults
9. Prayer in public schools
10. Drunk driving

6h

Exercise 4

Write two *different* introductions for a paper that would develop *one* of the thesis statements that you produced in Exercise 2 or Exercise 3 above. Which introduction do you like better? Why? Would the essays that followed these introductions be likely to differ? If so, how?

Exercise 5

Examine a chapter in one of your textbooks or an article in a magazine such as *Scientific American, Atlantic Monthly,* or *Natural History,* and consider the following points: (1) Are the introduction and the conclusion of the essay related? How? (2) Does the essay have a clear thesis? Where does it occur? (3) What are the main points with which the author develops the thesis? (4) What kind of support does the author present for each of these main points?

7 Paragraph Structure

The concept of a paragraph is no doubt familiar to you. Just about everything we read—from novels to newspapers, from textbooks to cookbooks—is printed with indentations that mark new paragraphs. And in most of your writing, you also probably adopt the tradition of using paragraphs to divide what you write into separate chunks. At the same time, you no doubt recognize that such divisions are not arbitrary, that paragraphs have a certain logic behind them. But how can we define more precisely what paragraphs are? And can we determine some principles for writing good paragraphs? These are among the questions to be explored in this chapter.

7a The paragraph as a unit

Try to imagine, for a moment, a world with no paragraph indentations. Every book, every newspaper, every magazine would present a solid page of type, with no white spaces inviting you to pause and rest, even momentarily. Reading under these circumstances would be tedious and tiring. But would removing printed indentations actually eliminate paragraphs, or would doing so only make identifying them more difficult for the reader? To find out, try reading the following short magazine article, printed without its original paragraph indentations. In particular, consider this question: without the indentations, has this text now become one long paragraph, or are the original separate paragraphs still here, and still perceptible, with a little extra work on your part?

In the course of almost four decades of research, Dr. Paul MacLean of the National Institute of Mental Health has determined that there is a zoo in the human brain. More precisely, there are in the human brain evolutionary holdovers from our animal origins, he says, that influence our behavior and thinking. In its evolution, the human forebrain has expanded in size while retaining three basic formations that reflect our ancestral relationship to reptiles, early mammals, and recent mammals. Radically different in size as well as chemistry, and in an evolutionary sense countless generations apart, the three formations constitute a hierarchy of three brains in one—a triune brain. The reptilian core, or "biological brain," which MacLean calls the R-complex, is involved in basic social behavior and preservation of the self and of the species. It contains built-in formats for the instinctual behavior of dominance and territoriality. As an example of human behavior that reflects that protoreptilian impulse, MacLean offers the "place preference" of lizards, which is no different, he says, from Archie Bunker's territorial attitude about his favorite chair. The limbic system, or "emotional brain," is a holdover from early mammals. Its integration of internal and external experiences accounts for the ineffable affective feelings required for self-preservation and for perpetuation of the species. Without the limbic system (a term that MacLean coined) there wouldn't be the kinds of behavior that distinguish mammals from reptiles—namely, nursing in conjunction with maternal care, vocalization for the purpose of maintaining contact, and play. The neomammalian formation, or "intellectual brain," is found only in the higher mammals. It makes language and rational thought possible for man and fosters cultural life. According to MacLean, the triune brain obliges us to view ourselves from three perspectives. As a further complication, there is evidence that the two older formations lack the necessary neural machinery for verbal communication. Despite [this] built-in incompatibility of the three brains, MacLean is not without hope for man. The continuing influence of our animal origins, millions of years strong, will not be easily transcended, but it can be, MacLean says in his forthcoming book, *The Triune Brain.*

—John White

Despite the way in which this passage is printed, you probably approached it by mentally dividing the text into separate chunks, in order to follow it more easily. When the author tells us in the introductory sentences that the human brain retains traces of three earlier formations, we expect him to discuss these three brains in the rest of the article. And that is indeed what he does in three middle paragraphs, each devoted to a different brain formation. After describing the three, he concludes with a paragraph commenting on the necessary conflict among them.

We look for these kinds of divisions whenever we read because, in order to read with understanding, we need to be able to identify the main ideas in the text before us and to perceive their relationship to one another. If we lived in a world where paragraphs were never marked, we would have to find them on our own as we read. To put it another way, if paragraphs were unknown in our world, we would simply have to invent them.

It should be evident from this discussion that the basic purpose that most paragraphs serve is to make a reader's work easier and more effective by dividing a text into its main parts and thus highlighting its main ideas. Underlying this concept of a paragraph are two other principles. First, a paragraph should ordinarily be unified around a single thought. If the function of paragraphing is to help point out a writer's main ideas, then it follows logically that separate ideas should be developed in separate paragraphs. On the other hand, all the paragraphs in a given piece of writing must also be related to one another in some clear way if the reader is to make sense of the text.

We might summarize these points by saying that paragraphs have a primarily *rhetorical* function. That is, they are intended by a writer to affect a reader in some way—in this case, to help a reader identify the writer's principal ideas and understand the relationship among them. Sometimes, of course, we create paragraphs almost unconsciously. When we are writing well, we find ourselves deeply involved in our subject and able to discover new ideas and connections as we go along. On such lucky occasions, we usually paragraph by the instinctive feeling that one section is complete and that we are ready to begin a new one. Later, during the revision of what we have written, we may expand or shorten a paragraph, or combine two paragraphs into one, or perhaps discover two paragraphs accidentally merged together that should be separated. We do all this so that our readers will be better able to follow our ideas.

7a

Exercise 1

Each of the following passages has been formed by printing two consecutive paragraphs without indentation. Separate each passage into two paragraphs again, and explain your reason for dividing them where you did. What is the main idea in each of the paragraphs you identified? Is the relationship between those ideas clear?

1.   Whoever said that people who do the least complain the most must have known my boss, Miss Eleanor. By hiding behind paperwork that takes the other store managers only a fraction of the time to finish, she is able to push the jobs she should be doing on whoever else is within earshot. Across the entire store one can hear her yelling for a clerk to bring her a file folder or a cash register tape lying only a few feet away. Her voice, fierce and commanding, together with her stony face and dark eyes, freezes everyone around her in fear. Eleanor is as vain as she is fearsome. In front of her desk she has a three-foot-square mirror in which we see her constantly making faces, admiring herself, and talking to herself. In her nearby "private" cabinet she has two cans of hair spray, a box of bobby pins, several combs and brushes, a set of electric curlers, enough makeup to make Frankenstein look acceptable, and half a dozen issues of *Vogue* magazine. It's no wonder Miss Eleanor is always so busy.

—Cathy Kwolik [student]

2.   The first thing you have to know, if you are going to be serious about Panama hats, is that genuine Panamas are not made in Panama at all and never have been. They are made in Ecuador—that is, the raw body of the hat is made in Ecuador, handwoven out of very thin strips of jipijapa palm leaves. Nor are they woven underwater, as many people seem to think; the leaves are simply woven while moist. The hat body is then sent off to hat makers around the world to be sized, blocked, and trimmed. But the important part, the weaving, has already happened in Ecuador. The misnomer is understandable: Sailors and traders first encountered the hat when they went ashore in Panama more than 150 years ago. Naturally, they called it a Panama hat, and the name they gave it stuck. All the more so when Teddy Roosevelt was photographed wearing a Panama hat at the construction site of the Panama canal. In the ensuing rush to buy Panama hats, no one took the trouble to straighten out the name, not even the Ecuadorians who had made Roosevelt's hat.

—John Berendt

3.   Medieval courtiers saw their table manners as distinguishing them from crude peasants; but by modern standards, the manners were not exactly refined. Feudal lords used their unwashed hands to scoop food from a common bowl and they passed around a single goblet from which all drank. A finger or two would be extended while eating, so as to be kept free of grease and thus available for the next course, or for dipping into spices or condiments—possibly accounting for today's "polite" custom of extending the finger while holding a spoon or small fork. Soups and sauces were commonly drunk by lifting the bowl to the mouth; several diners frequently ate from the same bread trencher. Even lords and nobles would toss gnawed bones back into the common dish, wolf down their food, spit onto the table (preferred conduct called for spitting under it), and blow their noses into the tablecloth. By about the beginning of the sixteenth century, table manners began to move in the direction of today's standards. The importance attached to them is indicated by the phenomenal success of a treatise, *On Civility in Children,* by the philosopher Erasmus, which appeared in 1530; reprinted more than thirty times in the next six years, it also appeared in numerous translations. Erasmus' idea of good table manners was far from modern, but it did represent an advance. He believed, for example, that an upper-class diner was distinguished by putting only three fingers of one hand into the bowl, instead of the entire hand in the manner of the lower class. Wait a few moments after being seated before you dip into it, he advises. Do not poke around in your dish, but take the first piece you touch. Do not put chewed food from the mouth back on your plate; instead, throw it under the table or behind your chair.

—Peter Farb and George Armelagos

7b The topic sentence

The main idea of a paragraph is often stated explicitly in a single sentence or two called the **topic sentence.** Just as a thesis statement identifies the central idea in an entire essay, a topic sentence helps to unify a paragraph around a single idea. Like a thesis, it usually introduces both a subject and a specific aspect of that subject, or focus. Like a thesis, too, a topic sentence is in some sense an arguable statement, one that leads to—in fact, demands—specific support or proof in the rest of the paragraph.

Consider for a moment the following two sentences:

a. Abraham Lincoln was born in what is now Larue County, Kentucky.
b. A food processor, as more and more good cooks are discovering, is an indispensable kitchen tool.

The first sentence here could not be a strong topic sentence, because instead of presenting an idea that needs support, it simply states a fact. The sentence is obviously about Lincoln, but it does not contain an idea that could be developed further into an entire paragraph. In contrast, the second sentence has both a clear subject, *food processor,* and a controlling focus, *indispensable.* This sentence naturally leads to a paragraph that will explain why a food processor is indeed indispensable in one's kitchen. What tasks does it do well? Does it save time? Or eliminate waste? Such a well-formulated topic sentence, with a clearly stated subject and focus, provides a writer with a kind of blueprint that directs the development of the rest of the paragraph. Organizing paragraphs around topic sentences in your first draft can help you determine the appropriate content for each paragraph in an essay, control the paragraph's focus, and eliminate irrelevant details. And keeping your topic sentences in view as you revise an essay is a way of checking that all the sentences in a paragraph really belong there.

7b

Topic sentences are often found near the beginnings of paragraphs. In this position, a topic sentence announces the writer's main idea and therefore establishes expectations about the development of the paragraph in the reader's mind. If you were to read a paragraph that began, "Traveling by train is once again becoming popular in the United States," you would expect that sentence to be followed by statistics or other evidence that demonstrated the rising popularity of rail travel. A good topic sentence near the start of a paragraph always arouses such expectations in the reader, and a good paragraph goes on to satisfy those expectations with relevant, specific, convincing information.

Although most writers naturally pause, reflect, and center their thoughts at the start of a paragraph, there is nothing sacred about beginning a paragraph with a topic sentence. A topic sentence may be placed anywhere—after a transitional sentence, in the middle, or at the end as a kind of conclusion. When a topic sentence comes in the middle of a paragraph, it usually links the sentences that precede it with the material that follows it, as in this example:

Topic sentence in middle

> In the Western world, the person is synonymous with an individual inside a skin. And in northern Europe generally, the skin and even the clothes may be inviolate. You need permission to touch either if you are a stranger. This rule applies in some parts of France, where the mere touching of another person during an argument used to be legally defined as assault. *For the Arab the location of the person in relation to the body is quite different.* The person exists somewhere down inside the body. The ego is not completely hidden, however, because it can be reached very easily with an insult. It is protected from touch but not from words. The dissociation of the body and the ego may explain why the public amputation of a thief's hand is tolerated as standard punishment in Saudi Arabia.
>
> —Edward T. Hall

The opening sentences in this paragraph provide a context for the writer's discussion of the Arab conception of the person. The topic sentence—the fifth sentence—introduces the paragraph's controlling idea, the contrast between Western and Arab attitudes.

When the topic sentence concludes a paragraph, it usually pulls together sentences that have led up to it. In these cases, the subject and focus of the paragraph are left implied until the reader reaches the topic sentence. The result is often a paragraph with an effective sense of climax, as in the following case.

Topic sentence at end

7b

Call it a clan, call it a network, call it a tribe, call it a family. Whatever you call it, whoever you are, you need one. You need one because you are human. You didn't come from nowhere. Before you, around you, and presumably after you, too, there are others. Some of these others . . . must matter. They must matter a lot to you and if you are very lucky to one another. Their welfare must be nearly as important to you as your own. *Even if you live alone, even if your solitude is elected and ebullient, you still cannot do without a clan or a tribe.*

—Jane Howard

Although the practice of constructing a paragraph around a focusing sentence is a valuable one, not *every* paragraph will have an explicit topic sentence. In some cases, a paragraph may be well unified without a topic sentence. But the paragraph's central idea or thought should still be evident to the reader. The following student paragraph, for instance, has no stated topic sentence, but its central idea is still clear.

Implied topic sentence

Classes at the medieval University of Paris began at 5 a.m. First on the agenda were the ordinary lectures, which were the regular and more important lectures. After several ordinary lectures and a short, begrudged lunch hour, students attended extraordinary lectures given in the afternoon. These were supplementary to the ordinary lectures and usually given by a less important teacher, who may not have been more than fourteen or fifteen years old. A student would spend ten or twelve hours a day with his teachers, and then following classes in the late afternoon, he had sports events. But after sports, the day was not over. There was homework, which consisted of copying, recopying, and memorizing notes while the light permitted. Nor was there much of a break. Christmas vacation was about three weeks, and summer vacation was only a month.

All of the details in this paragraph develop the same idea, which we might state in a sentence like "The long school day at the medieval University of Paris made heavy demands on students."

As you can see, an implied topic sentence works only when the development of your paragraph makes its point absolutely clear. Most of the time, you should probably make an effort to include a topic sentence somewhere in your paragraphs, rather than risk leaving your reader uncertain about your main point. Similarly, you can often make reading easier for yourself by locating, and perhaps underlining, the topic sentences in paragraphs you read. The great value of the topic sentence for reader and writer alike is its function of focusing on the main idea and giving a paragraph direction.

Exercise 2

Which of the following could make good topic sentences? Identify the subject and the specific focus of each. How might you develop those sentences into paragraphs?

1. Sunspots, magnetic storms on the sun's surface, are responsible for a number of important phenomena on earth.
2. Acquiring an inexpensive metal detector can be the start of a profitable hobby.
3. In most of the United States, the average annual rainfall is between 15 and 45 inches.
4. Montreal, the largest city in Canada, is also the second-largest French-speaking city in the world.
5. The most important requirement for a successful long-distance runner is not endurance but concentration.
6. Last July two friends and I went backpacking in the Smokey Mountains.
7. A person suffering from heatstroke must receive correct treatment swiftly.
8. The plays of Hrotswitha von Gandersheim, a tenth-century German nun, often suggest that she had a lively sense of humor.
9. Air mail service in the United States began in 1918.
10. *The Grapes of Wrath* is John Steinbeck's novel about dispossessed Oklahoma farmers.

Exercise 3

Identify the topic sentence in each of the following paragraphs. What subject and specific focus does it introduce? How do the rest of the sentences in the paragraph develop that idea?

1. Violence as a way of achieving racial justice is both impractical and immoral. It is impractical because it is a descending spiral ending in destruction for all. The old law of an eye for an eye leaves everybody blind. It is immoral because it seeks to humiliate the opponent rather than win his understanding; it seeks to annihilate rather than to convert. Violence is immoral because it thrives on hatred rather than love. It destroys community and makes brotherhood impossible. It leaves society in monologue rather than dialogue. Violence ends by defeating itself. It creates bitterness in the survivors and brutality in the destroyers.

    —Martin Luther King, Jr.

2. [C]ommercial interruption is most damaging during that 10 per cent of programming (a charitable estimate) most important to the mind and spirit of a people: news and public affairs, and drama. To many (and among these are network news producers), commercials have no place or business during the vital process of informing the public. There is something obscene about a newscaster pausing to introduce a deodorant or shampoo commercial between an airplane crash and a body count. It is more than an interruption; it tends to reduce news to a form of running entertainment, to smudge the edges of reality by treating death or disaster or diplomacy on the same level as household appliances or a new gasoline.

    —Marya Mannes

7c

3.   All is not well for caves or cave dwellers in Missouri. Many serious problems now exist in the effort to preserve caves in their original condition. Casual visitors often turn into vandals, breaking formations and chasing off the easily scared bat populations. In addition, holes and pits on the surface caused by natural cave collapses are being used as dumps, resulting in contamination of water systems in the caves. Another increasingly serious problem is the growing contamination of caves by septic tank drainage. The contamination of Devil's Icebox Cave by septic tanks. for example, has caused national groups such as the Sierra Club to organize a cave preservation program. Finally, the Army Corps of Engineers has been responsible for flooding hundreds of caves with its river-damming projects in the state.

—Scott Stayton [student]

4.   Children often transform what should be a matter of nutrition into a question of self-determination. For some youngsters the benevolence of their parents' assertions that carrots are good for you, that they help you to see in the dark, is lost in the suspicion that they are being tricked into tasting something nasty. Distrust flavors the carrots, they *do* taste unpleasant, and the child is even more adamantly opposed to eating them. The parents insist, the child resists, and battle lines are drawn. The issue is no longer whether vegetables are indeed good for you, but whose will power is to prevail. The ability to sustain her refusal becomes a matter of survival for the child. I recall that the longer I held out, the more I feared that giving in would topple my tower of autonomy. Those who would suggest that my parents simply were not authoritative enough underestimate the depth of my young conviction.

—Susan Young [student]

<u>7c</u> Paragraph length

Just as the structure of a paragraph is designed for the reader's benefit, so also the length of a paragraph is determined by its helpfulness to the reader. Indeed, we might say that the appropriate length of a paragraph is directly related to its structure. The key question is always: *How much evidence or other support do you need to develop the idea in your topic sentence?* Pages consistently cluttered by short, underdeveloped paragraphs scatter the reader's attention and give the impression of a writer unable to think an idea through completely. On the other hand, if too many sentences are combined without paragraph indentations, the reader will have a difficult time isolating the writer's main ideas. Paragraphs that run consistently to more than a page are little better than no paragraphing at all, since they force the reader to do work that is the writer's responsibility.

Ordinarily, then, we might say that a paragraph should be longer than one sentence but shorter than a page. But note that the length of paragraphs varies considerably in different kinds of writing. In formal, scientific, or scholarly writing, paragraphs may be four hundred words or longer. In magazine articles the average length is below two hundred words. In newspapers different rules of paragraphing apply, and indentations may come every fifty words or so. If you're in doubt about the length of a paragraph you're working on, ask yourself the questions about structure that we discussed above: What is the main idea in this paragraph? Are all of the sentences in the paragraph clearly related to it?

Occasionally, you may want to use a very short paragraph to call attention to an important shift in the line of thought or to emphasize a crucial point. A short paragraph will sometimes serve both of these purposes, but such paragraphs should be used sparingly. Notice in the following example that the student might have joined his short paragraph of rhetorical emphasis to either of the other paragraphs. He chose instead to make the two sentences into a separate transitional paragraph and thus to stress the importance of his early training and the shock he was to receive.

7c

Brief transitional paragraph

. . . I know from personal experience the truth of Erich Fromm's criticism that the American male is forced to repress his feelings. Our society does tend to suspect emotional outbursts in a man as signs of "abnormality." From childhood onward, I was taught to "control" my emotions. I was told constantly that good little boys don't cry; they act like big strong men. The little boy who fell off his tricycle and got up with a smile was admired and recommended as a model to be emulated by the rest of the tricycle set. Nor were feelings of pain the only emotion I was encouraged to suppress. Anger, hostility, envy, and melancholy were all taboo, and this training was almost impossible to resist.

By the age of thirteen, I was a true believer in this Spartan code. It was at this age that I was first startled into doubting it.

My uncle had been ill but had kept this fact secret from. . . .

Short paragraphs are also used for dialogue. In a narrative, any direct quotation, together with the rest of a sentence of which it is a part, is paragraphed separately. The reason for this convention is to make immediately clear to the reader the change of speaker.

Identified speakers paragraphed separately

"But 'glory' doesn't mean 'a nice knock-down argument,'" Alice objected.

"When *I* use a word," Humpty Dumpty said, in a rather scornful tone, "it means what I choose it to mean—neither more nor less."

"The question is," said Alice, "whether you *can* make words mean so many different things."

"The question is," said Humpty Dumpty, "which is to be master—that's all."

—Lewis Carroll

The same convention is usually observed in cases where the speaker is not named each time.

Unidentified speakers paragraphed separately

> "Hello," she said. "Are you awake?"
>
> "Where have you been?"
>
> "I just went out to get a breath of air."
>
> "You did, like hell."
>
> "What do you want me to say, darling?"
>
> —Ernest Hemingway

7d However, a short quoted speech that is closely united with the context is sometimes included in a paragraph of narration.

Short dialogue included in paragraph

> Now and then Mr. Bixby called my attention to certain things. Said he, "This is Six-Mile Point." I asssented. It was pleasant enough information but I could not see the bearing of it. I was not conscious that it was a matter of any interest to me. Another time he said, "This is Nine-Mile Point." Later he said, "This is Twelve-Mile Point." They were all about level with the water's edge; they all looked alike to me; they were monotonously unpicturesque. . . .
>
> —Mark Twain

<u>7d</u> Paragraphs and the whole essay

Rarely are we called on to write a single, isolated paragraph. Instead, effective writing usually means controlling individual paragraphs in the context of a longer composition. In the following essay, the student writer demonstrates such a firm sense of paragraph unity and appropriate paragraph length. Considered separately, each paragraph here makes a clear point, developed with specific details that interest and satisfy us. But the paragraphs of this essay also fit together neatly, leading us as readers through the writer's experiences and his reflections on them. The result is an effective piece of writing, well organized and complete. (The paragraphs in this essay have been numbered for easy reference in Exercise 4.)

I Surrendered

1.   Social order, it is said, can only be maintained through the restriction and prohibition of our often whimsical impulses (taking off from school or work, swimming nude, open sex), and we find ourselves inhibited by a civilization that was supposed to ensure our well-being. Parents, the law, and public opinion condition us to keep the lid tightly clamped on our drives for free and outward expression of inner needs: we are made to stop and evaluate our actions and thoughts and to feel guilty when they are not acceptable. And because this guilt often makes us tense and ill at ease, we give up and submit. This is what I understand Freud to be saying in *Civilization and Its Discontents,* and this is what I learned to be the melancholy fact when I went hitchhiking up the West Coast with my sleeping bag and thoughts of "doing my own thing."

2.   My hitchhiking trip with a white friend from Long Beach to Canada was plagued by social pressure even before it began. Two weeks before we started, reports over the news about hitchhikers being axed in their sleeping bags, as well as drivers being robbed, beaten, or killed, did not make our trip sound like a good idea to my family. My family was also concerned that reports like these make drivers hesitant of stopping for anyone unless they have a gun under the seat. That was just the beginning, though. I could have handled the fears others had for me, but the guilt I was made to feel was harder to cope with.

3.   My brother-in-law and I had a long discussion about the dangers of hitchhiking. The list was a frightening one that included the possibility I might be hassled and jailed by the police or be robbed and stranded. I felt quite guilty about running off and frolicking around while everyone worried about me, and this guilt took some of the pleasure—the thrill, day-to-day suspense, and excitement—out of the trip and made me wary.

7d

4.   My brother-in-law and I also discussed the fact that very few blacks hitchhike in the live-on-the-road manner I was about to, which means sleeping in forests, communes, or in freeway shrubbery, or going into strange towns and meeting all kinds of people. He suggested that if tension in any given situation forced a serious racial confrontation, my friend would surely turn to the safe side and against me. This kept me wondering all through the trip, and to my dismay, kept me looking for hints of racism in him, which took some of the pleasure out of the trip. It also made me feel guilty for suspecting him. My brother-in-law and I also talked about the fact that, instead of hitchhiking, I should be working to pay for college. Feeling all this guilt, and sensing the concern of my parents, I still set out with my friend.

5.   We carefully heeded (out of fear) California's policy on hitchhiking. Hitchhiking is illegal, but the law is not usually enforced if the hikers stay on the curb. We had no problems at all until just south of San Luis Obispo, where we were searched for weapons. There we were insulted by a pair of California Highway Patrol officers while they went over us. Among the many insults was the one directed at me, asking me who I was going to rape next. But, knowing how public opinion would side with the police if we retaliated, we kept our mouths closed. We knew that if the police reported subduing a couple of wandering, violent hippies, then the stereotype of the hippie (shiftless young bums begging for food and for money to buy drugs with) would justify the police in the public's view and set people's minds at ease. So we checked our natural impulse to fight back, but we were angry with ourselves for having to do so. We felt guilty for not standing up for our rights.

6.   Even with that episode behind us, the rest of the trip didn't bring me the pleasure I'd hoped for. The possible presence of dope in the cars of the young people who picked us up made me uneasy. But not my friend. He indulged heavily in marijuana all the way up the coast whenever he could get some. I knew that if we were arrested for dope it would go on my record, damage my chances in the future, and hurt my family badly. I would be ashamed and guilt-ridden. I was very worried about the presence of dope around me, even back in the deepest woods near Eureka, California. There, at one in the morning, my friend and another hiker who joined up with us smoked as much marijuana as they could hold. I was fearful that a band of night-roaming vigilantes would swarm on us and take us away. In Canada itself, I felt guilty the very first time I got in line for a feed-in. I was overly self-conscious because

7d

the food was paid for by Canadian taxpayers and was meant for needy people. We had enough money to buy food.

7.   It now seems that everything we did, beginning with the very thought of hitchhiking, was meant to prove we weren't as trapped as the people we left behind. But when it came to the wild, free expression of inner drives, I couldn't throw off the wet blanket of society. I couldn't even go skinny dipping in the Russian River because there were people around and I was afraid of what they might think if I stripped. We loved Canada and its forests, but we came back. Even though the air and water were like nectar in comparison to that of Los Angeles, we came back to the smog and noise and people. We discarded the forests, rivers, and meadows for the benefits and security of our social surroundings. I surrendered.

—Samuel Reece

Exercise 4

Reread Samuel Reece's essay "I Surrendered" (above) and consider the following questions.

1. What is Reece's thesis statement?
2. How do the final sentences of paragraph 2 provide a transition to paragraph 3? What other transitions between paragraphs can you identify in the essay?
3. Why has Reece separated paragraphs 3 and 4, both of which involve his brother-in-law's advice?
4. What is the topic sentence in paragraph 5? In paragraph 6?
5. How does Reece link his concluding paragraph with his introduction?

8 Paragraph Development

What happens in a paragraph—the shape and form it assumes—is often determined by the subject itself. If you are writing out a description of an automobile accident for your insurance company, you will probably let chronological order dictate the structure of your paragraphs (signaled left turn, waited for traffic light to change, started across intersection, suddenly saw other car coming through red light). On the other hand, if you are discussing two political candidates in your school newspaper, you might find your material falling easily into the form of a comparison. In short, in the words of American architect Louis Sullivan, "Form follows function."

Sometimes, however, the subject you are writing about may not arrange itself on your page with inevitable clarity and logic. For these occasions, it's useful to be acquainted with a number of basic patterns of paragraph development. Readers unconsciously expect to be able to discern such patterns and may be confused if the organization of a paragraph seems illogical or chaotic—for example, if a paragraph jumps back and forth in time for no clear reason. Controlling patterns of paragraph development, therefore, is simply another way of making your writing more effective by satisfying your readers' expectations.

Perhaps the most important thing to keep in mind about the methods of paragraph development described below is that, in actual practice, they are rarely used independently of one another. Instead, they naturally and inevitably overlap; development by examples, for instance, also implies development by detail. Thus, you should probably regard these patterns less as a set of alternatives for individual paragraphs than as a master list of techniques to select from and combine freely.

8a Development by specific detail

A paragraph lacking specific detail may strike a reader as dull and uninspired, even though its central idea is clear. Part of every writer's obligation is to supply the details necessary to support a paragraph's main idea; attempting to stress an idea simply by restating it is usually not sufficient. As a writer, you need to be able to distinguish between paragraphs that make effective use of detail and paragraphs that only seem to be developed specifically, but in reality offer little precise information that would move a reader to accept your argument or share your perspective.

8a

Writing with specific detail begins with recalling as precisely as possible the event to be described and then re-creating the taste, touch, sound, and sight with carefully chosen words. Often a paragraph can be dramatically improved by the simple substitution of specific details for generalities, without further revision. For example, in the two versions of the paragraph below, taken from a student essay about a senior class trip to Florida, notice how the writer has increased the effectiveness of his writing without adding significantly to its length, just by substituting specific details. The italicized passages indicate where changes have been made.

Vague original

When we left our high-school parking lot that Saturday morning, everybody was quite excited about the trip. We did a variety of things to pass the time, but monotony soon crept in. Also, I became cramped from sitting for long periods of time. When night finally came, we slept sitting up in our seats. Some slept on the aisle floors, where food and drinks had been spilled.

Revised with detail

When *the Greyhound bus roared out* of our high-school parking lot *at 6:30* that Saturday morning, everybody was excited about the trip. For a while we *sang songs and played cards* to pass the time, but monotony soon crept in. Also, after *seven or eight hours of sitting in the same seat,* I became stiff and cramped. When night finally came, most of us *dozed restlessly* sitting up in our seats, while others *huddled* on the *narrow* aisle floors, where *potato chips* and *Coke* had been spilled.

Of course, specific details in a paragraph must also be relevant to the writer's purpose. They must be *selected,* not merely inventoried. Details become boring—mere padding—when the writer confuses quantity with quality. For example, if an American student were asked by his Polish correspondent what a "drugstore" is, the American should not try to explain it by listing every type of cold tablet, sleeping pill, foot powder, lipstick, face cream, shaving lotion, writing implement, cigarette, candy, and magazine that it sells. But neither would it be helpful for him to write back simply that a drugstore fills prescriptions and sells medical supplies and cosmetics. Instead, the American might begin with such a definition and then explain that "medical supplies" *range from* cough syrups to allergy tablets, and that cosmetics *include* eye shadow, fingernail polish, and cologne. Such an approach could be used to suggest the variety and specialization of items available in a drugstore without having to rely on an exhaustive list.

8b Development by examples

Closely related to specific details are examples. An example is a member of a larger class or category, chosen to illustrate the class to which it belongs. Typically, the topic sentence of a paragraph developed by examples introduces the class that the writer wishes to develop. In this paragraph, for example, the class to be illustrated is "contaminants":

> Many contaminants contribute to air pollution inside offices, and they have a variety of sources. The worst offender, for smokers and nonsmokers alike, is ambient cigarette smoke, which contains benzene, formaldehyde and other carcinogens. Wet-process copiers give off odorless hydrocarbons, causing fatigue and skin irritations. Dry-process copiers leak ozone, an irritant to the eyes and respiratory tract. Computer screens exude low levels of radiation.
>
> —Susan Gilbert

8c

The pollutants mentioned here—cigarette smoke, hydrocarbons, ozone, and radiation—are not all of the office contaminants that could be mentioned. Rather, they are typical members of the class, presumably selected in this case because of their prevalence and importance.

Often examples are introduced in a paragraph with the transitions "for example" or "for instance." But even without these transitional markers, the structure of a paragraph developed by examples should be evident to a reader if the category that the examples illustrate is clearly stated at the outset. In the following paragraph, the illustrated category is "remedies [that] meet the test of modern scientific medicine."

> Undoubtedly many of the witch-healers' remedies were purely magical, such as the use of amulets and charms, but others meet the test of modern scientific medicine. They had effective painkillers, digestive aids, and anti-inflammatory agents. They used ergot for the pain of labor at a time when the Church held that pain in labor was the Lord's just punishment for Eve's original sin. Ergot derivatives are still used today to hasten labor and aid in the recovery from childbirth. Belladonna—still used today as an antispasmodic—was used by the witch-healers to inhibit uterine contractions when miscarriage threatened. Digitalis, still an important drug in treating heart ailments, is said to have been discovered by an English witch.
>
> —Barbara Ehrenreich and Deirdre English

8c Development by definition

In formal logic, definition involves referring a term to a general class of related elements (its genus), and then distinguishing it from others in that class. Before examining definition as a method of paragraph development, we should perhaps explain this basic use of the term.

To take a simple example, we would begin defining a pen by classifying it as a "writing instrument." However, since the class "writing instrument" also includes a number of other elements—pencils, felt markers, typewriters, to name just a few—we would have to go one step further and differentiate it from these and other members of the class. A pen, we might therefore continue, is "a writing instrument that makes use of a hard point and a colored fluid."

Term	Class	Differentiation
pen	writing instrument	makes use of a hard point and colored fluid
pencil	writing instrument	with a core of solid-state material like graphite inside a wooden or plastic case

8c

A description of an object can include all kinds of specific details—the pencil has a chewed end and is coated with yellow paint embossed with the motto "Quinn's Lumber Yard"—but these details are irrelevant to the definition of the term. Similarly, examples do not by themselves constitute a definition, although they may help to clarify one. To say that a Dixon Ticonderoga No. 2 Soft is an example of a pencil is not the same as specifying what the meaning of the term "pencil" is.

Informally, a writer can use simple apposition to define an unfamiliar term economically:

Definition by apposition

The X-ray showed a crack in the *tibia,* or *shinbone.*

Please analyze the importance of the *denouement—the final unraveling or outcome of the plot—*in *Lord Jim.*

Tonight the moon will be in *apogee,* that is, *at the point in its orbit farthest from the earth.*

But when writers are dealing with complex terms or terms used in a special sense, they may have to devote a paragraph or more to definition. The following student paragraph illustrates such an **extended definition.** The writer first classifies Sarah Woodruff and Clarissa Dalloway as belonging to the class of people whom she labels "heroic." Then, to differentiate her subjects' heroism from that of others in the class, she rejects one set of meanings for the term (control and domination) and presents another (sensitivity, endurance, independence). She closes the paragraph by explaining how each of her subjects meets this definition of "heroic."

The central characters in John Fowles's *The French Lieutenant's Woman* and Virginia Woolf's *Mrs. Dalloway* are women who embody certain heroic qualities that set them apart from what one character calls "the great niminypiminy flock of women in general." These two women, Sarah Woodruff and Clarissa Dalloway, are not heroic in the traditional masculine, aggressive sense of the word. They do not seek to control or to dominate but to cultivate a sensitivity, to endure, and to remain free of masculine narrow-mindedness. They possess a power that allows them to remain open to the compelling vitality of life. Their heroism is their ability to be responsive to reality, to feel even if it entails suffering and uncertainty; and this heroism spurs others on to live in the presence of life, with all its beauty and terror. Sarah is a free woman, and through her sensitivity, forbearance, and courage, she liberates Charles, a man caught in the petrifying forces of Victorian society, preoccupied with duty and piety. Clarissa Dalloway's radiant, vital presence at her party, a ritual of community, helps to liberate her guests from their shells of individual solitude and memory. It is in this sense and these ways that they are heroic.

8d

A few rules apply to the writing of all definitions, simple and extended. First, avoid circular definitions, that is, the use of the term being defined in the definition itself. "Democracy is the democratic process" and "An astronomer is one who studies astronomy" are both circular definitions. When words are defined in terms of themselves, no one's understanding is improved.

Second, avoid definition composed of long lists of synonyms. When a paragraph begins, "By education, I mean to give knowledge, develop character, improve taste, draw out, train, lead," the readers know they are in for the shotgun treatment. The writer has indiscriminately blasted a load of abstract terms at them, hoping one will hit. Precision and thoughtfulness are more important to a good definition than sheer volume.

Third, avoid loaded definitions, definitions which rely on evocative or inflammatory language. Their purpose is usually emotional impact rather than clarity. The negative phrasing of a definition like "Euthanasia is the outright murder of a helpless human being" makes the writer's bias unmistakable. Conversely, "By euthanasia I mean merciful intervention in a fellow human being's suffering" is a definition heavy with positive suggestions. Such judgments—for that is what they are—are sometimes used for powerful effect in persuasion, but they do not lead toward clarification if offered as definitions.

8d Development by classification

A writer using classification to develop a paragraph enumerates and describes the main divisions of a subject, either for clarification or as an introduction to further discussion. Underlying classification is the notion that the elements of any large group—classic cars, college students, home computers—can be collected into a number of subgroups ("There are three basic types of X"), and that the classification will better help us understand the category as a whole. In the following paragraph, for example, the noted anthropologist Margaret Mead uses classification to lead us to a new perspective on the concept of "culture."

> The distinctions I am making among *three* different kinds of culture—postfigurative, in which children learn primarily from their forebears, configurative, in which both children and adults learn from their peers, and prefigurative, in which adults learn also from their children—are a reflection of the period in which we live.

Primitive societies and small religious and ideological enclaves are primarily *postfigurative,* deriving authority from the past. Great civilizations, which necessarily have developed techniques for incorporating change, characteristically make use of some form of *configurative* learning from peers, playmates, fellow students, and fellow apprentices. We are now entering a period, new in history, in which the young are taking on new authority in their *prefigurative* apprehension of the still unknown future.

—Margaret Mead

Mead's paragraph illustrates a number of the principles of classification. First, a classification makes sense only if the things being classified are grouped according to some clearly understood principle or feature. For ease in record keeping, a college typically classifies its students according to a number of different principles: year of study, major, place of residence (dormitory, fraternity/sorority house, off-campus apartment, parents' home, etc.), to name just a few. Such classifications provide colleges with useful data about their student bodies, but a classification is usually worth writing about at length only if it also helps us understand something more fully or more clearly. Margaret Mead classifies cultures according to the sources of their members' education, and by doing so she gives us an important new perspective on some differences between our own culture and others that have preceded us.

The second feature of a successful classification is that it is exhaustive; that is, all the members of the larger group must fit into one or another of the categories of the classification. A college's students could not be classified sensibly as history majors, psychology majors, and music majors unless the college offered only these three fields of study. The three categories in Mead's paragraph illustrate the exhaustiveness necessary to a successful classification: the teachers in every society are either elders, or peers, or children; there are no other possibilities.

We routinely use classification every time we sort our laundry, plan a shopping trip, or organize the papers on our desk. Classification becomes an important pattern of organization for writing, though, when it helps us lead our readers to a new perspective on a complex subject.

8e Development by comparison or contrast

When we wish to point out the similarities or differences between two subjects, comparison or contrast is the logical method of development. The writer of an effective comparison/contrast paragraph indicates at the start the two subjects that will be treated and organizes the details related to each in a way that is easy for the reader to follow.

Comparisons are usually structured in one of two basic ways. In the first, known as an **alternating comparison,** the writer switches back and forth between two subjects throughout the paragraph, creating for the reader a point-by-point comparison based on specific aspects of the two subjects. The writer of the following paragraph, for instance, uses an alternating structure to compare books and films.

> There are other ways in which our freedom of choice is more limited with respect to film. While reading a book, we can imagine things quite freely even within the limits set by the description of the writer. Before *Gone with the Wind* was adapted to film, readers could picture Rhett Butler however they wished, although presumably basing that picture on the descriptions provided by Margaret Mitchell. But from the release of that movie on, Rhett Butler will always look like Clark Gable; indeed, that will be hardly less so even for readers who have never seen the film, so famous has that portrayal become. When we read Mary Shelley's novel *Frankenstein,* we may or may not be able to overcome the visual image imposed by all the movie *Frankenstein* monsters. But when we see the film *Frankenstein,* it is impossible for us to overcome the visual image; that is all there is, it is right in front of us, and we cannot make it any different. Moreover, a film can only show us what can be shown: the eye can only see what can be seen by the eye, a limitation not shared by the mind's eye.
>
> —Morris Beja

8e

The phrase "more limited" in the topic sentence indicates that a comparison is to follow, and the phrase "freedom of choice" indicates the issue on which the comparison will be based. Beja uses an alternating comparison in the rest of this paragraph because his point—that films impose limitations on the imagination which books do not—can best be illustrated by juxtaposing specific books and their film adaptations.

In the second type of comparison, called **divided comparison,** a writer deals fully with the first subject before turning to the second, thereby dividing the paragraph approximately in half. This approach works well when the subjects cannot be compared on a point-by-point basis and the writer is more interested in describing each at length. In the following divided comparison, the beginning of a longer paragraph, E. B. White reflects on one of the changes that have occurred at a favorite lake since he visited the place as a boy.

> Peace and goodness and jollity. The only thing that was wrong now, really, was the sound of the place, an unfamiliar nervous sound of the outboard motors. This was the note that jarred, the one thing that would sometimes break the illusion and set the years moving. In those other summertimes all motors were inboard; and when they were at a little distance, the noise they made was a sedative, an ingredient of summer sleep. They were one-cylinder and two-cylinder engines, and some were make-and-break and some were jump-spark, but they all made a sleepy sound across the lake. The one-lungers throbbed and fluttered, and the twin-cylinder ones purred and purred, and that was a quiet sound, too. But now the campers all had outboards. In the daytime, in the hot mornings, these motors made a petulant, irritable sound; at night, in the still evening when the afterglow lit the water, they whined about one's ears like mosquitoes. . . .
>
> —E. B. White

White's opening sentences introduce the subject of the paragraph, outboard motors, and suggest the comparison that is to follow ("only thing that was wrong now," "unfamiliar nervous sound"). Structurally, the paragraph hinges on the transition "but" at the beginning of the seventh sentence, which divides it into two parts, the first describing the agreeable sounds of the old inboard motors, the second expressing White's mild annoyance with the newer, noisier, outboards.

<u>8f</u> Development by analogy

One special type of comparison is analogy, a comparison between two essentially unlike things, one familiar to the reader, the other unfamiliar. As a method of illustration, a clever analogy can sometimes make a difficult concept easier to understand. In the following student paragraph, for example, the writer was faced with the problem of showing how the characters in William Faulkner's short story "Spotted Horses" could continue to admire and tolerate a man who continually fleeced them. To solve this problem, the student used the apt analogy of a game of pool with Willie Hoppe, for many years the world champion.

> "That Flem Snopes," says the narrator. "I be dog if he ain't a case now." The townspeople had respect for a good horse trader and Flem Snopes was that. Since money was of grotesque importance to these people who had to dig for every penny, they admired a man who could come by it easily and cleverly. Ironically, when Flem skinned someone of his last nickel and kept the fact to himself, the people would interpret Flem's silence as sheer modesty, while the victim laughed off as hopeless any thought of retribution. Their admiration and toleration of Flem is not hard to understand. It was like a game of pool in which you lose so decisively to Willie Hoppe that you feel no bitterness—merely a sense of pride and awe at having played the master at all. After Willie has beaten you and quietly taken off the stakes, you admit sheepishly to others you were licked before you started and put the cue back on the rack instead of taking it into some dark alley to wait for Willie. Most people didn't even try to beat the time-honored master, Flem Snopes, at his game of swindling.

Professional writers often use analogy to make difficult technical or abstract ideas accessible to the average reader, and they take care, while developing their paragraphs, to be sure that the reader regards the analogies as illustrations, not proofs. In developing the following paragraph on theories of gravitation, for example, Lincoln Barnett refers to his analogy as "this little fable."

> The distinction between Newton's and Einstein's ideas about gravitation has sometimes been illustrated by picturing a little boy playing marbles in a city lot. The ground is very uneven. An observer in an office ten stories above the street would not be able to see these irregularities in the ground. Noticing that the marbles appear to avoid some sections of the ground and move toward other sections, he might

assume that a [semi-magnetic] "force" was operating which repelled the marbles from certain spots and attracted them toward others. But another observer on the ground would instantly perceive that the path of the marbles was simply governed by the curvature of the field. In this little fable Newton is the upstairs observer who imagines that a "force" is at work, and Einstein is the observer on the ground, who has no reason to make such an assumption. Einstein's gravitational laws, therefore, merely describe the field properties of the space-time continuum. . . .

—Lincoln Barnett

8g Development by cause and effect

In a paragraph developed by cause and effect, a writer stresses the connections between a result or results and the preceding events. Some cause-and-effect paragraphs are primarily persuasive. Their purpose is to make the reader feel the forcefulness of the writer's conclusions, or at least see the grounds for those conclusions. Other cause-and-effect paragraphs are essentially explanatory. They are intended to help a reader understand a necessary relationship between causes and effects.

A cause-and-effect paragraph may begin by stating an effect and then explaining its causes, or it may open with a cause and go on to explore its various effects.

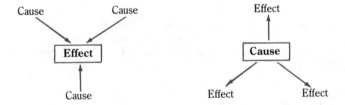

More often, however, causes and effects are intermingled in a subtler way, as in the following paragraph about television's influence on politics.

While the public and politicians are often blamed for being more concerned with images than with issues, the image bias may be inherent in the way we now get political information. Through television, we come to feel we "know" politicians personally, and our response to them has become similar to our response to friends and lovers. Just as we would not marry someone on the basis of a résumé or a writing sample, so are we now unwilling to choose Presidents merely on the basis of their stands on the issues. We want, instead, to know what they are "really like." However, the current drive toward intimacy with our leaders involves a fundamental paradox. In pursuing our desire to be close to great people or to confirm their greatness through increased exposure, we destroy the distance that enabled them to appear great in the first place.

—Joshua Meyrowitz

Two pairs of causes and effects are explored in this paragraph. The first sentence states an effect (our modern concern with politicians' images) whose cause (television's ability to make us feel close to politicians) is explained in the three sentences that follow. The last two sentences introduce a related issue: our desire for intimate knowledge of our leaders, Meyrowitz points out, is a cause whose ultimate effect is the collapse of their appearance of greatness. Such sophisticated analysis demands careful thinking as well as precise control of a paragraph's structure and organization.

8h Combining methods of development

As we said at the start of this chapter, most writers find themselves using a combination of the methods of development that we have been discussing. To illustrate this point, we have separated the following long paragraph into segments developed in turn by definition, contrast, and example.

Topic

I never have much confidence in people who talk a great deal about "their image" or "so-and-so's image": they make me wonder if they even care about what the real thing is.

Definition

By image, I don't mean an accurate copy or truthful likeness. I mean, rather, the same thing that PR types, bureaucrats, and political managers too often mean: a counterfeit, a phony projection, a manipulated picture intended to give the illusion of actuality.

Contrast

In daily situations where actual performances can be judged and experienced first-hand, rather ordinary ones like house painting or plumbing, no one spends much time worrying about the image of the performer. These performances are very different from the rigged ones on TV: either the walls are smoothly rolled and the faucets are fixed, or they aren't; the painter or plumber is competent or not so competent. But in some parts of our society, we are not even supposed to think about the reality as long as the image is "good."

Example

Recently, while watching a talk show, I was struck by one guest, a candidate for office, who kept harping on our need for "the image of strong leadership." The more he dwelled on his opponent's failure to project such an image, the more I wondered what policies the speaker stood for, what he would do if elected. And when he defended his expensive media blitz as part of "getting my image across" to the voters. . . .

A good paragraph is a "bounding line" which encloses its own distinct material. The phrase belongs to the artist and poet William Blake: "The great and golden rule of art, as well as of life, is this: That the more distinct, sharp, and wiry the bounding line, the more perfect the work of art. . . . How do we distinguish the oak from the beech . . . one face or countenance from another, but by the bounding line and its infinite inflexions and movements? . . . Leave out this line, and you leave out life itself: all is chaos again."

8h

Exercise 1

Write two different paragraphs on one of the topics below. In the first, make the diction as vague and general as you can. In your second paragraph on the subject, substitute specific detail to make your description vivid and interesting.

1. An ideal campsite
2. A teacher who cannot sit still or stay in one place
3. Subway or bus passengers after midnight
4. A public swimming pool on a hot day
5. The amusement section of a fair or carnival
6. A student trying to stay awake in class
7. Your best friend's room
8. A persistent salesperson
9. A man or woman shopping for clothes
10. A college dining room at noon

Exercise 2

Write a paragraph developed by examples on one of the subjects below, or another subject of your choice. Begin by listing points you might include and formulating a topic sentence.

1. The sameness of fast-food restaurants
2. Innovation in popular music
3. Lack of understanding among people
4. Overlooked problems in our society
5. Creativity

Exercise 3

Write a paragraph developed by definition on one of the subjects below, or another subject of your choice. Begin by listing points you might include and formulating a topic sentence.

1. Satisfaction
2. Commitment
3. Masculinity
4. Femininity
5. Concern for others
6. Propaganda
7. Caution
8. Neatness
9. Challenge
10. Anxiety

8h

Exercise 4

Write a paragraph developed by classification on one of the subjects below, or another of your choice. Begin by listing points you might include and formulating a topic sentence.

1. Relatives
2. Summer jobs
3. Extracurricular activities

4. Desires
5. Decisions

Exercise 5

Write a paragraph developed by comparison or contrast on one of the subjects below, or another of your choice. Begin by listing points you might include and formulating a topic sentence.

1. Discussing and arguing
2. Two close friends
3. Photography and painting
4. High-school and college computer courses
5. Yourself and your brother or sister

Exercise 6

Write a paragraph developed by cause-and-effect analysis on one of the subjects below, or another subject of your choice. Begin by listing points you might include and formulating a topic sentence.

1. Why I am frustrated by _____.
2. Why I prefer _____ to _____.
3. Why I usually refuse to _____.
4. Why I am always willing to _____.
5. Why I don't wear _____.

Exercise 7

Choose one of the subjects that you wrote about in the exercises above and write a paragraph on the same subject developed by a different method. For example, if you defined "commitment" (Exercise 3), now try *contrasting* it with a slightly different concept such as "fanaticism." If you classified summer jobs (Exercise 4), now try *describing* a particularly satisfying or distasteful summer job that you have had. If you analyzed the cause of one of your frustrations (Exercise 6), now try *classifying* all the things that frustrate you. Pay attention to the way in which the choice of a method of development may determine how you think about a subject.

Exercise 8

Closely examine the paragraphs of several articles in a magazine such as *The New Yorker, Psychology Today, Rolling Stone,* or *Scientific American.* What methods of paragraph development can you identify? How often do the paragraphs seem to be developed by a combination of methods? Based on your findings, write a paragraph about paragraph development in published writing.

9 Sentence Structure

We all know that a sentence in grammar is a series of spoken or written words which forms the grammatically complete expression of a single thought. On the page, such a unit of discourse begins with a capital letter and ends with the appropriate end punctuation mark. Spoken aloud, the sentence is marked by voice inflection and pauses, the longest of which signals its completion. We have a well-developed, intuitive sense of the sentence because we have been hearing and speaking and writing and reading sentences most of our lives.

In English this grammatical term also names a judicial pronouncement. If we look up the word in the *Oxford English Dictionary,* that historian of our language, we find that "sentence" is one of those words that has contracted over the centuries: it had more meaning in Shakespeare's time than it has in ours. Some of these meanings, such as "opinion" and "way of thinking," are listed in the dictionary as obsolete and are not available to contemporary writers. Nevertheless, they point the way back to the Latin origin of the word, *sentire,* to feel, to be of the opinion, to perceive, to judge. The word "sentence" shares the same root as "sensation" and "sense," and appropriately so, for the construction of a sentence, even the simplest two-word kind, requires sensing and thinking, perceiving and judging. Good sentences are written by a vigilant observer prepared to judge and to declare.

9a Elements of a sentence

For any kind of grammatical analysis, it is necessary to classify the words and groups of words that make up a sentence. To classify means simply to group together words that are alike in some respects and to give names to the classes thus formed.

Let's start with a kind of classification you may never have thought of, though structural linguists use it all the time. *Pen, telephone, tax,* and *fluid,* for example, are alike in that they often appear after words like *the, a,* or *this: a pen, the telephone, this tax.* Words of this class also take inflectional endings to indicate the plural, usually a suffix including the letter *s: telephones, fluids, taxes.* Another class is made up of words to which inflectional suffixes like *-ed* can be added: *ask, asked; cry, cried; walk, walked.* A third class consists of words to which *-er* and *-est* can be added: *happy, happier, happiest; swift, swifter, swiftest.*

As names for these classes, let's adopt the ones used by traditional grammar: we'll call the first class **nouns** (words that name something), the second class **verbs** (words that assert something), and the third class **adjectives** (words that describe or limit the meaning of a noun). However, as we go on to classify more and more words, it will become apparent that these classes must be broadened. Traditional grammar will suggest that a word like *man* should be put in the first class, even though the plural is *men,* not *mans.* Similarly, in the second class we will want to put such a word as *weave,* even though, instead of taking an *-ed* ending, it is inflected *wove.* The third class will be widened to include some words which do not add *-er* and *-est,* like *beautiful,* which is inflected *more beautiful, most beautiful.*

In widening the classes, traditional grammar makes use of another set of similarities: it puts words into classes not merely by their position in a sentence or by their forms (the way they can be inflected), but by their functions in a sentence. That is, traditional grammar says that *man, pen,* and *tax* belong together in a class because they name something, whereas *rich* and *beautiful* and *cold* belong together in another class because they modify (that is, describe or limit) something.

Modern linguists have proposed alternative classifications which may well provide a more accurate and complete analysis of grammatical structures and relationships than the categories of traditional grammar do. But for the limited sort of analysis needed in a handbook, which tries merely to explain why certain constructions are "grammatical" without offering a complete system of grammar, the traditional classifications and the old names have the advantage of simplicity and familiarity. And they can be made consistent enough to-be relevant and usable.

Many of the supposed inconsistencies of traditional grammar are caused by the fact that most English words can function in more than one way, and hence fit into more than one class. The word *poor* belongs in the class with *happy* and *swift* because it can take the suffixes *-er* and *-est* to make *poorer* and *poorest.* But the sentence "The poor usually eat poor food" shows that *poor* can also be used like words of the first class described above. *The poor* belongs with *the telephone, the pen,* etc., even though it does not take an *-s* suffix like *telephones.*

Into what class, then, do we put the word *poor?* The answer is no class, until we see the word used in a sentence. In a sentence, the form and position will indicate the word's meaning and grammatical function. *The poor* names an economic class; in this construction, the word belongs with other names like *telephone* or *fluid.* In the construction *poor food, poor* describes the quality of food; it belongs in the class with *rich, hot,* and *good.*

Once it is clear that grammatical analysis deals not with isolated words but with words used in sentences, various systems of classification are possible.

For the present purpose, classifying words by their functions in a sentence provides a simple and usable tool.

There are four functions of words in sentences: to name things, to assert things, to modify (describe, identify, or limit) other words, and to connect other parts of a sentence. Groups of words (what linguists call **constructions**) may have the same functions as single words; such groups are called **phrases** or **clauses.**

Class	Function	Types
substantive	to name	nouns, pronouns, gerunds
predicative	to assert	verbs
modifier	to describe or limit	adjectives, adverbs, participles
connective	to join elements	conjunctions, prepositions

9a

Infinitives, gerunds, and participles are verbals, that is, verbs that function as other parts of speech. They will be discussed more fully later in the chapter.

Sentences ask questions or answer them, issue commands or requests, express strong feeling, and, most often, make statements. The **syntax** of the sentence, its arrangement of words, tells us immediately what kind of a sentence it is.

What a ridiculous assignment!	Exclamatory
Write the paper.	Imperative
Are you writing the paper?	Interrogative
I have written the paper.	Declarative

1. Subject and predicate

A statement says something about something, and to make a statement you need to *name* what you are talking about and *assert* something about it. The grammatical term for the word or words that name what you are talking about is the **subject.** The **predicate** is the assertion you make about the subject.

Subject	Predicate
Edison	invented the light bulb.
The storm	cut off our lights.
A coyote	howled all night.
I	like spices.
My younger brother	does not like spices.

The subject is usually a noun or **pronoun** (a word used in place of a noun), though it may be a phrase or clause, as will be explained later. The predicate may contain a number of different words used in different ways, but the essential part is a verb, a word that asserts something.

2. Modifiers

It is possible to make a complete sentence of two words, a subject and a verb:

Rain fell.

Few sentences, however, are as simple as this. We usually add other words whose function is to describe the subject or the verb:

A gentle rain fell steadily.

Here *gentle* describes *rain* and *steadily* describes how it fell. Such words are called **modifiers,** and they may be attached to almost any part of a sentence. Although modifiers usually describe, they may also indicate how many (*three* books, *few* books), which one (*this* pencil, *the* pen, *my* pencil), or how much (*very* gently, *half* sick, *almost too* late).

Modifiers are divided into two main classes: **adjectives** and **adverbs.** Any word which modifies a noun, pronoun, or gerund is an adjective in function; an adverb is any word which modifies a verb, an adjective, or another adverb.

Very hungry men seldom display good table manners.

In this sentence, *hungry, good,* and *table* are adjectives, describing or indicating what kind of men and manners. *Very* is an adverb since it modifies the adjective *hungry; seldom* is an adverb modifying the verb *display*.

Adjectives and adverbs have different forms to indicate **relative degree.** In addition to the regular, or "positive," form (*slow, comfortable, slowly*), there are the **comparative** (*slower, more comfortable, more slowly*) and **superlative** (*slowest, most comfortable, most slowly*) **degrees.** The examples illustrate the rule: adjectives with more than two syllables form the comparative and superlative degrees by the words *more* and *most,* instead of the suffixes -*er* and -*est.* All adverbs ending in -*ly* use *more* and *most* to indicate degrees of comparison (see Chapter **29**).

3. Identifying subject and verb

The analysis of any sentence begins with the identification of the simple subject and the verb. Look first for the verb: a word or group of words that often states an action or happening. Some forms or tenses of a verb are really phrases, including one or more **auxiliary verbs**—*He was hit, he has been hit; you had taken, you will have taken.* Verbs which do not add -*ed* to form the past tense are called **irregular verbs**—*swim, swam, swum; eat, ate, eaten,* etc.

I *sprained* my wrist.

Joe Miller *wrote* me a letter.

The fire *burned* out.

He *has* never *painted* landscapes before.
[In this sentence the two parts of the verb are separated by the adverb *never.*]

Some verbs merely assert, with varying degrees of certainty, that something is—or looks or sounds or seems or appears to be—something. These are called **linking verbs,** or **copulas.**

9a

> She *is* a good mechanic.
>
> He *seems* intelligent and dependable.
>
> There *were* two reasons for believing their story.
>
> The troops *looked* weary.

When you have found the verb, ask yourself the question, "Who or what _____?" putting the verb in the blank space. The answer to the question is the subject, and if you strip away the modifiers you have the **simple subject.**

> A long, dull speech followed the dinner.
> [What followed the dinner? *A long, dull speech.* But *long* and *dull* are adjectives describing *speech;* the simple subject is *speech.*]

This method of identifying the subject is especially helpful when the normal order of the sentence is inverted (that is, when the subject comes after the verb).

> Half a mile away *rose* the spires of the cathedral.
> "No," *said* his father firmly.
> [What rose half a mile away? The answer is the subject, *spires.*
> Who said "no"? The answer is the subject, *father.*]

In a sentence that asks a question, the subject often follows some form of the verb *have* or *be,* or a form of an auxiliary verb.

verb	subject		
Have	*you*	the time?	
Is	*he*	qualified?	

auxiliary	subject	verb	
Have	*you*	read	this novel?
Did	*she*	write	it?
May	*they*	borrow	it?

	auxiliary	subject	verb
What kind of story	did	*he*	tell?

In an imperative sentence the subject is not expressed. Since a command or request is addressed directly to someone, that person need not be named.

	subject	verb	
(	)	Come	in.
(	)	Return	the books no later than Monday.
Please (	)	take	these books to the library.

Since we can make one assertion about several persons and things, a sentence may have several nouns as its subject. Such a construction is called a **compound subject.**

compound subject

The trees and plants	were dying.
Jane Austen, George Eliot, and Emily Brontë	are my favorite novelists.

9a

Similarly, we can make several assertions about one subject. Such a construction is called a **compound predicate.**

She *wrote, revised, copied,* and *proofread* the manuscript.

Exhausted, she *went* to bed and *slept* for twelve hours.

Exercise 1

Pick out the simple subjects and the verbs in the following sentences. Note that either the subject or the verb may be compound.

1. After locking the door, the flight attendant sat down at the rear of the plane.
2. Invisible to us, the pilot and copilot were checking the instruments.
3. Signs warning passengers not to smoke and to fasten their seat belts flashed on.
4. Directly beneath the signs was a door leading to the pilot's compartment.
5. Altogether there were about sixty passengers on the plane.
6. In a few moments the plane moved, slowly at first, and then roared into life.
7. After taxiing out to the airstrip, the pilot hesitated a moment to check the runway.
8. Then with a sudden rush of speed the plane roared down the runway and gradually began to climb.
9. Below us, at the edge of the airport, were markers and signal lights.
10. The football field and the quarter-mile track enabled me to identify the high school.

4. Complements

Some verbs, called **intransitive** verbs, require nothing to complete them; that is, in themselves they make a full assertion about the subject.

After meeting all the relatives, my cousin *left.*

In a heavy rain, cabbage *may explode.*

Transitive verbs, however, are incomplete by themselves. If one says only "I bought," the reader is left hanging in mid-air and is likely to ask "What did you buy?" Words which answer such a question, and thus complete the assertion, are called **complements** of the verb.

subject	verb	complement
I	bought	*a scarf.*

The commonest type of complement is the **direct object** of a transitive verb, illustrated in the sentence above. The direct object is usually a noun or pronoun, though it may be a phrase or a clause, and it usually names the thing acted upon by the subject.

subject	verb	direct object
My niece	built	*a water clock.*
They	chased	*the soccer ball.*

The easiest way to identify a direct object is to say the simple subject and verb and then ask the question "What?" My niece built what? The answer, *clock,* is the direct object of the verb *built.* Note that the direct object may be compound.

9a

subject	verb	direct object
I	borrowed	*a tent, a sleeping bag, and a gas stove.*

In addition to the direct object, certain verbs (usually involving an act of giving or telling) may take an **indirect object,** a complement that receives whatever is named by the direct object.

> The award gave the young photographer encouragement.
> [What did the award give? *Encouragement* is the direct object. Who received the encouragement? *Photographer* is the indirect object—the receiver of what is named by the direct object.]

The same meaning can be expressed by a phrase beginning with *to*:

> The award gave encouragement *to* the young photographer.
>
> He offered me his pen.
>
> He offered his pen *to* me.

Direct and indirect objects are called **object complements.** A **subject complement,** in contrast, follows a linking verb and completes the predicate by giving another name for the subject or by describing the subject.

> My mother was the *mayor* of our town.

Mayor cannot be called the direct object of the verb since it is merely another name for my *mother,* and it can be made the subject of the sentence without changing the meaning. "The mayor of our town was my mother." To appreciate the difference between object and subject complements, substitute a transitive verb.

> My mother *scolded* the mayor.

The direct object, *mayor,* now names a person other than the subject, one who is acted upon by *my mother.* Making *mayor* the subject of this sentence would change the meaning considerably.

A noun that serves as a subject complement of a linking verb is called a **predicate noun.** Linking verbs may also be completed by an adjective that describes the subject. Such a subject complement is called a **predicate adjective.**

> The mayor was *attractive and popular.*

Attractive and *popular* describe the subject, *mayor,* but instead of being directly attached to the noun ("an attractive, popular mayor"), they are joined to it by the linking verb *was* and become predicate adjectives.

Exercise 2

Pick out the subjects and verbs in the following sentences. Identify direct objects, indirect objects, predicate nouns, and predicate adjectives.

1. As a wedding present, my uncle gave us a picture.
2. It was an original sketch by Dufy.
3. The technique was interesting, since Dufy had used only a few simple lines.
4. It seemed an early work, according to a friend to whom I showed it.
5. We hung it in the living room and it looked good.
6. I wrote my uncle a note and thanked him for the picture.
7. We enjoyed it for several months, until my friend told us its value.
8. Then we worried about burglars, and we wrote my uncle again asking if he would give us a less valuable picture.

5. Phrases

A group of words may have the same function in a sentence as a single word. For example, in the sentence "The train to Boston leaves in ten minutes," the group of words *in ten minutes* modifies the verb *leaves* in exactly the same way as an adverb like *soon.* Similarly, *to Boston* functions like an adjective: it describes and identifies *train.* Such groups of words, which do not make a complete statement but which function like a single word, are called **phrases.** Phrases may be named for the kind of word around which they are constructed—prepositional, participial, gerund, or infinitive. Or they may be named by the way they function in a sentence—as adjective, adverb, or noun phrases. *To Boston* in the sentence above is a prepositional phrase used as an adjective.

Prepositional phrases

A **prepositional phrase** consists of a preposition joined to a noun or a pronoun, which is called the object of the preposition. Such phrases usually modify nouns or verbs, and they are described accordingly as adjective or adverb phrases.

	adjective		adverb
The leader	*of the band*	swayed	*in the sun.*
The walk	*from the church to the cemetery*	lasted	*over an hour.*

Verbals and verb phrases

A **verbal** is a form of a verb that functions as some other part of speech. It is important to distinguish between verb forms ending in *-ing* and *-ed* when they function as part of the verb, as in "I was turning around," and such forms when they function as adjectives to modify a noun, as in "a turning point" or "a turned ankle." A verbal that modifies a noun is called a **participle.** Note that a participle may be in the past or in the present tense—"a *used* car with *splitting, worn* upholstery."

A verb form that functions as a noun is called a **gerund:** "*Writing* is his passion." In this sentence, *writing* is the subject of the sentence. Gerunds may also be used as the objects of verbs or of prepositions.

object of verb		object of preposition
He loves *writing*	and amuses himself by	*scribbling dull verses.*

A third type of verbal is the **infinitive,** the present form of the verb preceded by the preposition *to: to write; to scribble.* Infinitives are frequently used as nouns—as subject or object of the verb.

subject	object
To err is human, but remember	*to apologize.*

Since they are verb forms, participles, gerunds, and infinitives may take objects, and they may be modified by adverbs or by prepositional phrases. A verbal with its modifier and its object, or subject, makes up a verbal phrase and functions as a single part of speech, but it does not make a full statement.

Participial phrase	*Moved by the spirit of his life and the dignity of his death,* my friend proposed that the town build a monument to my uncle. [Here the participle *moved,* modified by a prepositional phrase, describes *my friend.*]
Gerund phrase	*Selecting an inexpensive and appropriate site* took considerable time. [Here the phrase—gerund, object, and the modifiers of the object—is the subject of the sentence.]
Infinitive phrase	The task required us *to walk for hours.* [The infinitive has a subject, *us,* and a modifying prepositional phrase, *for hours.*]

Absolute phrases

An **absolute phrase** is a group of words that has a subject but no verb and is not grammatically connected to the rest of the sentence. The subject of an absolute phrase is frequently followed by a participle.

The site having been selected, we met to choose a sculptor.

A tree, *all things considered,* is a better monument than a statue.

His brow creased with anger, his hands clenched on the table, the speaker insisted on having his way.

The subject of an absolute phrase may also be followed by an adjective or a prepositional phrase:

She recounted the incident, *her voice angry, her face pale, her eyes tearful.*

We listened quietly, *our hearts in our mouths.*

We left the room, *all hopes of a peaceful settlement in shambles.*

Because absolute phrases are formed by the suppression of connecting elements—prepositions (*"with* our hearts in our mouths") or subordinating conjunctions and the finite verb (*"when* all things *are* considered")—they have a toughness and economy that can be a virtue in writing.

9a

Appositive phrases

An **appositive** is a noun, or noun substitute, added to explain another noun: "My mother, *the mayor,* was the subject of controversy all her life." Appositives with their modifiers make up phrases, since they function as a unit to give further information about a noun.

The memorial she wanted, *a grand magnolia tree,* now stands in the center of town.

The townspeople, *wise and practical citizens,* made the decision, *a radical one for that time and place.*

Appositives, like absolute constructions, compress connections by eliminating words. The last sentence could have been written, "The townspeople, who were wise and practical citizens, made the decision, which was a radical one for that time and place," but the result would have been a less economical and far less effective sentence.

Exercise 3

Pick out the phrases in the following sentences. Identify them as prepositional, participial, gerund, infinitive, or appositive, and be ready to describe their function in the sentence.

1. On Tuesday I came home expecting to drive my car, a shiny new convertible, into the garage.
2. To my surprise, I found a ditch between the street and the driveway.
3. A crew of men had begun to lay a new water main along the curb.
4. Hoping that I would not get a ticket for overnight parking, I left the car in the street in front of the house.
5. For three days a yawning trench separated me from my garage.
6. Finding a place to park was difficult, since all the neighbors on my side of the street were in the same predicament.
7. By Friday the workmen had filled up the ditch, but my car, stained with dust and dew, looked ten years older.
8. I had to spend the weekend washing and polishing it.
9. My wife, a strong advocate of justice, suggested sending the city a bill for the job.
10. My refusal convinced her that men are illogical, improvident, and easily imposed upon.

6. Clauses

A **clause** is a group of words that contains a subject and a predicate and that makes a statement. Except for elliptical questions and answers, every sentence must contain at least one clause.

Independent and dependent clauses

Although all sentences must contain a clause, not all clauses are sentences. Some clauses, instead of making an independent statement, serve only as a subordinate part of the main sentence. Such clauses, called **dependent** (or **subordinate** or **relative**), perform a function like that of adjectives, adverbs, or nouns. **Independent clauses,** on the other hand, can stand alone as complete sentences. They provide the framework to which modifiers, phrases, and dependent clauses are attached in each sentence. Any piece of connected discourse is made up of a series of independent clauses.

"She heard the news" is a clause because it has a subject, *she,* and a verb, *heard.* It is an independent clause because it is complete in itself and can stand alone as a sentence. "When she heard the news" is also a clause because it has a subject and a predicate, but it is a dependent one. The addition of the word *when* creates a condition of incompleteness or dependency. Any reader will expect to be told what happened when she heard the news.

dependent clause	independent clause
When she heard the news	she was delighted.

Dependent clauses are usually connected to the rest of the sentence by **relative pronouns** (*who, which,* or *that*) or by **subordinating conjunctions** such as *while, although, as, because, if, since, when* or *where.* The terms "relative" and "subordinating" remind us that clauses introduced by these words are not self-sufficient: they are related or subordinated to the main or independent clause of the sentence. Written separately, they are fragments.

Dependent clauses function like parts of speech. They can be subjects and objects (like nouns), and (like adjectives and adverbs) they can be modifiers.

Noun clauses

A **noun clause** functions as a noun in a sentence. It may be a subject or a complement in the main clause, or the object of a preposition or of a gerund.

Noun clause as subject of the sentence

That she was considered for the position at all is remarkable.

Noun clause as direct object of the verb

She said *that she would accept only under certain conditions.*

9a

9a

Noun clause as object of the preposition

We will give the job to *whoever is best qualified.*

Noun clause as object of a gerund

We do best for ourselves by asking *what we can do for others.*

Adverb clauses

An **adverb clause** is a dependent clause used to modify a verb or an adjective or an adverb in the main clause.

Adverb clause

We ate *whenever we felt like it.*
[*Whenever we felt like it* modifies the verb *ate.*]

Adverb clause

The trip was as pleasant *as we had hoped.*
[The clause *as we had hoped* modifies the adjective *pleasant.*]

Adverb clause

The train arrived sooner *than we had expected.*
[The clause *than we had expected* modifies the adverb *sooner.*]

Adjective clauses and relative pronouns

A dependent clause used to modify a noun or pronoun is called an **adjective clause.**

Adjective clause

The salesman *we met yesterday* showed us his library, *which includes all the first editions of Dorothy Sayers.*
[The adjective clause *we met yesterday* modifies the noun *salesman;* the adjective clause *which includes all the first editions of Dorothy Sayers* modifies the noun *library.*]

Adjective clauses are usually introduced by relative pronouns, which serve both as pronouns and as subordinating conjunctions. The following sentences illustrate how they work.

Dorthy Sayers wrote many books; the books were widely read.
[This sentence consists of two independent clauses. It would be more idiomatic, however, if we substituted a pronoun for the second *books.*]

Dorothy Sayers wrote many books; *they* were widely read.
[If, instead of using the pronoun *they*, we now substitute the relative pronoun *that*, the second clause becomes dependent, and the sentence itself becomes more tightly subordinated.]

Dorothy Sayers wrote many books *that* were widely read.
[*That were widely read* no longer will stand as an independent sentence. Joined to the first clause, it functions as an adjective, modifying *books.*]

The relative pronouns *who* (and *whom*), *which,* and *that* always have two simultaneous roles: they serve as subordinating conjunctions, connecting dependent clauses to independent ones, but they also function like nouns, as subject or complement in the dependent clause. Often, relative pronouns can be omitted: "She is a person I cherish." But just as often, they need to be expressed. "He thought to be educated we should read good books" is awkward, but "He thought that to be educated we should read good books" is not.

9b

Exercise 4

Find the simple subject and verb of each clause in the following sentences. Point out the main clauses and the dependent clauses, and be prepared to state the function in each sentence of each dependent clause.

1. The movie director who did much to perfect the one-reel Western as a distinct genre was D. W. Griffith.
2. Shortly after he had entered movies in New York, Griffith achieved immediate success with his first film, which he directed in 1908.
3. Between 1908 and 1913, while he was directing Westerns, Griffith continually worked with techniques which, though they had been introduced by others, were developed and refined by him.
4. Griffith was delighted by the Western because it offered opportunities for spectacle and scope.
5. He found that the Western was an ideal genre in which to experiment with close-ups and with cross-cutting, the techniques he employed to build narrative suspense.
6. Some critics have pointed out that Griffith was more interested in dramatic situations which lent themselves to lively visual treatment than he was in the details of plot or conventional justice.
7. He would willingly let the villains go free whenever he felt the dramatic situation warranted it.
8. The close-up of the outnumbered settlers grimly hanging on and the panoramic view of the battle seen from afar were characteristic Griffith shots.
9. In 1915, Griffith produced *The Birth of a Nation,* the first great spectacle movie.
10. It made use of many of the techniques he had developed while he was making one-reel Westerns.

9b Types of sentences

Sentences are traditionally classified according to their structure as simple, compound, complex, and compound-complex.

1. Simple sentences

A **simple sentence** consists of one independent clause with or without modifying words or phrases but with no dependent clauses attached.

9b

	subject	verb
Simple	Harvey	despaired.

Simple

modifying phrase
Nervously biting his fingernails,

subject / verb
Harvey despaired

modifying phrase
of ever learning grammar.

Simple

modifying phrase
Nervously biting their fingernails,

compound subject
Harvey and his girlfriend, Zelda,

modifying phrase
puzzled once more by the red marks on their papers,

compound predicate with modifying phrase
despaired of ever learning the fine points of grammar and longed for the simple beauty of differential calculus.

Obviously, simple sentences can be quite elaborate when the subject or the verb is modified with verbals and appositives. Still, such sentences can be reduced to a simple kernel and, as such, are limited in expressing complicated ideas or showing the relation of one idea to another. Simple sentence following simple sentence leads to tedious writing at best, at worst to what in writing is called a "primer style." The straightforward thrust of the simple declaration should be modulated by the careful use of other types of sentences.

2. Compound sentences

The **compound sentence** consists of two or more independent clauses joined by a coordinating conjunction or by a semicolon.

Compound

independent clause
He wrote for hours, and

independent clause
his hunger vanished.

Compound

independent clause
His style was graceful;

independent clause
his sentences were lively and varied.

Compound

independent clause
His roommate left the shower running, but

independent clause
Al did not notice.

The compound sentence offers the advantage of possible balance and antithesis. Skillfully used, it creates effective parallelism and coordination.

3. Complex sentences

The **complex sentence** contains one independent clause and one or more dependent clauses, which express subordinate ideas.

9b

dependent clause
Complex   Because he was tired and hungry and discouraged,

independent clause
he did not want to rewrite the paper.

independent clause   dependent clause
Complex   Still, ideas for writing come   when we least expect them.

independent clause   dependent clause
Complex   Reluctantly, he put pen to paper,   while his roommate sang in the shower.

The complex sentence has the advantage of flexibility; it can be arranged to produce a variety of sentence patterns and to indicate subtle relationships between ideas. It also provides selective emphasis, since the subordination of dependent clauses throws the weight of the sentence on the main clause. Understanding when and how to subordinate is a fundamental writing skill.

4. Compound-complex sentences

When a compound sentence contains one or more dependent clauses, the whole is described as a **compound-complex sentence.**

independent clause
Compound-complex   He was surprised

dependent clause
when the water rose above his tennis shoes,   but

independent clause
he went on writing.

dependent clause
Compound-complex   Although he was drenched to the bone,

independent clause
he typed up the paper,   and

dependent clause
while his roommate bailed out the room,

independent clause
he read the finished manuscript with undampened satisfaction.

9b

Classify the following sentences as simple, compound, complex, or compound-complex. Identify the subject, verb, and complement, if any, of each clause. Describe the function of each dependent clause.

1. When Renaissance physicians began to study human anatomy by means of actual dissection, they concluded that the human body had changed since the days of antiquity.
2. Galen, an ancient Greek physician, was generally accepted as the authority on anatomy and physiology.
3. His theory of the four humors, blood, phlegm, bile, and black bile, was neat and logical, and authorities had accepted it for centuries.
4. Similarly, his account of the structure of the human body, revised by generations of scholars and appearing in many printed editions, was generally accepted.
5. If dissection showed a difference from Galen's account, the obvious explanation was that human structure had changed since Galen's time.
6. One man who refused to accept this explanation was Andreas Vesalius, a young Belgian physician who was studying in Italy.
7. Asked to edit the anatomical section of Galen's works, Vesalius found many errors in it.
8. Galen's statement that the lower jaw consisted of two parts seemed wrong to Vesalius, who had never found such a structure in his own dissections.
9. He finally concluded that Galen was describing the anatomy of lower animals—pigs, monkeys, and goats—and that he had never dissected a human body.
10. When he realized that Galen could be wrong, Vesalius began a study which came to be recognized as his major work: a fully illustrated treatise on the human body based on actual observation.

10 Sentence Style

When we speak of style in writing, we mean the distinctive effects that a writer creates with language. The precise sources of a writer's style may be as difficult to isolate as the components of a professional basketball player's style or the elements that characterize the style of service at a fine restaurant. But the study of style repays our effort. Through it we are able not only to appreciate more fully the mastery of other writers but also to enlarge our own repertoire of stylistic skills.

This chapter focuses on several basic writing strategies that many readers regard as the mark of an agreeable and satisfying style. If concentrating on your sentence style is a new experience for you, you may at first find it difficult to experiment with new sentence patterns; they may seem strange and unnatural coming from your pen, and you may believe that they make your writing sound stilted or false. But you cannot increase your stylistic fluency if you do not take at least a few risks. The process of developing your own distinctive prose should involve trying out new stylistic devices. Some, you will discover, have an appeal that will win them a place in your instinctive writing habits; others, perhaps, you may never be entirely comfortable with. Like proficiency in all skills, stylistic skill comes with practice and experience. If you seek out appropriate opportunities to use the strategies below in your prose, you may be surprised by your writing's new confidence and sophistication.

10a Parallel structure

The human eye and the human ear lean toward balance and harmony. We like matchings and pairs, equity, pattern, order. Once a major chord is struck in a piece of music, we expect to hear it again, just as we appreciate looking at surfaces where planes and colors complement one another. In writing, this ordering of like element with like element is called **parallelism,** or **parallel structure.** Parallel structure balances word with word, phrase with phrase, subordinate clause with subordinate clause. It is one of the most basic of stylistic devices, one that is appropriate in many writing situations.

Parallel words and phrases

It is often the failure who is the pioneer in   new lands,
                                          new undertakings,
                   and   new forms of expression.

—Eric Hoffer

We are joined by   highways,
                      networks,
         and   slogans,
      not by   imaginative acts.

—Wright Morris

And he yearned to package for each of the children,
                             the grandchildren,
                 for   everyone,
     that   joyous certainty,
     that   sense of mattering,
              of moving and being moved,
              of being one and indivisible
                    with   the great of the past,
                    with   all that freed, ennobled man.

—Tillie Olsen

Parallel clauses

Where She Danced is the story of two generations of American dancers:
                how they were educated,
                what gave them the courage, the insight, the foolhardiness to say
                   they had found a new art form,
     and   what gave them the drive to insist on its ultimate seriousness.

—Elizabeth Kendall

The *Iliad* is only great because all life is a battle,
     the *Odyssey* because all life is a journey,
 and   the Book of Job because all life is a riddle.

—G. K. Chesterton

Parallel sentences

Children begin by loving their parents.
After a time they judge them.
Rarely, if ever, do they forgive them.

—Oscar Wilde

The scientist anatomizes, someone must synthesize; the scientist withdraws, someone must draw together. The scientist particularizes, someone must universalize.

—John Fowles

Although the following sentences are a rather extreme example of parallel structure, they offer a good illustration of the effects that can be created with parallelism. To appreciate the way in which parallel structure works in this passage, try reading it slowly out loud:

> The cunning and attractive slave women disguise their strength as womanly weakness, their audacity as womanly timidity, their unscrupulousness as womanly innocence, their impurities as womanly defencelessness; simple men are duped by them, and subtle ones disarmed and intimidated. It is only the proud, straightforward women who wish, not to govern, but to be free.

—Bernard Shaw

10a

The first independent clause of Shaw's compound sentence states its subject and predicate simply. The phrases functioning as the direct objects of the verb (*what* do these slave women disguise?) have exactly the same construction because they are grammatical equals in the sentence. We might illustrate their parallel relationship by diagramming them like this:

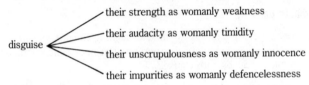

The parallelism of Shaw's sentence does not end there. In the independent clause following the semicolon, *simple men* are balanced against *subtle ones,* and *disarmed* and *intimidated* form parallel elements in the predicate of the second clause:

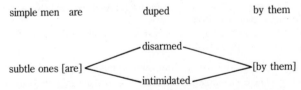

The sections of the sentence on either side of the semicolon are themselves contrasted in parallel fashion. The active voice of the verb in the first clause (*disguise*) is balanced against the passive voice of the verbs in the second (*are duped . . . disarmed and intimidated*); aggression is balanced against passivity.

The brisk second sentence introduces parallel objects of the verb *wish* with the correlatives *not . . . but.*

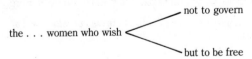

The initial pair of adjectives (*cunning* and *attractive*) defining the subject of the first clause (*slave women*) is here paralleled by a new pair of adjectives that describe the different women in this second sentence (*proud, straightforward*). Shaw ingeniously suggests the inequality between the two types of women by replacing the *and* which connnects the adjectives in the first sentence with a comma in the second. A new rhythm is established.

This analysis of just two sentences suggests the concentration of ideas and the range of effects that a writer can create using parallel structure. Parallelism both compares and contrasts, affirms (*both . . . and*) and negates (*neither . . . nor*) by putting like or different elements in similar constructions. Perhaps the fact that we have two eyes, two legs, two sides of the brain, two hands (*on the one hand . . . on the other hand*) accounts for our pleasure when elements in a sentence are balanced, and our dissatisfaction when they are askew. Whatever the reason for our attraction to equality and balance, parallelism is indispensable for good writing. Below are some guidelines for fashioning parallel sentences.

1. Coordinate pairs

All sentence elements joined by the coordinating conjunctions *and, or, nor, for, but* should be in like grammatical structures. Balance nouns with nouns, phrases with phrases, clauses with clauses.

> **Faulty** He likes reading all the books he can lay his hands on and to write whenever the mood strikes him.

The reader is jarred by the faulty parallelism of the gerund *reading* with the infinitive *to write*. Rewriting them in the same form creates parallel structure.

> **Parallel** He likes *to read* all the books he can lay his hands on and *to write* whenever the mood strikes him.
> **Parallel** He likes *reading* all the books he can lay his hands on and *writing* whenever the mood strikes him.

In the first sentence below, the conjunction *and* connects an infinitive phrase and a subordinate clause beginning with *that*—two structures that are not parallel. The second sentence presents one way of revising for parallelism.

> **Faulty** Students in composition classes are taught to read with attention and that coherent essays must be written.
> **Parallel** Students in composition classes are taught *to read* with attention and *to write* coherent essays.

The sentence could be rephrased to emphasize the parallelism even more.

> **Parallel** Students in composition classes are taught *to read attentively* and *to write coherently.*

Sometimes the part of a sentence that should be parallel to another part is so far away that the writer forgets to balance both.

Faulty I try to stay awake in chemistry class, fortifying myself with coffee, pinching myself at intervals, hanging by my fingernails on the professor's every word, but falling asleep nonetheless.

The *but* at the end of this sentence must be followed by an independent clause, to balance the clause that begins this compound sentence.

10a

Parallel *I try* to stay awake in chemistry class, fortifying myself with coffee, pinching myself at intervals, hanging by my fingernails on the professor's every word, but *I fall asleep* nonetheless.

2. Elements in a series

Like coordinate pairs, three or more elements in a series must be grammatically parallel to each other.

Faulty I concluded that she was intelligent, witty, and liked to make people feel at home.

The first two elements after the verb *was* are adjectives; the third is another verb. The lack of parallelism is clearly revealed if we construct a diagram of the sentence:

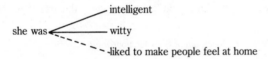

The faulty parallelism can be corrected by making all three elements adjectives:

Parallel I concluded that she was *intelligent, witty,* and *hospitable.*

The sentence might also be rewritten by inserting another *and* in order to create two parallel relative clauses.

Parallel I concluded *that she was* intelligent and witty, and *that she liked* to make people feel at home.

3. Repetition of words

Sometimes it is necessary to repeat a conjunction, preposition, or other preceding word to make a parallel construction clear.

Unclear My adviser told me that I spent far too much time worrying about what was expected of me and I needed more confidence in myself.

Clearer My adviser told me that I spent far too much time worrying about what was expected of me and *that* I needed more confidence in myself.

Unclear	Because she had been teaching for twenty years and she could remember being a student herself, I listened to her advice.
Clearer	Because she had been teaching for twenty years and *because* she could remember being a student herself, I listened to her advice.

Occasionally, the absence of such a preceding word can significantly distort the meaning of a sentence:

Unclear	The vineyard is often visited by tourists who sample grapes and connoisseurs of wine.
Clearer	The vineyard is often visited by tourists who sample grapes and *by* connoisseurs of wine.

10a

4. Correlatives

Conjunctions that occur in pairs are called **correlatives:** *either . . . or, neither . . . nor, not only . . . but also, both . . . and.* The rule to follow when you use correlatives is that the parts of speech immediately following each conjunction must be identical.

Faulty	William Blake is not only famous for his poetry but also for his illustrations.

Not only in this sentence is followed by the adjective *famous; but also,* however, is followed by a prepositional phrase beginning with *for.* In this case, the faulty parallelism can be corrected simply by rearranging the words in the sentence:

Parallel	William Blake is famous *not only for* his poetry *but also for* his illustrations.
Faulty	He either is a liar or a remarkably naive person.
Parallel	He is *either a* liar *or a* remarkably naive person.
Parallel	*Either he is* a liar, *or he is* a remarkably naive person.
Faulty	The legislature hoped both to raise taxes and stimulate business.

Placing *both* after *to* in this sentence would make the two verbs parallel, but it would produce the awkward split construction *to both raise.* A smoother sentence would result from adding another *to:*

Parallel	The legislature hoped *both to* raise taxes *and to* stimulate business.

5. Subordinate clauses

A subordinate clause is never parallel to the main clause in a sentence, and it should therefore not be connected to the main clause by *and* or *but.*

Faulty	She is a woman of strong convictions and who always says what she thinks.

The clauses can be put into proper relationship to one another by omitting the coordinating conjunction:

Correct She is a woman of strong convictions who always says what she thinks.

Another alternative is to rewrite the sentence with two parallel subordinate clauses:

Parallel She is a woman *who has* strong convictions and *who* always *says* what she thinks.

10a

Faulty parallel constructions like those in the following sentences are corrected in a similar way.

Faulty In the middle of the sleepy village is a statue dating from 1870 and which depicts General Lee on horseback.

Parallel In the middle of the sleepy village is a statue *which* dates from 1870 *and which* depicts General Lee on horseback.

Faulty He appeared before the committee with a long written statement, but which he was not allowed to read.

Parallel *He* appeared before the committee with a long written statement, *but he* was not allowed to read it.

6. Sequence of ideas

Elements that are parallel in grammatical structure should also be parallel in sense. Used carelessly, a parallel construction can lead to an illogical series or an awkward sequence of ideas, as in the following sentence.

Illogical Her many friends, her promising marriage, and her slumping business could not offer Amy the happiness she had known while in college.

The items in this series are not parallel in meaning. A person might reasonably be expected to find happiness in friends and marriage, but not in a slumping business. Only the first two of these ideas can be expressed in a parallel construction.

Correct Neither her many friends nor her promising marriage could offer Amy the happiness she had known while in college.

A similar juxtaposition of positive and negative ideas in the following sentence creates a puzzling effect:

Illogical During his last year in law school, David rose to the top of his class, worked on the law review, and decided not to enter law practice.

Correct During his last year in law school, David rose to the top of his class and worked on the law review. However, he decided not to enter law practice.

10a

Exercise 1

Revise the following sentences to eliminate faulty parallelism.

1. On their annual hunting trips, Sam teaches his son patience, endurance, and how to shoot accurately.
2. If you feel ambitious, you might play golf on the club's eighteen-hole course, go bowling in the air-conditioned alleys, or you might swim laps in the fifty-meter pool.
3. In the reading clinic, Allen learned how to coordinate his eye movements, how to scan for information, and how frequent reviewing for key ideas helps.
4. Applicants for the position must be United States citizens, willing to work abroad, and qualify under security regulations.
5. The opera's opening performance was spirited, colorful, and with many people attending.
6. During the summer, they planned to hitchhike along Route 40, to stop at interesting places, and take sidetrips whenever they wanted to.
7. Joan of Arc was regarded either as a patriotic martyr or a crazed fanatic.
8. The flasks were difficult to fill, not only because their necks were narrow but also they were slippery and hard to hold.
9. The bumper crop of rice neither helped the farmer nor were the customers helped.
10. At the campground we met a Mr. and Mrs. Olson from somewhere near San Francisco and who had their eleven children with them.

Exercise 2

Create at least one parallel construction in each of the following sentences by adding appropriate words, phrases, or clauses. Change the original sentence slightly if necessary.

Example

The afternoon sunlight filtered through the trees.

Parallel words added: The afternoon sunlight filtered through the *leaves and branches* of the trees.

Parallel phrases added: The afternoon sunlight filtered through the trees, *casting shadows* on the blanket *and making reading* difficult.

Parallel clause added: The afternoon sunlight filtered through the trees, *and a light wind brushed across the grass.*

1. I understood what had made Jean angry.
2. The pizza was smaller than we had expected.
3. International relations must be improved if our children are to have a future on this planet.
4. For those who have room in their homes, antique furniture is a wise investment.
5. The car began to lose power as we approached the state line.
6. Vince's pictures of the fire were the start of his career as a professional photographer.

7. Students who volunteer as campus guides meet a number of interesting visitors to the college.
8. Fast-food restaurants have become hallmarks of suburban America.
9. When I can find the time, there is nothing I like to do more than sail in the Gulf of Mexico.
10. Synthesizers, which only a decade ago were considered exotic equipment, have completely changed popular music.

10b Cumulative and periodic sentences

Sentences are sometimes characterized as **cumulative** or **periodic,** depending on where their main ideas occur. A cumulative sentence states its main idea first and then follows it with modifying words, phrases, or clauses.

> *I began to keep a journal* when I discovered that my life was interesting, my dreams colorful, and my thoughts rather remarkably profound.

> *My brother stared at the unopened letter,* trembling, pale, oblivious of the students who crowded past him in the stairwell.

Both of these cumulative sentences open with the main idea, to which are added phrases and clauses that provide supplementary information. Cumulative sentences offer a writer two advantages. First, they are clear, direct, and relatively easy to control. We generally speak in cumulative sentences, making a statement and then adding, almost as afterthoughts, reasons and qualifications for what we said. Every writer who can identify the main idea of a sentence has the beginning of a possible cumulative sentence. Second, such sentences are wonderfully flexible. Once the main idea of a sentence is on the page, a writer can freely arrange modifiers after it, varying its length and rhythm.

Periodic sentences are opposite in structure from cumulative sentences. In a periodic sentence, the main idea is held until the end—until the period—and the sentence begins instead with all the subordinate details. A periodic sentence can very effectively engage the attention of the reader, who is made to continue reading until the point of the sentence is revealed.

> When I discovered that my life was interesting, my dreams colorful, and my thoughts rather remarkably profound, *I began to keep a journal.*

> Trembling, pale, oblivious of the students who crowded past him in the stairwell, *my brother stared at the unopened letter.*

Periodic sentences are suspenseful and conclusive, since the weight of their statement falls on the long-awaited predication. And because they are artful and deliberate, such sentences give the reader an impression of thoughtful arrangement. Placed strategically after a series of cumulative sentences, the periodic sentence, surprising the reader by reversing the expected pattern, has an emphatic effect.

But periodic sentences also present a writer with certain hazards. For one thing, since they are less characteristic of contemporary prose than are cumulative sentences, periodic sentences used excessively give writing a slightly old-fashioned ring. Moreover, a periodic sentence whose main idea is not important enough for the emphasis that it inevitably receives may sound anticlimactic or even ridiculous:

> As the rainy night grew darker and the mysterious banging and howling in the attic stairway increased, I decided to make a peanut-butter sandwich.

No one can prescribe when to use a cumulative sentence, when a periodic one. Such a choice must grow out of your subject, the surrounding sentences in your prose, and your instinctive sense of appropriateness. But only when you have mastered both forms will you be able to choose between them consciously and deliberately.

Exercise 3

By adding different sets of appropriate modifiers, rewrite each of the following sentences first as a cumulative sentence and then as a periodic sentence. Do you prefer one version of your sentence over the other?

Example

No one seemed to be living in the house.

Cumulative version: No one seemed to be living in the house, which loomed darkly against the stormy sky, its broken window panes and rotten siding suggesting years of neglect.

Periodic version: Although the grounds were neatly cared for and lights burned within the curtained windows on the second floor, no one seemed to be living in the house.

1. David looked across the room at Sandra's empty chair.
2. I took a firm position against the proposal.
3. Laws are intended to protect all the citizens.
4. My house plants always die.
5. Jerry's classic 1965 Mustang had begun to develop rust.
6. Books were what really interested Lisa.
7. You will have a difficult time removing those bloodstains.
8. We realized that we should not have invited the Wilsons.
9. The screeching car barely missed the pedestrian.
10. Rita offered honest advice to every student who saw her.

10c Sentence variety

When the sentences in a passage are all approximately the same in length and structure, as in this opening passage from a published article, the result can be tedious reading:

> Nonsense bears the stamp of paradox. The two terms of the paradox are order and disorder. Order is generally created by language, disorder by reference. But the essential factor is their peculiar interplay. Elizabeth Sewell, in a penetrating analysis of nonsense, stresses the idea of dialectic. Yet her analysis deals almost exclusively with the formal structure of order. . . .

No reader can be expected to maintain interest in such prose for very long. Most of us, after all, read for pleasure as well as for information, and we expect writers to appeal to our desire for prose that satisfies and delights. The kind of monotonous prose in the example above can be revised effectively simply by varying the length and structure of the sentences:

10c

> Nonsense bears the stamp of paradox, whose two terms are order and disorder. Although order is generally created by language and disorder by reference, the essential factor is their peculiar interplay. Elizabeth Sewell stresses the idea of dialectic in a penetrating analysis of nonsense, yet her analysis deals almost exclusively with the formal structure of order. . . .

The six sentences of the original, each approximately ten words long, have here been combined into three sentences of thirteen, eighteen, and twenty-five words. Related ideas are joined more clearly, and the second sentence's opening adverbial clause (*Although order* . . .) eliminates the monotony caused by a series of sentences that all begin with their subjects. Moreover, the progressively increasing length of these three sentences leads the reader more smoothly into the rest of the article. Variety, in short, has the same beneficial effects on writing that it has on life itself.

Becoming familiar with the English sentence structures described in Chapter **9** is the first step toward developing variety in your writing. Experiment with prepositional and verbal phrases; look for opportunities to use subordinate clauses; try to mix simple, compound, complex, and compound-complex sentences in your prose. At the same time, vary the length of your sentences. Remember that a string of long sentences is just as tiring to a reader as a series of short ones. It's the mixing of sentences of different lengths that keeps most readers engaged in a text.

One important way of giving your prose new sophistication is by varying the first elements in your sentences. Many of us think of the main idea in a sentence first and are therefore inclined to place it first in the sentence. But when every sentence in a piece of writing begins with its subject, as in the first passage quoted above, the effect is wearying dullness. Try experimenting with some of the alternative ways of opening sentences described below. (See Chapter **9** for further information about each of these constructions.)

1. Single modifiers

When a modifying word is placed at the start of a sentence, rather than buried somewhere else, it inevitably draws attention. The result is an emphatic sentence opening.

Fay checked through the reports carefully, despite distracting noises coming from the office next door.

Carefully, Fay checked through the reports, despite distracting noises coming from the office next door.

The exhausted street musician began to pack up his collection of instruments.

Exhausted, the street musician began to pack up his collection of instruments.

2. Prepositional phrases

Like single modifiers, prepositional phrases can often be pulled from a later position in a sentence and placed at its beginning for variety and greater emphasis.

The weather in this city is completely unpredictable.

In this city, the weather is completely unpredictable.

U.S. auto manufacturers have begun to reestablish their credibility with American consumers during the past five years.

During the past five years, U.S. auto manufacturers have begun to reestablish their credibility with American consumers.

3. Appositives

Though usually placed after the nouns they refer to, appositives can precede them and may be used to begin a sentence.

Those stained glass windows, a gift of the college's first graduate, are irreplaceable.

A gift of the college's first graduate, those stained glass windows are irreplaceable.

David, an unwilling partner in the scheme, feared that he would lose more money than he would make.

An unwilling partner in the scheme, David feared that he would lose more money than he would make.

Some readers would say that both of these sentences have been improved by beginning with the appositive, which in each of the original versions interrupts the flow of the sentence in its position between the subject and predicate.

4. Verbal phrases

Look for opportunities to convert verbs in a sentence into participial or gerund phrases as beginning elements.

Alina was worried about the legal implications of the document and refused to sign it.

Worried about the legal implications of the document, Alina refused to sign it. [participial phrase]

I considered many ways of using my medical training and finally decided to work
    in the field of public health.

After considering many ways of using my medical training, I finally decided to
    work in the field of public health.
[preposition with gerund phrase]

5. Absolute phrases

    An absolute phrase—usually made up of a noun plus an adjective or
participle—is a distinctive sentence opener. Use it for emphasis and economy.

Mark tried to attract Julie's attention by waving his arms wildly.

His arms waving wildly, Mark tried to attract Julie's attention.

Jill's patience was exhausted, and she began to raise her voice.

Her patience exhausted, Jill began to raise her voice.

6. Adverbial clauses

    Moving an adverbial clause from the end of a sentence to its beginning
shifts emphasis, and changes a cumulative sentence into a periodic one.

The mayor refused to sign the proclamation, because most of the city council
    members advised against it.

Because most of the city council members advised against it, the mayor refused to
    sign the proclamation.

Sometimes an independent clause can be reduced to an adverbial clause and
used as a sentence opener.

Service at the oldest restaurant in town has been declining, but the prices have
    steadily risen.

Although service at the oldest restaurant in town has been declining, the prices
    have steadily risen.

    Ultimately, you must decide which of these strategies best suit your
writing. Read your prose aloud, experiment with new stylistic techniques, and
work toward developing a style that reflects your own personality.

Exercise 4

The following sentences all begin with the subject. Rewrite each so that some other
element functions as the sentence opener. Add new material as necessary.

Example

    Lydia typed up the report, making changes where she found they were needed.

    As she typed up the report, Lydia made changes where she found they were
        needed.

1. High-speed film enables you to shoot pictures in poor light, but it produces
    somewhat grainy prints.

10c

10c

2. Judy's red hair was barely visible behind the piles of paper on her desk.
3. The declining price of electronic equipment such as home computers threatens the financial stability of several major electronics manufacturers.
4. The water that surrounds New Orleans prevents the evening temperatures from dropping in the summer.
5. Louise is an excellent secretary and also a person with an unusually dry sense of humor.
6. Biological research is more attractive to many students than a career in medicine.
7. I consider international peace the most important issue of our time, and I've organized a group of students and faculty who share my concern.
8. Procrastination is a vice that most people are surprisingly willing to acknowledge.
9. Jane's office was very small, but she saw several dozen clients each day.
10. Professor Adamson's popularity was due in part to his scrupulous fairness in grading student papers.

Exercise 5

Most of the sentences in the paragraph below are of about the same length, and all begin with the subject. Rewrite the paragraph to increase variety in sentence structure and sentence length. Add new material as necessary.

Selecting an apartment in a strange city is a task full of unknowns. The first step is finding the apartments you want to inspect. You will probably need a recent city map to guide you. A city map, however, doesn't give you all the information you need. It doesn't tell you that there's a noisy factory across the street from the apartment you saw advertised. You have to arrive at the apartment to discover that. The reliability of your new landlord is another very important question. Your landlord may seem friendly when you first meet. He or she must be available when your pipes begin to leak. Acquiring information about your new neighbors may also be difficult. An apartment complex may be quiet when you visit it during the day. You may not meet your neighbors until after you have moved in. They may have a state-of-the-art stereo system that keeps you awake nights. It may even rattle the dishes in your cupboard. Your signature on a lease may condemn you to a year of frustration.

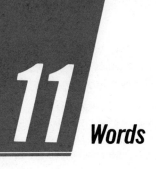

11 Words

Like all languages, English is constantly changing. New words are added as names are required for new inventions, discoveries, and ideas: *laser, meson, transistor, cybernetics, tagmeme.* Old words acquire new meanings as they are used in new ways: *half-life* (physics), *snow* (television), *hardware* (computers), *cartridge* (stereo recording). And some words disappear as the need for them vanishes; such is the case, for example, with a whole vocabulary dealing with horse-drawn vehicles. Words gain or lose prestige: *strenuous* and *mob,* once considered slang, are now in standard usage. As all of these examples suggest, an important part of being a writer is developing a genuine curiosity about words.

11a Using the Dictionary

A dictionary is an attempt to record the current uses and meanings of words. Although many people believe that a dictionary tells them what a word *ought to* mean or how it *should be* used, a modern dictionary tries to be an accurate and objective record of what is actually being said and written. It discriminates among the current meanings of a word and tries to indicate the ways in which each is used. Since words and constructions differ in prestige value, a conscientious lexicographer will also try to record the current status of words, usually by labels such as *Dialectal* or *Regional, Obsolete* or *Archaic, Informal, Colloquial, Nonstandard,* or *Slang.*

A good dictionary can be a trustworthy aid in your dialogue with those who will read your writing. Large, unabridged dictionaries include a history of the meanings of words, biographical and geographical data, guides for pronunciation, spelling, and punctuation, and a variety of other useful information. The large dictionaries in established widespread use in most college libraries include the following.

The *Oxford English Dictionary,* 13 volumes and 4 supplements (in progress), Oxford University Press, New York, 1933, 1972, 1976, 1982.
[This is the standard historical dictionary of the language; it traces and illustrates the development of each word from its earliest appearance to the present.]

11a

Webster's Third New International Dictionary, Unabridged: The Great Library of the English Language, Merriam-Webster, Springfield, Mass., 1981.
[This dictionary gives few usage labels.]

The Random House Dictionary of the English Language, New York, 1979.

Webster's New Twentieth Century Dictionary of the English Language, Second Edition, William Collins Publishers, New York, 1979.

Unabridged dictionaries are invaluable for occasional reference, but more practical for the student are the following abridged desk dictionaries. All are reliable, but some instructors may have preferences.

The American Heritage Dictionary of the English Language, Houghton Mifflin, Boston.

Funk & Wagnalls Standard College Dictionary, Harper & Row, New York.

The Random House College Dictionary, New York.

Webster's New Collegiate Dictionary, Merriam-Webster, Springfield, Mass.

Webster's New World Dictionary, Simon & Schuster, New York.

To use a dictionary effectively, you must understand the abbreviations and symbols it uses. These are explained in its introductory section. Below are entries from four collegiate dictionaries, followed by notes on the information they provide.

spelling & syllabication   etymology

¹**im·ply** (im·plī′) *vt.* **-plied′, -ply′ing** [ME. *implien* < OFr. *emplier* < L. *implicare,* to involve, entangle < *in-,* in + *plicare,* to fold < IE. base **plek-,* to plait, wrap together, whence Gr. *plekein,* to braid: cf. FLAX] **1.** to have as a necessary part, condition, or effect; contain, include, or involve naturally or necessarily [drama *implies* conflict] **2.** to indicate indirectly or by allusion; hint; suggest; intimate [an attitude *implying* boredom] **3.** [Obs.] to enfold; entangle —*SYN.* see SUGGEST

usage label

pronunciation   part of speech   meanings

²**im·ply** (im·plī′) *v.t.* **·plied, ·ply·ing 1.** To involve necessarily as a circumstance, condition, effect, etc.: An action *implies* an agent. **2.** To indicate or suggest without stating; hint at; intimate. **3.** To have the meaning of; signify. **4.** *Obs.* To entangle; infold. **—Syn.** See INFER. [< OF *emplier* < L *implicare* to involve < *in-* in + *plicare* to fold. Doublet of *EMPLOY.*]

11a

    —Syn. 1. *Imply* and *involve* mean to have some necessary connection. *Imply* states that the connection is casual or inherent, while *involve* is vaguer, and does not define the connection. **2.** *Imply, hint, intimate, insinuate* mean to convey a meaning indirectly or covertly. *Imply* is the general term for signifying something beyond what the words obviously say; his advice *implied* confidence in the stock market. *Hint* suggests indirection in speech or action: our host's repeated glances at his watch *hinted* that it was time to go. *Intimate* suggests a process more elaborate and veiled than hint: she *intimated* that his attentions were unwelcome. *Insinuate* suggests slyness and a derogatory import: in his remarks, he *insinuated* that the Senator was a fool.

full discussion of synonyms

inflected forms
³**im·ply** (ĭm-plī′) *tr. v.* **-plied, -ply·ing, -plies. 1.** To involve or suggest by logical necessity; entail: *His aims imply a good deal of energy.* **2.** To say or express indirectly; to hint; suggest: *His tone implied a malicious purpose.* **3.** *Obsolete.* To entangle. –See Synonyms at **suggest.** –See Usage note at **infer.** [Middle English *implien, emplien,* from Old French *emplier,* from Latin *implicāre,* infold, involve, IMPLICATE.]

⁴**im·ply** im-′plī *vt* **im·plied; im·ply·ing** [ME *emplien,* fr. MF *emplier,* fr. L *implicare*] (14c) **1** *obs:* ENFOLD, ENTWINE **2:** to involve or indicate by inference, association, or necessary consequence rather than by direct statement < rights ~ obligations > **3:** to contain potentially **4:** to express indirectly < his silence *implied* consent > *syn* see SUGGEST *usage* see INFER

      illustration of use   synonym   usage

Spelling and syllabication

When more than one spelling is given, the one printed first is usually to be preferred. Division of the word into syllables follows the conventions accepted by printers.

Pronunciation

A key to the symbols used to indicate pronunciation of words is usually printed on the front or back inside cover of the dictionary. Some dictionaries also run an abbreviated key to pronunciation at the bottom of each page or every other page. Word accent is shown by the symbol (') after the stressed syllable or by (ˈ) before it.

Parts of speech

Abbreviations (explained in the introductory section of the dictionary) are used to indicate the various grammatical uses of a word: for example, *imply, v.t.* means that *imply* is a transitive verb.

Inflected forms

Forms of the past tense and past and present participles of verbs, the comparative or superlative degree of adjectives, and the plurals of nouns are given whenever there might be uncertainty about the correct form or spelling.

Etymology

The history of each word is indicated by the forms in use in Middle or Old English, or in the language from which the word was borrowed. Earlier meanings are often given.

Meanings

Different meanings of a word are numbered and defined, sometimes with illustrative examples. Some dictionaries give the oldest meanings first; others list the common meanings of the word first.

Usage labels

Descriptive labels, often abbreviated, indicate the level of usage: *Archaic, Obsolete, Colloquial, Slang, Dialectal, Regional, Substandard, Nonstandard,* and so on. Look up the meanings of these words in the dictionary you use. Sometimes usage labels indicate a special field rather than a level of usage: for example, *Poetic, Irish, Chemistry.* If a word has no usage label, it may be assumed that, in the opinion of the editors, the word is in common use on all levels; that is, it is *Standard English.* Usage labels are often defined and illustrated in the explanatory notes in the front of a dictionary.

Synonyms

Many words have closely related or nearly identical meanings and require careful discrimination. A full account of the distinctions in meaning among synonyms (for example, *suggest, imply, hint, intimate,* and *insinuate*) may be given at the end of the entry for each word, or cross references to its synonyms may be provided.

Exercise 1

11a

In looking up the meanings of words, try to discover within what limits of meaning the word may be used. Read the definition as a whole; do not pick out a single synonym and suppose that this and the word defined are interchangeable. After looking up the following words in your dictionary, write sentences that will unmistakably illustrate the meaning of each word.

anachronism	innocuous	precocious
eminent	materiel	sinecure
fetish	misanthropy	sophistication
hedonist	nepotism	taboo
imminent	philanthropy	travesty

Exercise 2

Look up each of the following words in the *Oxford English Dictionary,* in an unabridged dictionary, and in an abridged one, and write a brief report explaining how the larger dictionaries explain the use of each word more carefully and clearly than the smaller one. Give the title, the publisher, and the date of each dictionary.

Bible	color	idealism
catholic	court	liberal
Christian	evolution	

Exercise 3

How may the etymologies given by the dictionary help one to remember the meaning or the spelling of the following words? (Note that when a series of words has the same etymology, the etymology is usually given only with the basic word of the series.)

alibi	insidious	privilege
capitol	isosceles	sacrilegious
cohort	magnanimous	sarcasm
concave	malapropism	subterfuge
denouement	peer (noun)	thrifty

Exercise 4

Most dictionaries put abbreviations in the main alphabetical arrangement. Locate the following abbreviations and their meanings.

at. wt.	Ens.	LL.D.
CAB	ff.	OAS
colloq.	K.C.B.	PBX
e.g.	l.c.	Q.E.D.

Exercise 5

Consult the dictionary for the distinction in meaning between the members of each of the following pairs of words:

neglect—negligence
ingenuous—ingenious
fewer—less
admit—confess
infer—imply

instinct—intuition
nauseous—nauseated
eminent—famous
criticize—censure
increment—addition

11b

Exercise 6

In each sentence, choose the more precise of the two italicized words. Be able to justify your choice.

1. Many in the class were *disinterested, uninterested* and went to sleep.
2. His charming innocence is *childlike, childish.*
3. The problem is to assure the farm workers *continuous, continual* employment.
4. She is *continuously, continually* in trouble with the police.
5. I am quite *jealous, envious* of your opportunity to study in Europe.
6. She is so *decided, decisive* in her manner that people always give in to her.
7. If we give your class all of these privileges, we may establish *precedents, precedence* which are unwise.
8. She always makes her health her *alibi, excuse* for her failures.

Exercise 7

Find the precise meaning of each word in the following groups, and write sentences to illustrate that meaning.

1. abandon, desert, forsake
2. ludicrous, droll, comic
3. silent, reserved, taciturn
4. meager, scanty, sparse
5. knack, talent, genius
6. anxious, eager, avid

11b Levels of usage

Every good dictionary tells you the contexts in which the use of a word is appropriate, its customary usage. **Standard English** includes the great majority of words and constructions that native speakers would recognize as acceptable in any situation or context, whether spoken or written. All words in a dictionary that are not otherwise labeled are, in the judgment of the editors, Standard English and acceptable for general use. A good many other words and constructions, which have, for various reasons, a more limited use, are commonly labeled in various ways. For example, words used in some sections of the country but not in all, such as *carry* in the sense of "escort" (as in "He carried his sister to the movies") will be labeled *Regional* or *Dialectal.* If the usage is even more localized, such as *arroyo* (a dry gully), the word will be labeled *Southwestern U.S.* or *New England* or whatever. Other labels identify words still found in books but no longer in common use, such as *Obsolete* (for example, *deer* used in the sense of "any small animal," as in Shakespeare's "Rats and mice and such small deer") or *Archaic* (for example, *olden* and other such old words preserved for historical or poetic reasons).

Appropriateness of usage depends upon a number of interacting factors. Some words and phrases are associated only with particular groups, whether ethnic (for example, black English), professional (legal language), generational (the speech of teenagers), or economic. Dictionaries use such terms as *nonstandard, substandard, colloquial, jargon,* and *slang* to distinguish such words and phrases from Standard English. Level of formality is another factor that affects usage. We use some constructions solely with intimate friends and relatives, others only on the most formal of occasions. Thus most people would find it as out of place to greet a family member with "May I help you, sir?" as to ask a customer, "What do you want, darling?"

11b

1. Edited English

Edited English, the usual written form of the language, is relatively formal Standard English. It is the language of books from reputable publishers, good magazines, and most newspapers. Edited English is defined not merely by choice of words, but by widely accepted conventions of spelling, punctuation, grammatical pattern, and sentence structure. The general subject of this book is Edited English, the normal means of official communication in the professions and in business and industry.

Authorities, it must be admitted, often differ among themselves, particularly where the language seems to be changing. For example, many handbooks deplore the use of *contact* as a verb meaning "to get in touch with." But the most recent editions of five leading dictionaries differ widely: two accept the usage, with no label, as Standard English; one accepts it but labels it as an *Americanism;* two others label it *Informal* and discourage its use in Edited English.

Faced with such disagreement, what practical conclusion can we draw? If you use *contact* as a verb and someone challenges it, you can certainly defend yourself by citing *Webster's Ninth New Collegiate Dictionary* or the *Random House College Dictionary,* both of which make no objection to it. Of course, being challenged is a nuisance, and controversial usages may be distracting for readers. If the main purpose of your writing is to get something said, be wary of usages that need lengthy defense.

2. Formal English

Formal English appears in scholarly or scientific articles, formal speeches, official documents, and any context calling for scrupulous propriety. It makes use of words and phrases, such as "scrupulous propriety," which rarely occur in conversation and which would seldom appear in casual writing.

As another example, consider the verb *endeavor.* This is a perfectly good word that everyone knows, but its use is almost entirely limited to formal, written English, and even there it is not common. It is likely to give a bookish flavor to casual writing, and it is almost never used in speech. (Try to imagine yourself handing a friend a piece of writing with the request, "Endeavor to read this.") Formal English also includes technical language—the specialized vocabularies (sometimes called *jargon*) used in such professions as law, medicine, and the sciences. Technical language can be very precise and economical, but it is Greek to the ordinary reader and out of place in most Edited English, except in such special circumstances as legal documents, medical reports, and scientific papers. The basic principle of good usage is to fit the level of your language to the situation and to the expected reader. The most formal English is for the most formal occasions, such as commencement or a funeral, or for official personages, such as college presidents in their public speeches and writing. In the most formal English, one might *endeavor to assuage one's consternation;* less formally the writer might say *attempt to calm* (or even *try to end*) *your fears.* But only in informal (or colloquial) speech or in a personal letter might one *take a whack at wiping out your hang-ups.*

Levels of usage, like the language itself, undergo changes from generation to generation. Such changes have been especially rapid in recent decades. During the past seventy years, the center of Edited usage has moved away from the formal level toward greater informality. Especially in magazines and newspapers, good writers are more likely to use *colloquialisms* and even *slang* rather than risk the stilted pomposity of Formal English in a commonplace context.

3. Colloquial English

Colloquial English means, literally, conversational English. Everyone's language is more casual and relaxed among friends than in public speech or writing. Colloquial expressions may be jarringly out of place in formal contexts or in serious writing. Examples are adjectives such as *steep* for "expensive," verbs like *get away with* something, and adverbs such as *sure* in the sense of "certainly" (*I sure would like . . .*). When words and constructions are labeled *Colloquial* (some dictionaries use *Informal* for the same purpose), you should consider their possible effects on a reader before writing them. If in doubt, look for an accepted synonym.

4. Regional English

The label **Regional** refers to usage that is common only to speakers in a limited geographical area. These words are often standard in speech and informal writing in the regions where they are found, and sometimes they are useful additions to the local vocabulary. But for general public writing, including most college writing, they should be avoided when equivalent words in national currency are available. Some examples of regional words and expressions are *gumband* for *rubber band, yuz* and *y'all* for *you,* and *stand on line* for *stand in line.*

5. Dialect and nonstandard English

A **Dialect** is a variety of a language spoken in a particular region of the country or by a socially identifiable group of persons. Speakers of a dialect may use not only special vocabulary, but also distinct grammatical structures that differ from those of Standard English. All dialects—including Standard—retain words and linguistic rules that have died out in other dialects (*reckon* and *yonder,* for example, in the Southeast). Other dialect forms are new to the language, as when the Southeasterner says *You might could say that* rather than *Maybe you could say that,* or the Midwesterner *Tom smokes a lot anymore* where most speakers of English would have to say *Tom smokes a lot these days.* Speech forms which are restricted to a particular social dialect are often labeled *Nonstandard* (sometimes *Substandard*) in dictionaries. The use of *learn* for *teach* or *she don't* for *she doesn't* are Nonstandard in this sense. So, too, is the use of *be* for *is,* characteristic of black folk speech.

To the modern linguist, all the dialects spoken by different groups in American society are equally expressive varieties of English, even though many of their most obvious forms are not appropriate in Edited English. However, the social prestige and broad acceptability associated with Standard English make it important for educated persons to be able to distinguish this form of English from other types. Since a regional or social dialect's grammatical rules may differ from the rules of Standard English, students who are bi-dialectical have two sets of grammatical rules to keep in mind. They must be aware of those areas where their spoken English and written English conflict, and they may have to proof-read their written work with special care to make certain that it follows the conventions of Edited English.

The labels *Nonstandard* and *Substandard* are also used to indicate a wide variety of usages not accepted by most educated readers but not necessarily associated with dialects at all: misspellings, unconventional punctuation, idio-syncratic grammatical constructions, and certain widespread usages that edu-cated people have qualms about writing. Examples are words such as *irregardless* for *regardless, imply* for *infer,* and *flaunt* for *flout,* and grammatical errors such as *between you and I* (where *me* is correct). Many other common problems of this nature are listed in the Glossary of Usage. Expressions labeled *Nonstandard* have no place in serious Edited English, unless in direct quotation.

6. Slang

Slang is the label given to words with a forced, exaggerated, or humorous meaning used in extremely informal or colloquial contexts.

To call a man whose ideas and behavior are unpredictable and unconventional *a kook* and to describe his ideas as *for the birds* or *out to lunch* certainly satisfies some obscure human urge toward irreverent, novel, and vehement expression. Some slang terms remain in fairly wide use because they are vivid ways of expressing an idea that has no exact standard equivalent: *stooge, lame duck, shot* of whiskey, a card *shark*. Such words are becoming accepted as Standard English. *Mob, banter, sham,* and *lynch* were all once slang terms. It is quite likely that, eventually, such useful slang words as *honky-tonk* and *snitch* will also be accepted as Standard.

A good deal of slang, however, reflects nothing more than the user's desire to be colorful, outrageous, or part of a particular in-group, and such slang has little chance of gaining complete respectability. Sports commentators and disk jockeys, for example, often use a flamboyant jargon intended to show off their ingenuity and cleverness and to establish their credentials as members of a select group or inner circle who keep up with the times. For centuries criminals have used a special, semisecret language, and many modern slang terms originated in the argot of the underworld: *gat, scram, squeal* or *sing* (confess), *push* (peddle).

Whatever the motive behind it, slang should be used with discretion. On the other hand, its incongruity in a sober, practical context makes it an effective way of achieving force and emphasis.

Acceptable slang

His book is so intelligently constructed, so beautifully written, so really acute at moments—and so *raunchy*.

But slang terms are too jarring to fit comfortably into most Edited English. Furthermore, most slang goes out of fashion very quickly, and dated slang sounds more quaint and old-fashioned than Formal English. *Smashed* has worn well, but *tight, crocked, bombed,* and *plastered* may soon be museum pieces. In the 1950s, to call someone a *square* identified the speaker as a youthful, up-to-date person; today, the term has been replaced in collegiate slang.

The chief objection to the use of slang is that it so quickly loses any precise meaning. Calling a person a *nerd*, a *twerp*, or a *bozo* conveys little more than your feeling of dislike. *Cool* and *bummed out* are the vaguest kind of terms, lumping all experience into two crude divisions, pleasing and unpleasing. Try to get several people to agree on the precise meaning of *nerd* and you will realize how vague and inexact a term it is. The remedy is to analyze your meaning and specify it. What exactly are the qualities that lead you to classify a person as a *twerp* or a *nerd?*

If, despite these warnings, you must use slang in serious writing, do it deliberately and accept the responsibility for it. Do not attempt to excuse yourself by putting the slang term in quotation marks. If you must apologize for a slang term, do not use it.

Exercise 8

With the aid of a dictionary and your own linguistic judgment (that is, your ear for appropriateness), classify the following English words as *Formal, Informal, Colloquial,* or *Slang.*

1. crank, eccentric, (a) character
2. hide, sequester, sneak
3. irascible, cranky, grouchy
4. increase, boost, jack [up the price]
5. decline, avoid, pass [up]
6. pass [out], faint, swoon
7. necessity, [a] must, requirement
8. inexpensive, [a] steal, cheap
9. snooty, pretentious, affected
10. crib, steal, plagiarize, pilfer

11b

Exercise 9

For each of the following Standard English words supply one or more slang terms and, to the best of your ability, judge which are so widespread that they have already begun to creep into highly informal writing (for example, letters to friends, college newspaper columns) or seem likely to do so in the near future.

Example: to *sleep* [to *crash,* slang]

1. money
2. to relax
3. a skilled performer
4. to be going steady or to be in love
5. failure
6. to tell off
7. pleasant or enjoyable
8. to vomit
9. liquor
10. to ignore or disregard
11. complaint
12. a dull person
13. an unconventional person
14. to be unfairly treated
15. puzzling

Exercise 10

Pick five or six slang terms widely used around campus and ask at least five people to define the meaning of each term in Standard English. Write the results and your conclusions.

Part III

Revising

12 Revising the Essay

From childhood on, we spend much of our time learning to ask others what they think and to pay attention to what their opinion is of what they see. Serving on the committee for the spring prom or some other school project, exchanging views on recent films or books, sorting out tangled relationships with friends, relatives, or lovers—in these and dozens of other situations we depend on others to deepen our understanding. We count on others to help us focus; we need others to test or probe our initial conclusions, to add perceptions and details, to help us notice what we might otherwise forget or ignore. At our best, when our ego does not intrude or we don't feel threatened, we realize how vital the insights of others can be, how much we enjoy collaborating. Such moments are possible in writing, especially in the stages of revision. Presenting one's views, experience, or research to others, submitting them for criticism, discussion, and modification is the process of effective communication.

Revision is "seeing again," the chance to rethink the argument, reconsider the evidence, rearrange the ideas. As such, revision is best accomplished a day or two after a first draft has been written. Usually, writers need to detach themselves from their work, to put a little distance between themselves and their enthusiastic first efforts, and gain objectivity. Like rehearsals for the final production, revision is the occasion for catching omissions, errors, ambiguities, and clumsy staging. And, like the director, the writer must try to see the work through the audience's eyes while still preserving his or her vision of the whole. The point is to be open. Rethinking your paper later, you are not bound to accept all criticisms as equally valid, but every criticism should tell you something. Even the occasional silence, where a roommate or a classmate seems indifferent and has little to say, could imply that the paper needs complete redoing because it is too cautious, obvious, or impersonal.

To begin with, we can identify at least two types of revisions: those that writers themselves see the need for and make on their own, and those that others suggest or request. In principle, the aim of any composition course is to make students their own editors—their own instructors, as it were—who can see what is necessary and revise accordingly. In practice, most writers, from the most professional to the mere beginner, depend on the comments of others to improve their work. Revision can (and should) be the ideal occasion to

12

improve skills, to gain confidence, to discover that one makes sense and is understood by others. As you may have discovered from your own experience, revision takes various forms: often, the writer will simply mark up the text and make insertions and revisions between the lines; sometimes, especially if the manuscript has been heavily edited, the writer will begin afresh; on other occasions, the writer will recopy substantial parts of the draft, making changes in wording and sequence in the light of his or her own comments or those of others; on still other occasions, particularly if the paper is long, the writer will cut and paste or return to the word processor. Only rarely, however, can one revise simply by changing the occasional misspelling and fiddling with a few commas. Cosmetic revision that involves merely the correction of the most obvious errors is largely a waste of the brief time spent. Genuine revision usually requires at least as much time as the drafting of the original.

In the examples that follow, note how each student has tried to revise on several levels simultaneously. These levels include the most general one of the paper's overall structure as an argument, the more specific levels of individual paragraphs and sentences, and the quite concrete level of individual words and problems in grammar and punctuation. For purposes of clarity, we have divided Part III so that each level is treated separately. In actuality, however, revision is a complex process of moving back and forth between larger and smaller elements of the work, and able writers often revise several times. Chapter **12** concerns itself with revising the essay as a whole.

Our first set of examples typifies the usual college experience—the student's manuscript after the teacher has gone over it, and the revised paper. Normally, you will be expected to look up the grading symbols in the key at the front or back of your handbook, read the relevant discussions in the text, reflect on the written comments, and see your instructor about anything you don't understand or don't agree with. Some teachers will use the symbols we have employed (inside back cover); others will use a numbering system (2b, 9c, and the like) that refers you to particular handbook sections. In reading the following example, notice *how* the teacher's summary comments direct the student's attention to the primary strengths and weaknesses in the paper.

Wanted Dread and Alive

In different cultures or contexts, the same word can take on different meanings. To understand these meanings, one must know this culture or context. Consider the word "dread." In America, we associate it with negative connotations.

awk. ref

But <u>this</u> need not be the case. Ninety miles south of Cuba in the Caribbean lies a green and <u>shimmering island</u> where the concept of "dread" has taken on new meanings. In Jamaican society, "dread" implies something completely different from our <u>understanding of the word</u>. It is my intention to explore the Third World's interpretation of "dread" and expand our limited notion of (it's) meaning.

Jamaica?

how so?

How do you know? Specify basis of your evidence

logic Jamaica = the Third World?

abrupt transition

The Rastafarians, concentrated in Jamaica but with many followers among the large <u>Jamaican</u> immigrant population centers such as New York and London, are a religious cult that has become a political movement within Jamaica. One of the true marks of a true Rastafarian is the way he wears his hair. The most visible characteristic of the Rastafarian is his long dreadlocks ( ) or "dreads" ( ). Even if the cult is unconscious of <u>it</u>, there are some <u>deep social implications</u> to dreadlocks. Hair style in Jamaica is often used as an index of social differences, for example fine and silky hair has always been considered "good," while woolly or kinky hair is frowned upon. <u>It is generally thought that the Rastafarian's hair style ridicules the ambivalence of the society.</u> Long hair worn by Jamaican men is a symbol of defiance. The Rastas will not adhere to society's codes unless there is <u>radical change</u>. Nearly all conservative Jamaicans "dread" the locks of the Rastafarians; and the stronger <u>the</u> revulsion, the longer the Rastas cause their locks to grow. Today, some

rep

combine sentences

why parens?

ref

wordy & unclear

cs

wordy & unclear

what?

their

12

Rastafarians sport "dreads" as long as twenty inches.

Members of this Jamaican religious/political cult wear dreadlocks as a sign of their commitment to the Rasta path of knowing themselves and leading a righteous life. The Rastafarians consider themselves to be Nazarites, and as holy men they follow the ancient commandments of the Bible. In Maccabean times, the Nazarites were distinguished by their mass of uncut hair. The word "Nazarites" means "to separate" or "to dedicate" in ancient Hebrew. The Nazarites were dedicated and set apart by their individual exemplification of pure and holy living. The Nazarite vow stated that one was not to cut his locks, drink alcohol, or deal with any form of death. The locksman follows the "dread" path by continuing his commitment to an ancient Biblical tradition. Some Rastas even referring to their locks as antenni through which they receive inspiration from God. They believe that the early Israelites and prophets, as well as Christ and the early Christians, must have worn dreadlocks. To them, dreadlocks are a natural hair style with deep cultural meaning, representing their Biblical commitment. The unshaven man is the natural man, who typifies in his appearance the unencumbered life.

The concept of "dread" has taken on new meanings in Jamaican society. To the elite, it refers to a dangerous and dirty appearance; to

This ¶ is repetitious Can you tighten it up?

meaning?

what? develop

combine sentences

meaning?

this

frag

sp

transition a bit abrupt

12

the Rastafarians, it signifies power and freedom. "Dread" means rebellion or a certain
behavior pattern outside of society. Recently,

vague and dead

"dread" has become an established word closer to
our meaning among the youth. For example, if a
teacher is severe that teacher is known as
"dread." Subject such as mathematics and science are "dread." If a man is good at a sport, he
is "dread." As one can see, the word has become
routinized in the society in a value-free way.

jargon

Undoubtedly, though, the Rastafarians have
caused the term "dread" to assume new meanings in

rep

the Jamaican vocabulary.

As I have tried to show, one must know the
culture and context in order to understand how
and why a word gains new connotations. In

conclusion is brief

Jamaica, from the Rastafarian point of view, it
makes sense to say, "Wanted dread and alive."

do they say this?

This essay has real promise. It develops an interesting thesis with some good detail. But the essay is also wordy and unclear in places, and it needs tighter coherence within and among paragraphs. In revising, try to make the connections tighter, the diction clearer, and the logic sharper. Also look up sentence fragments, comma splices, and the other errors for corrections.

Before looking at the student's revision, let us consider what the teacher has said and suggested. She finds the essay promising because it has an interesting thesis and because it is sustained by good detail in places. But she also finds the essay wordy and unclear in places and sometimes lacking coherence within and among the paragraphs. The student's primary challenge in revision is not the correction of mechanical errors, though there are several that need attending to. Rather he has been asked to rethink—to see afresh—his logic, his evidence, and his phrasing. In the final version below, notice how he has revised his opening paragraph to clarify his focus and to make a smooth transition to his second paragraph. In addition, notice how he has reworked each of the subsequent paragraphs to combine ideas and cut down on the passive voice, to eliminate meaningless or repetitive phrases, and to sharpen his analysis by more detail and tighter connections.

Wanted Dread and Alive

In different cultures or contexts, the same word can take on different meanings. To understand these meanings, one must know this culture or context. Consider, for example, the word "dread." In America, we associate it with negative connotations. As students, we "dread" to take exams. As taxpayers, we "dread" April fifteenth. As human beings, we "dread" death. But ninety miles south of Cuba in the Caribbean lies the green and shimmering island of Jamaica where the concept of "dread" has taken on new meanings. During my three months there, I came to understand the cultural significance of the term, especially its connections with the Rastafarians.

Concentrated in Jamaica but with many followers among the large immigrant centers in New York and London, the Rastafarians are a religious cult that has become a political movement. The true mark of a Rastafarian is the way he wears his hair: his long dreadlocks, or "dreads," are his most visible characteristic. Dreadlocks have specific cultural implications because Jamaicans often use hair style as an index of social differences. For example, they have always considered fine and silky hair to be "good" and frowned on woolly or kinky hair. Long hair worn by Jamaican men is a symbol of defiance. Nearly all conservative Jamaicans "dread" the locks of the Rastafarians; and the stronger their revulsion, the longer the Rastas cause

their locks to grow. Today, some Rastafarians sport
"dreads" as long as twenty inches.

Members of this cult wear dreadlocks as a sign of their
commitment to the Rasta path of the righteous life.
Rastafarians consider themselves to be Nazarites, holy men
following God's Biblical commandments to Moses and the
children of Israel (Numbers 6:5): "As long as he is bound by
his vow, no razor shall touch his head; until the day of his
consecration to Yahweh is completed, he remains under vow
and shall let his hair grow free." Distinguished in Maccabean times by their mass of uncut hair, the Nazarites were
dedicated to and set apart by their exemplification of pure
and holy living. ("Nazarite" comes from the ancient Hebrew
which means "to separate" or "to dedicate.") Nazarites also
vowed not to drink alcohol or touch corpses. The locksman
follows the "dread" path by continuing his commitment to
this ancient Biblical tradition. Some Rastas even refer to
their locks as antennas through which they receive inspiration from God. They believe that the early Israelites
and prophets, as well as Christ and the early Christians,
must have worn dreadlocks. To them, dreadlocks are a
natural hair style that represents their Biblical commitment. The unshaven man is the natural man, who typifies the
unencumbered life in his appearance.

Thus, the concept of "dread" has taken on new meanings
in Jamaican society. To the elite, it refers to a dangerous
and dirty appearance; to the Rastafarians, it signifies
power and freedom. Recently, among the youth, however,
"dread" has become an established word closer to our
meaning. For example, if a teacher is severe, he is known as
"dread." Subjects such as mathematics and science are
"dread." If a man is good at a sport, he is "dread." As one

12

can see, the word has become routinized in its connotations. Undoubtedly, though, the Rastafarians have
caused the term "dread" to assume new associations in the
Jamaican vocabulary.

As I have tried to show, one must know the culture and
the context in order to understand how and why a word gains
new connotations. In one society and for one group of
people, "dread" signifies dedication and change. In
Jamaica, from the Rastafarian point of view, it might make
sense to say, "Wanted dread and alive."

While the student could make still further changes, he at least has improved
the economy and clarity of his paper. The revision, as a whole, is more direct and
precise than the original. His revision also suggests a few useful questions that
you can ask about your own papers.

Revision checklist for the overall argument or analysis

1. Does your essay have a clear thesis that restricts your topic and indicates
   the main stages or direction of your analysis?
2. Do your paragraphs support or develop your thesis clearly, fully,
   coherently?
3. Are the connections among the paragraphs and within each paragraph
   smoothly and adequately made?
4. Are your major assertions soundly argued and persuasively detailed?
5. Is your tone appropriate for your audience?

Like the first paper, the essay below grew out of an assignment to discuss a
word's connotations in its social context. Here, with some gentle assistance
from her instructor, the writer has edited her own paper before submitting a
final version. She has begun to meet the greatest challenge of revision—to see
one's work through the eyes of others. She has paid special attention to
questions 2 and 5 because they pinpoint recurrent problems in her essays: the
clear, coherent development of her thesis in her paragraphs, and the appropriateness of her tone for her audience. Notice how she has regrouped her ideas
and how she has controlled the tone.

Aloha

I find it sad that so often words with
originally serious meanings become the slang so
lightly used in our everyday language. Take, for

example, the Hawaiian word "aloha." Today, aloha
is a chic way for saying "hello," especially
around the little beach towns in Southern California. Used in other contexts, it sometimes
means nothing more than "Hawaiian." Aloha has
also become a meaningless ~~word~~ *term* that tourists ~~in
Hawaii~~ proclaim, ~~not knowing its meaning, but~~
thrilled that they know (but cannot pronounce) a
Hawaiian word. Aloha has become ~~a fun word~~, an
empty expression, but to the people of Hawaii it
is a warm, ~~friendly, sincere~~ word that includes a
multiplicity of feelings.

examples?

12

   Aloha in Hawaiian is a term of endearment.
Although there is no equivalent English meaning, the closest and most accurate ~~English~~
translation would be "love." To give someone
your aloha is to give them your ~~deepest~~, heartfelt feelings of "best wishes and love." Many
times you will hear someone say, "My aloha goes
out to you." You know that you are someone
special ~~and dear~~ if this is said to you, for
aloha embraces strong ~~feelings~~ *affection.* ~~The term is not
used lightly, but expresses the most sincere
feelings of the heart~~.

   Aloha used in a different context comes
close to the English words "blessing" or
"consent." For example, when a couple decides to
get married, their parents will either give
their aloha, or will oppose the marriage. If the
parents give their aloha, they give the couple
their blessing by opening up their hearts to the
event. ←

The term is not used lightly; it expresses what is deepest.

   ~~Aloha in Hawaiian is also a term of appre-~~

12

Aloha has other shades of meaning

~~ciation, much like "thank you" in English. When someone does something nice that you greatly appreciate, you might send them a card, expressing your aloha, in the same way that someone sends you a thank you note.~~

→ In conjunction with the Hawaiian words for morning, afternoon, and night, ~~aloha also~~ *it* becomes a greeting. If ~~a~~ friend say~~s~~ *-s*, "Aloha kakahiaka" to you, they are saying "Good morning." Paradoxically, aloha is also a salutation. You would use it in the same way that you use "sincerely" to close a letter, or say "good—bye" when leaving people behind. Often I end my letters with aloha, or a phrase like "much love and aloha." Used as "good—bye," aloha means that you are leaving a little of ~~your love~~ *yourself* with the person. In other contexts, it can show gratitude. Queen Liliuokalani expressed both her love and her gratitude when, on the eve of the annexation of the Hawaiian Islands she wrote the song "Aloha Oe." It expresses her love for the islands and their people, her gratitude for so much, as well as her sorrow at the overthrow of the monarchy. The song was her farewell address, her last aloha to the people of Hawaii.

The multiplicity and complexity of aloha's meanings make it ~~a~~ difficult ~~word~~ to define, ~~for in no other language is there a word completely or closely synonymous to aloha. It seems that~~ To truly understand its meaning, you must grow up learning it and feeling it. ~~The word should not be used~~ *When* as slang fo~~r~~ it loses the beauty of its meaning that is so ~~special and~~ dear to the

Hawaiian people. It should be used sincerely,
seriously, warmly. I hate to hear it abused.

To restructure her essay, the writer has combined two paragraphs and cut one out, transposed one sentence and rephrased it, and inserted clearer transitions. To modulate her tone, she has edited out a number of adjectives and adverbs, deleted a glittering generalization (". . . in no other language is there a word. . . ."), and used "love" and "feelings" more sparingly. She has also added more detail in the first paragraph to exemplify the kinds of usage of "aloha" she deplores. Her revised version below is a more orderly essay, and it places more trust in its words and in the reader.

12

Aloha

I find it sad that so often words with originally serious meanings become the slang so lightly used in our everyday language. Take, for example, the Hawaiian word "aloha." Today, aloha is a chic way for saying "hello," especially around the little beach towns in Southern California. Used in other contexts, it sometimes means nothing more than "Hawaiian," as in all those phrases like "aloha attire," "aloha shirt," and "aloha print." Aloha has become a term that tourists proclaim, thrilled that they know (but cannot pronounce) a Hawaiian word. Aloha has become an empty expression, but to my people it is a warm word that includes a multiplicity of feelings.

Aloha in Hawaiian is a term of endearment. Although there is no equivalent English meaning, the closest and most accurate translation would be "love." To give someone your aloha is to give them your heartfelt feelings of "best wishes and love." Many times you will hear someone say, "My aloha goes out to you." You know that you are special if this is said to you, for aloha embraces strong affection. In another context, aloha signifies "blessing" or "consent."

For example, when a couple decides to get married, their parents will either give their aloha, or will oppose the marriage. If the parents give their aloha, they give the couple their blessing by opening up their hearts to the event. The term is not used lightly; it expresses what is deepest.

Aloha has other shades of meaning. In conjunction with the Hawaiian words for morning, afternoon, or night, it becomes a greeting. If friends say "Aloha kakahiaka" to you, they are saying "Good morning." Paradoxically, aloha is also a salutation. You would use it in the same way that you use "sincerely" to close a letter, or say "good-bye" when leaving people behind. (Often I end my letters with aloha, or a phrase like "much love and aloha.") Used as "good-bye," aloha means that you are leaving a little of yourself with the person. In other contexts, it can show gratitude. Queen Liliuokalani expressed both her love and her gratitude when, on the eve of the annexation of the Hawaiian Islands, she wrote the song "Aloha Oe." It expresses her love for the islands and their people, her gratitude for so much, as well as her sorrow at the overthrow of the monarchy. The song was her farewell address, her last aloha to the people of Hawaii.

The multiplicity of aloha's meaning make it difficult to define. To truly understand its meaning, you must grow up learning it and feeling it. When used as slang, it loses the beauty of its meaning that is so dear to the Hawaiian people. It should be used sincerely and warmly. I hate to hear it abused.

One remaining question you may have is the obvious one: How do I go about editing my papers? How can I correct problems that I don't even see in my work? While there is no single answer, there are several commonsensical guidelines. First, go back over earlier papers and study your instructor's comments and criticisms; use these, along with the revision checklist suggested earlier, to focus your attention. Deficiencies that have shown up in your work before are likely to show up again. Second, read your papers aloud, *slowly and accurately,* and mark all passages that sound vague or disunified, all sections that sound repetitive or clumsy. Skimming by eye alone usually results in hasty, superficial revisions: you need to compel yourself to attend to what you have written. Third, work closely with your instructor. Make full use of your teachers; if your college offers a writing clinic or lab, by all means go whenever you can or feel you need help.

Exercise 1

This exercise is constructed to give you practice in editing papers.

1. Keep a copy of a paper you submit for class and mark it up as you imagine your instructor will; pay special attention to the kinds of problems you have had in earlier essays. When your paper is returned, compare your criticisms with your instructor's. How many had you anticipated? Had you, while writing the paper, been aware of any of the problems but decided to fudge a bit by ignoring them?
2. Find a classmate and exchange drafts of an assignment you are both submitting. Go over each other's papers as you imagine the instructor will. Then compare your comments and criticisms with the instructor's. How frequently have you agreed with the instructor? How frequently have you disagreed or concentrated on different things?
3. Using the revision checklist, analyze several graded papers you have written for other courses. Do these papers need the same kinds of revisions as those you have written for your composition course? What kinds of revisions can you find that your instructors did not comment on or call for?

Exercise 2

This exercise is constructed to help you see papers as completed wholes.

1. Summarize aloud to a friend or classmate the contents of a paper you are planning to write. As you talk together, do you find needed changes in the thesis, evidence, or stages of the analysis?
2. Repeat this procedure, this time summarizing a draft you have already written.
3. Pair off with a classmate writing on the same topic that you are and *exchange written summaries* of the papers you have in mind. Discover what problems you have in common—for example, the implications of the assigned topics, the issues you will need to address, the pertinent evidence or details.

12

13 *Revising Paragraphs*

Paragraphs are the timber writers use to construct papers. Depending on the writer's blueprint, they can be cut into various sizes and shapes and planed down or nailed together, and they can serve as doors, joists, or flooring. Problems occur, however, when a beam is too thin to support the weight it must bear, or when it is cracked and knotty or too loosely fastened on. The beam must be solid; the tongue and groove must match. To put it another way, effective paragraphs have the thickness of evidence needed to sustain their ideas; they are unsplintered and intact; and they are firmly joined together. Effective paragraphs are fully developed and have coherence. Here, we will discuss two of the most common weaknesses in paragraphs—lack of development and lack of coherence—and some means of repair. (To be sure that you understand the main characteristics of effective paragraphs, you may wish to read or review Chapters **7** and **8**.)

13a Inadequate development

Although its central idea may be clear, an underdeveloped paragraph may be too brief, general, thin, or dull. Developing a paragraph requires that the writer take time to see clearly and say accurately what his or her generalities signify. It means filling out the bare statement with specific detail. It certainly does not mean padding out a simple statement or repeating the same idea in different words. Unless the writer shows how his generalities apply in detail to particular cases, how his conclusions differ from someone else's, or what specifically has led him to his view, the reader remains uninformed and unpersuaded. Underdeveloped paragraphs are among the most common and most irritating weaknesses in student writing. In reading the following student essay, concerned with small groups of freshmen meeting their advisors and having dinner together, notice the thinness of the paragraphs:

> Mr. Miller was not what I had expected of a faculty member. He was not over fifty years old. He was not wearing thick glasses. He was, in contrast, about twenty-six, rather athletic looking, and a very interesting conversationalist, not only in his own field, but in every subject we discussed.

My classmates, most of whom I had not met before, were also a surprise. There were no socially backward introverts, interested only in the physical sciences, as I had feared. I found instead some very interesting people with whom I immediately wanted to become friends. Some were interested in sports, some in hobbies, some in card games, and all in sex. Each individual had something to offer me.

The Millers did a marvelous job of preparing the dinner. We did a marvelous job of eating it. However, the real purpose of the dinner was to become acquainted with at least two of our faculty members and about ten of our fellow students. In this endeavor we were also quite successful, for the discussions begun during the meal lasted for a long time after and as a matter of fact, some of them were continued the next day.

This year's advisor dinner was very rewarding and I believe it should remain a tradition. The students really get to know each other, and a few of the faculty are pleasantly surprised.

13a

A reader might well wonder why the dinner should be continued as a tradition. Nothing the writer says carries real conviction because nothing is developed concretely. These paragraphs raise more questions than they answer: (1) Why should the writer have expected the faculty to resemble his caricature of them as ancient, nearsighted bores? (2) What was Mr. Miller's "field" and what did he talk about as a "very interesting conversationalist"? (3) What "sports," "hobbies," and "card games" was the writer so pleased to discover he shared in common with his classmates? (4) If the meal was so memorable, what was it and how many servings did he have? (5) What was talked about so enthusiastically and "for a long time after" the meal?

The writer has substituted jargon ("very interesting conversationalist," "socially backward introverts"), vague generalities ("some were interested in sports, some in hobbies, some in card games"), and unexplained events (the dinner discussion) for specific detail. The paragraphs are not developed; they merely repeat the same idea unconvincingly—that the advisor's dinner was a good chance to discover that faculty and students were in some vague way "interesting" and "rewarding," not what the writer "had expected."

Concrete diction cuts out fuzziness and gives a paper sharpness and depth. Consider these sentences: "The Millers did a marvelous job of preparing the meal. We did a marvelous job of eating it." Do they mean that the Millers barbecued two dozen hamburgers and tossed a spicy bean salad for a delicious buffet meal on paper plates? Or do they mean that the Millers gave a sit-down dinner, complete with white linen, silver setting, and candlelight, and served roast turkey, hot rolls, and two vegetables? Either of these alternatives is better than the empty generality of the original. A buffet dinner for thirteen people implies a relaxed host and hostess, students going for several helpings, and comfortable informality. A sit-down dinner for thirteen people implies a busy host and hostess, reserved freshmen, hushed requests for the gravy, and long, earnest discussion as the coffee lingers in cups and the candles melt. Whatever the case was, specific wording would help readers see the event and prepare them for the writer's conclusion about it.

To get specific detail by specific wording, writers think in concrete images to recall and re-create the taste, touch, sound, and sight as clearly as possible. In doing do, writers are trying to give the reader as much relevant information as they can. For example, in the following two versions of the same paragraph the student has improved the second by more complete information. Her revision is not much longer than the original but it tells far more. It is the choice of words, not the number of words, that creates an image. The italicized passages indicate the places where she has made her major changes.

Vague original

13a

Though the air was *uncomfortable,* the sand was *soothing* and warm, and I dug a *hole* into it and piled it up *until it half-covered* me from the air. I sat there, shivering in the *air,* until the sand *began falling away* from me. I tried to *bury my legs* again, but the sand *was dry and it would not stay in place.* I tried to find damp sand near me, but in a short time it also dried out and *wouldn't stay in place.* So I rested for *a while* and watched the sea rise and fall and the various objects it threw onto the beach. *Seaweed* and *other things* were washed up, then carried back in a regular rhythm.

Revision for detail

Though the air was *cold,* the sand *felt soft* and warm, and I dug a *damp trough* in it and piled it up around my *legs until I had a body only from the waist up.* I sat there, shivering in the *cool mist,* until the sand began to *crumble* down around me. I tried to *gather it back up* on my legs, but it *had dried* and *kept slithering down again in little shifting rivers. I dug with my hands beside me* until I came to damp sand which I piled on my legs, but in a short time it too *dried and slipped away.* So I rested *my head on my knees* and watched the sea rise and fall and *rise and fall, bringing with it,* to the beach, something new each time: a *loop of rust-colored* seaweed, *a shell, a rock, a small jellyfish. And falling away,* it would *often take with it* what it had *just brought.*

Notice that the writer has done more than make the diction specific. She has developed her paragraph by adding extra detail and slowed down the tempo of the narrative. She has tried to make the reader see and feel what happened.

If your instructor comments that your paragraphs are inadequately developed, you can do several things. First, examine the paragraph or paragraphs carefully for vague generalities, needlessly abstract words, and clichés, and underline them. For instance:

When they are young, children are free and can be themselves. They are protected from nature's hardships by our modern-day society and by our complex technology. They only have to keep out of trouble. Mostly they are free to do whatever they want. But as they get older, they have more and

more <u>duties and responsibilities</u> put upon them. They begin
to <u>lose their freedom and become conformists</u>.

Such phrases as "When they are young" may be changed to "Before they start elementary school"; "free and can be themselves" to "playful, spontaneous, and imaginative"; "protected from nature's hardships" to "protected from hunger, disease, and the weather." Underlining may also reveal that certain generalities, if they mean anything at all, are untrue or need extensive qualification: Do children who bike to school, who roam where they wish afterward, and who spend time in the evenings with their friends really "lose their freedom and become conformists"? Or, to take a very different view, is it true that our "modern-day society" and our "complex technology" "protect" a ghetto child from rats, crime, poverty, sickness, and dilapidated firetraps?

Many undeveloped paragraphs result from a writer's failure to distinguish between fact and opinion. Did the writer of the paragraph about children ever bother to ask what factual basis he had for his opinions? He assumes as self-evident that young children lose their identity and freedom as they grow up. But is it true to say that a child of three or four has a wider range of choices or a more clearly defined individuality than a child of nine or eleven? Clearly, in handling topics of any complexity, writers need to examine their underlying assumptions and to question the external evidence and authority for their views. If they take the time to do this, they are more likely to spot the flaws in their own generalizations and to discover how much more there is to be said.

13a

Another useful device is making a list of the concrete images, details, and examples you want to include. One way is outline form:

I. Drama in Robert Frost's Imagery
  A. Natural Settings
     For example, a boy climbing to top of birch tree
  B. Domestic Settings
     For example, wife crouching on stairs in "Home Burial"

If you find this method too technical, at least jot down the specific items that can illustrate and deepen your generalizations. In the footnotes to the following example, notice how the writer has visualized the concrete details to give the generalizations some real content:

> Working as a door-to-door magazine salesman in and around St. Louis last summer gave me more than just extra spending money. It gave me a chance to meet types of people* I might otherwise never have known, and some practical experience* I am glad I had.

The last two generalizations could stand expansion.

*Young wives of construction workers living in trailers, retired jazz musicians and newsstand operators living in boarding houses, electronic engineers in suburbs.

*How to keep temper when insulted, how to walk through a neighborhood not showing fear, how to size up a person's tastes by the way he keeps lawn or TV show she's watching.

An excellent way to get depth is to practice building up examples that contribute to the dominant idea or impression, the topic sentence. Cutting is usually easy, and you can always thin out in revising. In this next example, notice how the student has marshaled details to sustain a complex comparison and argue a complex thesis.

Sustain development by detail

13b

One section of Golding's *The Inheritors* demonstrates how science fiction can incorporate the materials of ritual. *The journey of Lok's primitive people to their summer home on the cliff is a model of the rite of renewal and contains many of the themes associated with it in religious traditions* [Topic sentence]. Mal, as leader, makes the choice of direction when faced with a fork on the trail, picking the harder but quicker way in order to reach the comfort of the terrace cave sooner. Lok, not concentrating on the path but preoccupied with food, slips and falls when he turns to what he thinks is the smell of the fire the old woman is carrying. Along the trail, the tribe stops and stands in awe of an "ice woman," frozen snow that resembles their mother earth goddess Oa. All these images—the ageless choice between two paths, the stumbling caused by wordly hunger, and yet the knowledge that deity is ever-present—portray components of the ritual passage witnessed for thousands of years, as for example in the Judeo-Christian tradition. Once the people arrive at the terrace, they believe they are protected and safe, like travelers who have passed through the guarded gates. And to complete their journey, they must sanctify their home by rekindling the fire the old woman has carried as coals. The transport and the revival of the hearth fire by Lok's people are just as necessary as the transport of the Ark of the Covenant and the building of an altar were to the Hebrew people as they moved. For Lok and his people believe they have reached their promised land.

13b Lack of coherence

Within every paragraph the sentences should be arranged and linked in such a manner that readers can easily follow the thought. It isn't enough for readers to know what each sentence means; they must also see how each sentence is related to the one that precedes it and how it leads into the one that follows. The connections may be clear enough to the writer but not at all clear to readers. Coherence demands continuity within and between paragraphs. The means of securing coherence are, first, the arrangement of sentences in a logical order and, second, the use of special devices such as the repetition of key words to link sentences. Chapter 7 discusses the various ways to arrange paragraphs to ensure a logical order. Here, we will discuss the use of special devices.

These special devices of achieving coherence include *transitional words, linking pronouns, the repetition of key words,* and *parallel structure.* Usually, experienced writers employ all these means, and they are not much interested in the label attached to the method they use. Instead, they are concerned to achieve coherence accurately and gracefully. But here it will be helpful to discuss separately each technique available to you for improving paragraphs that lack coherence. What happens when the available means are not fully employed can be seen in the following paragraph:

Disjointed

> In Tillie Olsen's story "I Stand Here Ironing," a young woman attempts to love and help her oldest daughter, Emily. The mother's own problems and responsibilities prevent her. The mother was young. Her husband abandoned her. She was forced to work. This separated her from Emily. Emily had to be left with others, and the mother lost touch with her. The mother was able to find a new husband. She was soon forced to concentrate on her other children. Her other daughter, Susan, is the most notable example. Susan became everything Emily was not. Susan was blonde, pretty, quick, and articulate. Emily was dark, slow, and sickly. The mother looks back with guilt. She says, "I was a young mother, I was a distracted mother."

13b

Although it has unity and development, the paragraph generally lacks coherence because the writer too often leaps and jumps erratically from one sentence to the next, as reading aloud will make especially clear. Revised by slight rephrasing and the addition of connecting words, the paragraph becomes easier to follow:

More coherent

> In Tillie Olsen's short story "I Stand Here Ironing," a young woman attempts to love and help her eldest daughter, Emily, *yet her own* problems and responsibilities prevent her from fulfilling *these goals. As a young mother, abandoned by her husband,* she was forced to work, *separating her from her daughter. Forced to leave* Emily with others, the mother lost touch with her. *Although* the mother was able to find a new husband, she was soon forced to concentrate on her other children, *most notably* her other daughter, Susan. Susan became everything Emily was not—blonde, pretty, quick, and articulate. Emily was dark, slow, and sickly. *Looking back in guilt,* the mother says, "I was a young mother, I was a distracted mother."

In the revised passage, the writer is no longer thinking in single sentences only. Instead, he has looked for the continuity among his ideas and for the most accurate means of showing this continuity in each case.

Transitional words and phrases serve to indicate different relationships. Here is a list of relationships and appropriate transitional words:

1. Result or consequence: *hence, consequently, as a result, therefore.*
2. Comparison or contrast: *similarly, likewise, however, on the other hand, yet, still, nevertheless.*

3. Example or illustrations: *as an illustration, for example, specifically, for instance.*
4. Additional aspects or evidence: *moreover, furthermore, also, too, next, besides, in the second place.*
5. Conclusion or summary: *in conclusion, to sum up, to conclude, in short.*

Notice the careful use of transitional words in the following passage:

Relationships indicated

13b

Past and future are two time regions which we commonly separate by a third which we call the present. *But* strictly speaking, the present does not exist, *or* is at best no more than an infinitesimal point in time, gone before we can note it as present. *Nevertheless* we must have a present; *and so* we get one by robbing the past, by holding on to the most recent events and pretending that they all belong to our immediate perceptions. If, *for example,* I raise my arm, the total event is a series of occurrences of which the first are past before the last two have taken place; *yet* I perceive it as a single movement executed in one instant of time.

—Carl Becker

Sentences also may be connected by pronouns that have clear antecedents. This technique is an effective way of avoiding needless repetition. Notice in the following example how Henry James substitutes "it" for "symbolism" and later for "this suggestion," and how he uses the phrase "this suggestion" to point back to the entire preceding sentence.

Linking pronouns

In *The Scarlet Letter* there is a great deal of symbolism; there is, I think, too much. *It* is overdone at times, and becomes mechanical; *it* ceases to be impressive, and grazes triviality. The idea of the mystic *A* which the young minister finds imprinted upon his breast and eating into his flesh, in sympathy with the embroidered badge that Hester is condemned to wear, appears to me to be a case in point. *This suggestion* should, I think, have just been made and dropped; to insist upon *it,* and return to *it,* is to exaggerate the weak side of the subject. Hawthorne returns to *it* constantly, plays with *it,* and seems charmed by *it;* until at last the reader feels tempted to declare that his enjoyment of *it* is puerile.

—Henry James

Paragraph coherence is also maintained by the repetition of key words that are related to a central idea. In the following passage, notice the key words *darkness, deep sea,* and *blackness* and the words related to them by contrast such as *sunlight, red rays,* and *surface:*

Key words repeated

Immense pressure, then, is one of the governing conditions of life in the *deep sea; darkness* is another. The unrelieved *darkness* of the *deep waters* has produced weird and incredible modifications of the *abyssal* fauna. It is a *blackness* so divorced from the world of the *sunlight* that probably only the few men who have seen it with their own *eyes* can visualize it. We know that *light fades out rapidly with descent below the surface*. The *red rays* are gone at the end of the first 200 or 300 feet, and with them all the *orange and yellow warmth of the sun*. Then the *greens* fade out, and at 1,000 feet only a *deep, dark, brilliant blue* is left. In *very clear waters* the *violet rays* of the spectrum may penetrate another thousand feet. Beyond this is only the *blackness* of the *deep sea*.

—Rachel Carson

Continuity can also be sustained by parallel structure, which calls attention to similar ideas. This coordination of equally important ideas is often useful with introductory or summary paragraphs, although its use is by no means confined to such paragraphs. In the following example, the first paragraph is taken from the beginning of a chapter, the second from near its conclusion.

13b

Parallel structure

To "become a pueblo" *meant to adopt* many of the ways and political forms and ambitions of townspeople. *It meant to accept* the tools, leadership, and conceptions of progress which were then being offered to the villagers of Yucatan by the leaders of Mexico's social revolution. *It required* the inhabitants *to give up* some of the isolation which was theirs in the remote and sparsely inhabited lands that lay apart from the goings and comings of city men. In future they would be a part of the political and economic institutions of Yucatan, of Mexico, and—though of course they would not have put it so—of the one world that was then in the making.

• • •

Chan Kom had attained its loftiest political objective. *It had become* the head of its own municipality. *It had made* itself into a pueblo, a community of dwellers—some of them—in masonry houses. *It had* a municipal building, with a stone jail; a school building, also of masonry; a masonry church—and a masonry Protestant chapel. *It had* two gristmills and four stores. *It had* two outdoor theatres and a baseball diamond.

—Robert Redfield

Notice how the parallel structure in the first three sentences of the second paragraph restate what it meant for Chan Kom to achieve its "loftiest political objective." Notice how the parallel structure in the last three sentences of the second paragraph lists equally important features in a "community of dwellers." And notice how the parallel structure of the second paragraph harks back to the parallel structure of the first paragraph—from what Chan Kom "had attained" back to what "it required" to become a pueblo.

The main devices for providing coherence among paragraphs are the same as those for providing coherence within a paragraph—transitional words, linking pronouns, key words repeated, and parallel structure. Probably more important than any of these devices is the *arrangement* of the material so that a paragraph begins with some reference to the idea that has come before, or ends with some reference to the idea that is to be taken up next. In the following example, taken from an essay by Ursula K. Le Guin, notice how continuity is sustained by the theme of "the open universe," "that huge and drafty house."

Continuity by arrangement of material and focused thesis

If science fiction has a major gift to offer literature, I think it is just this: the capacity to face an open universe. Physically open, psychically open. No doors shut.

What science, from physics and astronomy to history and psychology, has given us is the open universe: a cosmos that is not a simple, fixed hierarchy, but an immensely complex process in time. All the doors stand open, from the prehuman past through the incredible present to the terrible and hopeful future. All connections are possible. All alternatives are thinkable. It is not a comfortable, reassuring place. It's a very large house, a very drafty house. But it's the house we live in.

And science fiction seems to be the modern literary art which is capable of living in that huge and drafty house, and feeling at home there, and playing games up and down the stairs, from basement to attic.

I think that's why kids like SF, and demand to be taught it, to study it, to take it seriously. They feel this potential it has for playing games with and making sense and beauty out of our fearfully enlarged world of knowledge and perception. And that's why it gripes me when I see SF failing to do so, falling back on silly, simplistic reassurances, or whining Woe, woe, repent, or taking refuge in mere wishful thinking.

So I welcome the study and teaching of SF—so long as the teachers will criticize us, demandingly, responsibly, and make the students read us demandingly, responsibly. If SF is treated, not as junk, not as escapism, but as an intellectually, aesthetically, and ethically responsible art, a great form, it will become so: it will fulfill its promise. The door to the future will be open.

—Ursula K. Le Guin

Revision checklist for paragraphs

1. Is the main idea of each paragraph clearly stated or implied?
2. Does each paragraph have enough details and examples to support or develop the main idea adequately?
3. Does each paragraph have a clear, logical order and the necessary connections for coherence?

Exercise 1

This exercise is for practice in working with concrete detail and diction.

1. List as many details as you can for describing one of the following subjects. Then write two paragraphs about the subject, the first as complete as you can make it, the second edited to include only the most relevant details.

A cat stalking a moth or grasshopper

A crowded airport terminal

Runners in a marathon

A college party

An audience at the late showing of a horror film

2. Plan a tentative outline for an upcoming paper and list as many concrete examples or details as you can for each major idea or stage in the analysis. Write a rough draft using all of your evidence. Then study your rough draft with the following questions in mind: Do all the examples and details warrant inclusion? If some are more effective than others, why are they? Do some of the examples or details bring others to mind that you had not included? If so, is any of the new material more effective than your original evidence? How or why?

Exercise 2

This exercise is for practice in improving paragraph coherence.

1. Analyze the paragraphs of a recent paper you have written to determine what specific devices you have used most frequently for coherence. If you still have the rough draft, compare it with the final version. What changes, if any, did you make to improve coherence? If you made changes, were they to improve the order used (for example, making time sequence clearer), to supply more specific links, or to sharpen up the thrust of the whole argument? Or were they a combination of these?

2. Exchange rough drafts for an assigned paper with a classmate and go over each other's work for paragraph coherence. Mark every passage that lacks coherence and suggest revisions. Then discuss these proposed changes. Which do you find helpful? Why? Which do you reject? Why?

Exercise 3

This exercise is for practice in improving paragraph development and coherence.

1. Pick a topic below and write *one* paragraph on it as rapidly as you can for about twenty minutes. Then revise the paragraph by adding, expanding upon, or trimming detail as needed, and by using whatever devices you decide will improve coherence. If you find that you need more than one paragraph in revising, make the necessary transitions and division(s).

A case for or against banning smoking in public places

A case for or against an import quota on foreign cars

A film or book you especially liked or disliked

A singer or musical group you especially like or dislike

A person you are glad you met, or wish you had not

A place you would like to return to or never visit again

A skill you wish you had learned or don't care to learn

2. Revise the revision you produced above. Then compare all three revisions and answer the following questions: What are the most noticeable improvements in paragraph development and coherence, especially between the first and third drafts? While writing the revisions, did you change your mind or modify your views? Is the last version the best you can do? Or would still another revision improve the detail and coherence?

13b

14 *Revising Sentences*

If paragraphs are the timber for building papers, then by analogy sentences are the kinds of wood chosen for the paragraph. Each kind of wood has its own texture, color, and strength; some are harder to work with than others; some are more likely to warp than others. Pine is soft, common, cheap, and serviceable, rather like the ordinary sentence using the verb "to be." Maple is hard, close-grained, and highly finished, like the complex sentence with parallel elements. Most oak is heavy, durable, and strong, like the long, formal periodic sentence. Each kind has its own qualities and advantages. Problems occur, however, when one uses unseasoned or wet wood or oversized nails, or when one tries to cut against the grain. The flooring buckles or cracks; the board splits or splinters. So, too, with sentences—unseasoned or handled wrongly, they can warp or fracture.

To put this in other terms, sentences are often crudely shaped during the preliminary stages of writing. Trying to maintain the creative flow of ideas, we slap down the words as they come. Fragments and fused sentences, mixed constructions and faulty parallelism—these may be the rough materials that confront us when we begin revising. And because revising entails rethinking, the job is challenging. For rethinking demands that we examine each statement to see if it says exactly what we want it to say. Few sentences will survive this scrutiny intact. Testing what we think, we grope for words and stumble over structures, but in rethinking we cross out and rearrange, shift parts, polish and hone to make each sentence coherent, concise, and unified.

Revising sentences entails more than repairing them for coherence and conciseness, however. Because different words—like different woods—have their particular textures, colorings, and associations, writers usually have to revise their diction. For sentences may be clear and concise yet still alienate the reader through their inappropriate tone, inflated phrasing, or unfortunate connotations. Consider three examples from college papers:

Inappropriate tone   The last novel we had to read made me vomit; it was disgusting. Only a sick person could finish it without throwing up. It was pure garbage!
[The sentences are certainly clear, but the writer's vehemence, however sincere, leaves no room for discussion or honest differences of opinion.]

Inflated phrasing   Cultural and socioeconomic variables are important
factors in determining taste.
[Through jargon, the sentence puffs up a simple idea—that
background influences taste.]

Inappropriate connotations   Many of us appreciate the freedom college gives.
Even as freshmen, we are making choices that we
never had to make before. But some kids abuse this
freedom.
[Given the writer's intent and context—gratitude for being
treated as an adult—the word *kids* demeans all students, not
just those students who can't handle this freedom.]

As these examples suggest, your choice of individual words crucially affects
the statement as a whole. Because these relationships are complex, we have
necessarily and somewhat arbitrarily divided our discussion into two chapters.
The first chapter, this one, stresses ways that you can revise *structures* that are
awkward, confusing, or misleading. The second chapter, "Revising Diction,"
stresses ways you can revise to *name* more concretely and felicitously. But our
division is for convenience only: the effective strategy for all rewriting takes all
elements of the sentence into account. We begin with sentence unity.

14a

14a Sentence unity

A well-organized sentence makes a main point and produces a single
effect. It can contain many details if their subordinate relationship to the major
idea is made clear by the grammatical structure. Here are the details that a good
writer gathered into one clear and efficient sentence:

> The barber's pole originally represented an arm or leg wrapped in bandages. Barbers
> were also the surgeons in those days. The jars of colored water in a chemist's shop
> represented the medicines and elixirs offered for sale. Three gold balls are the
> traditional sign of a pawnbroker. They originally indicated the shop of a banker or
> moneylender. Most villagers in those days could not read. The signs indicated where
> these essential services could be found.

Here is the final product:

> The barber's pole (originally intended as a limb swathed in bandages), the chemist's
> coloured jars, the banker's three gilt balls, were marks of identification for those (and
> they were most of the village) who could not read.
>
> —Louis Kronenberger

A sentence is not a container designed to hold all the available information on a
subject, although some sentences read as if their authors had that impression:

> The earliest known examples of sculpture date from the Old Stone Age, which was
> more than 20,000 years before the time of Christ and is sometimes called the
> Paleolithic Period, making sculpture one of the oldest arts known to man, many

pieces of ancient sculpture having been found in caves or old burial grounds in various parts of the world.

The main point of this sentence seems to be the great antiquity of the art of sculpture. The following revised sentence stresses that idea and subordinates or eliminates all other details:

Improved   Sculpture is one of the oldest arts known to man: the earliest examples, found in caves or burial grounds, go back to the Old Stone Age, more than 20,000 years ago.

It is easy to lose sight of the main point in first-draft sentences and to allow unrelated ideas to intrude. Unified writing requires the cutting of everything that does not contribute to the central point.

14a

Disunified   Inexpensive word processors, which first became available to the public in the 1970s and which, like other technological innovations such as television and computer chips are part of what sociologists call the "post-industrial revolution," have made a real dent in the manual and electric typewriter market, which includes secretaries, students, and teachers, among others.

The period when inexpensive word processors first became available may or may not be related to their popularity; in any case the idea belongs in another sentence. So also does the information about computer chips, sociologists, and the "post-industrial revolution"; while interesting, it is not immediately relevant to the main idea—the increased sales of word processors. The clause about students and secretaries is merely an afterthought. Revised for unity, the sentence makes a simple and direct point.

Unified   Inexpensive word processors have made a real dent in the manual and electric typewriter market.

A sentence should relate to the thought it expresses as a map does to the terrain it describes. Often in unsuccessful sentences the relationship between two ideas is obscured or only implied by the structure. The reader of such a sentence fails to see connections and gets lost, much as the reader of a faulty map does.

Obscure   Being from Honolulu, I am not used to putting on a parka and putting up an umbrella the minute it starts raining.

The sentence suggests the interesting if unintended generalization that all people living in Honolulu are averse to parkas and umbrellas, which would be difficult, even pointless to prove. The writer has omitted a logical step in the cause-and-effect relationship, which the rewritten version includes:

Clear   Since I come from Honolulu, where the rains are warm and refreshing, I am not used to putting on a parka and putting up an umbrella the minute it starts raining.

A writer can also assume connections that the sentence should make explicit:

> **Obscure**   Maturing faster because of parents' divorcing does not hold true in all cases, and a child may become timid and insecure.

The causal relationship between a child's shock at divorce and his or her emotional maturity needs to be clearly stated:

> **Clear**   The shock of a divorce may contribute to the maturity of a child or retard that maturity by making the child timid and insecure.

1. Excessive detail

Some sentences are very long, some short, some of moderate length. A sentence should be constructed to hold compactly what it has to say in as many words as it needs to say it.

> When the cry for women's suffrage was first heard, there was immediate opposition to it, which continued for a long time until men finally began to realize that women were entitled to the vote, and in 1920 the Nineteenth Amendment was ratified.

This sentence tries to say too much. It should be broken down into at least two sentences.

> When the cry for woman's suffrage was first heard there was immediate opposition to it, and this opposition continued for a long time. Gradually, however, men realized that women were entitled to the vote, and in 1920 the Nineteenth Amendment was ratified.

2. Primer sentences

Earlier we described the habitual use of simple, declarative sentences as "primer style." The term is derived from the primer books that taught us how to read in the early grades. Most of us can still chant by heart, "See Dick throw the stick to Spot. Spot is chasing the stick. Run, Spot, run!" Seldom do such naive patterns turn up in college writing, but some apprentice writers have the tendency to rely on short, uncomplicated sentences that put every detail and idea in a main clause. But all ideas and facts are not of equal weight, and the structures we choose should reflect this disparity. Less important elements should be put into subordinate constructions—dependent clauses, participial phrases, or appositives. Ideas of equal importance should be put into coordinate constructions.

3. Coordination and subordination

The prefixes of these two important grammatical terms explain the different sort of ordering each construction provides: *co* (with) and *sub* (under) *ordinare* (to arrange in order). Coordinate arrangements express equality, sameness, or balance by means of the coordinating conjunctions, *and, but, or, for, yet, nor.* Subordinate arrangements express inequality among sentence parts and rank these parts in relation to each other by means of such subordinating conjunctions as *since, when, unless, because, while.* The term subordination also refers to all those sentence elements—phrases, clauses—which modify by tucking into the sentence additional, elaborating information.

Many sentences deftly combine coordination and subordination.

> There seems something else in life besides time, something which may conveniently be called "value," something which is measured not by minutes or hours, but by intensity, so that when we look at our past it does not stretch back evenly but piles up into a few notable pinnacles, and when we look at the future it seems sometimes a wall, sometimes a cloud, sometimes a sun, but never a chronological chart.
>
> —E. M. Forster

Within the frame of this complex sentence, the writer has placed a number of coordinate or balanced elements.

14a

> There seems
>> something else in life besides time,
>> something which may conveniently be called "value,"
>> something which is measured
>>> not by minutes or hours,
>>> but by intensity,
>> so that when we look at our past
>>> it does not stretch back evenly
>>> but piles up into a few notable pinnacles,
>> and when we look at the future
>>> it seems sometimes a wall,
>>>> sometimes a cloud,
>>>> sometimes a sun,
>>>>> but never a chronological chart.

Readers feel a sense of balance when they read such a sentence and (better still for the writer) the inclination to agree with it. (See Chapter **10** for a complete discussion of parallel structure.)

4. Faulty coordination and subordination

The more a writer practices, the more the habits of coordination and, especially, subordination become easy, even automatic. There are, however, hazards along the way to finding the best arrangement in words for our thoughts. The coordinate or subordinate constructions we select must be suitable to the ideas they are expressing. If not, the reader will sense a discrepancy between the subject of the sentence and its form. We must be careful not to coordinate elements that are not equal to each other, thus leaving the reader with a false sense of parity between ideas.

> **Faulty** In English courses we had to learn many rules of grammar, and few of these rules are taken seriously today.

The writer of this sentence is hedging on the important question of what these two ideas have to do with one another. One or the other deserves more emphasis, which can be shown through subordination.

Correct In English courses we had to learn many rules of grammar, few of which are taken seriously today.

Correct Few of the many rules that we had to learn in English courses are taken seriously today.

Each of these sentences subordinates in a different direction, but each avoids the mistake of the first sentence, which implied, with the coordinator *and,* that the ideas are balanced. Equally distracting is the sentence that ranks its main idea in a subordinate position as a dependent clause or a modifying phrase.

Faulty Ruth Benedict is the author of *Patterns of Culture,* in which she praises the Zuni Indians for their ceremonial life and its cooperative attitude toward the natural world.

14a

That Benedict wrote a book, *Patterns of Culture,* is clearly not the main idea of this sentence, but the predication of the independent clause implies as much. What she does in the book is the important idea of the statement, and the sentence should be phrased to reveal that.

Correct In her *Patterns of Culture* Ruth Benedict praises the Zuni Indians for their ceremonial life and its cooperative attitude toward the natural world.

The title of the book is subordinated in the introductory phrase to the important asssertion, which is that Benedict praises a certain manner of life.

The context finally determines which ideas are important and which are secondary. A personal journal might well subordinate otherwise significant facts to the experience of the writer.

> I read recently that Erik Erikson, a major thinker about the life cycle, considers adolescence the stage in which "the promise of finding oneself and the threat of losing oneself" are most closely allied. His discussion of youth, that crucial period when one is torn between intense fidelity and angry rejection, reminded me of my own adolescent moments of great elation and confidence and of total rebellion and hostility, when I was such a trial to my family.
>
> —Personal Journal

A more formal analysis of Erikson's ideas, of his views about adolescence, would require the subordination of personal experience to a summary of his argument.

> Erik Erikson, a major thinker about the life cycle, considers adolescence the stage in which "the promise of finding oneself and the threat of losing oneself" are most closely allied. His discussion of youth, which reminded me of my own, stresses it as a crucial period when one is torn between intense fidelity and angry hostility.

The initial phrasing of a statement may bury the real subject in a subordinate part of the sentence. After discovering in the first or second draft the purpose and thrust of your essay, go over each sentence to see if the real subject is the grammatical subject.

> We can readily see how fame was achieved by Chief Joseph of the Nez Perce Indians whose famous surrender statement—"I will fight no more forever"—proves that language does not have to be grammatical to be eloquent.

The independent clause that begins this sentence is simply a windy windup to what the writer finally manages to say in the last subordinate clauses. The sentence should begin where it ends.

> The famous statement by Chief Joseph of the Nez Perce Indians—"I will fight no more forever"—proves that language does not have to be grammatical to be eloquent.

14a

Exercise 1

Revise the following sentences by putting the main ideas in main clauses and less important ideas in subordinate clauses. Be prepared to explain why you have chosen certain ideas as the main ones and to explain the form of subordination you have used.

1. An especially big wave rolled in, when I finally managed to get my line unsnagged.
2. The ocean was choppy, causing the fishermen to have little luck and to return to the pier disappointed.
3. The population of Latin America, ranging from Indians who live as their ancestors did hundreds of years ago to highly educated women and men in the modern cities such as Buenos Aires and Rio de Janeiro, is varied.
4. He was trying to kill a bee inside the car, driving off the road as a result.
5. Contact lenses are worn next to the eyeballs and have advantages over ordinary glasses, since contact lenses are invisible, are kept unfrosted by the eyelids, and correct faulty corneas.
6. The horse came to the first jump, where he stumbled and threw Janet off.

Exercise 2

Revise the following sentences by subordinating the less important ideas. Be prepared to explain the choices you make and the form of subordination you have used.

1. The potter must roll the clay out on a flat surface, and a surface that the clay will not stick to.
2. Five hundred citizens were too many to meet at one time, and so instead the Council was divided into the ten smaller groups.
3. The job was interesting, and the pay was good, but finally I decided not to accept it and I regretted my decision later.
4. Gertrude Stein and Hemingway are contemporaries, and Stein was one of the first to recognize Hemingway's genius as a writer.
5. Scientists are continually developing new photographic equipment, and now they have devised ways of photographing planets as far away as Saturn by rockets that relay the pictures back to Earth.
6. I got the note from my parents, and I gave it to my teacher, but he just scowled at me, but finally he said I could take the afternoon off.

Exercise 3

Revise the following sentences by eliminating the excessive subordination.

1. In 1666 when he sent a beam of white light through a glass prism which broke the beam up into bands of colored lights which resembled a rainbow, Isaac Newton showed that what we normally think of as white light is actually made up of light that consists of different colors, a discovery that revolutionized the science of optics, which was in its infancy before Newton.
2. When I bought my parrot from the pet store on the Mall, where I had visited several times and spent hours gazing at the cages because I so badly wanted a bird of my own, I was so excited that I could hardly contain myself as I rushed home to begin training him from the booklet which I had also bought at the store.
3. At the beginning of the story, which takes place in Sicily at some unknown time in the past, Verga makes us realize that the main character is called "La Lupa," which means the wolf, because the villagers are superstitious people who believe in the devil and other evil forces that can take human form.
4. When the gymnasts who had been practicing for weeks and who were in excellent condition were ready to enter the gym which was filled with people who were shivering in the unheated room were finally called in, the excitement grew because of the the long wait that everyone had endured while they were waiting in the cold.

14a

Exercise 4

Revise the following sentences to improve their unity. Be prepared to explain the changes you have made.

1. I usually enjoyed an appointment with my dentist, and she would make me feel good because she complimented me on my teeth.
2. The swimming pool was intended for college students only, but is now open to townspeople as well.
3. The train was late, causing me to miss my appointment and lose the client.
4. The picture that won first prize was in water color. It was an abstract painting. Most people criticized it, but the judges liked it.
5. The first book I consulted lacked an index, and next I tried an almanac.
6. The Greek word *papyros* originally meant thin sheet of paper made from a certain Egyptian reed, from which we have borrowed our modern word *paper* and which now means any kind of writing material.
7. The United Nations, which was founded in San Francisco more than forty years ago when many of the major diplomats of the world were there, has increased greatly in size, many of the new members being the small nations which have recently gained their independence.
8. Freud grew up in Vienna, doing some of his most creative psychoanalytic research in that city.
9. There were about ten women out for field hockey, and we only had four weeks before our first match, so we worked very hard to get in condition, but three of our best players caught the flu and so we didn't do well against our opponents.
10. The match burned his fingers. He tried to light his pipe in the wind, and he dropped it on the ground when he burned himself.

14b Concise sentences

Waste in writing, as in anything else, dilutes and weakens. A sentence that spills more words on the page than its sense justifies pollutes a reading environment that is already littered. There is a difference, of course, between brevity and conciseness. Brevity is not always a virtue; conciseness always is. Any statement can be made brief by omitting detail, but details are often essential and must be included. Concise writing states the necessary details without wasting words.

Brief   The market dropped.

Concise   The stock market fell fifteen points today, the sharpest decline in seven years.

Wordy   By the time trading stopped on Wall Street, the stock market had fallen down fifteen points, which was significant because it was the sharpest decline since a similar drop seven years ago.

Wordy constructions flourish in free-writing and in first drafts as we find out what we want to say and the most efficient means of saying it. No harm is done if we can recognize what is deadwood and ruthlessly cut it away. Phrases used in casual speech as fillers between thoughts are as unconscious as clearing one's throat, but, like the distracting noises made during a recording, they should be erased in editing. Here are some common examples of deadwood and the ways to prune them:

Deadwood	Revision
proceeded to show	showed
the field (or *area*) *of* engineering	engineering
a person by the name of Anita Wildman	someone named Anita Wildman *or* Anita Wildman
at this point in time	now
in order to prove	to prove
due to the fact that	because
because *of the fact that*	because
for *the purpose of*	for
on the occasion when	when
was of the belief (or *opinion*) *that*	believed
in the event that	if
in a great many cases	often
during the period when	when or while
to *have the ability* to	to be able to

Answering a young man's question about how to become a good stylist, the

English writer Sydney Smith once said, "You should cross out every other word. You have no idea what vigor it will give your style." The advice, though exaggerated, makes a fine point. Notice how the deadwood in the following passage blocks the reader's way:

> Because *of the fact that* I wanted to major in *the field of* business I *proceeded to* take several courses in *the area of* accounting in *the period of* my sophomore year. *During the time* when I was a junior, I *was* still *of the belief* that business was my best choice for *the purpose of* making a living.

Imagine having to read such stuff, page after page. Revised, the sentences become ordinary but tolerable:

> Because I wanted to major in business, I took several accounting courses in my sophomore year. While a junior, I still believed that business was my best choice for making a living.

14b

1. Redundant phrases and clauses

The word **redundancy** means "overflowing"; words that carelessly repeat what has already been said are redundant. Readers are seldom misled by such writing, but they are certainly bored and irked by it.

Wordy	When the poet writes in his poem that the character was never "odd in his views," he means to imply that the man was a conformist, accepting the standards of his society in all aspects.
Concise	When the poet writes that the character was never "odd in his views," he implies that the man was a conformist.

Much redundant phrasing results from spelling out the meaning of a word that can and should stand alone. "Conformist" means "accepting the standards of society."

Wordy	Over the years, she became suspicious that she was being exploited *by people who wanted to take advantage of her and use her.*
Wordy	The criticisms I will make are major ones *which ought to be given careful consideration because of their importance.*
Wordy	We like to be appreciated and admired for our talents *which we possess* and we hope to be praised for our achievements *that we have attained as individuals.*

In the last sentence the writer wasted nine words defining the pronoun "our." Some other redundant phrases include:

attractive *in appearance*	refer *back to*	small (or large) *in size*
connected *up together*	repeat *again*	tall (or short) *in height*
cooperate *together*	rectangular (or	young *in age*
perplexing *in nature*	square) *in shape*	
red *in color*	several *in number*	

2. Unnecessary repetition

Repetition is not necessarily a flaw in writing. In fact, as you have seen in the discussion of parallel structure, writing that gracefully repeats phrases and words pleases the ear and reminds the reader of what is being said. However, unnecessary repetition sounds awkward and looks cumbersome.

Wordy   The question *of* who is to be considered needy is *a* hard *question* to answer.

Concise   The question who is to be considered needy is hard to answer.

Wordy   If one examines the *story* carefully, *one* will find that the hidden symbolism in the *story* makes the *story* stand for something more than *one* first found in the *story*.

Concise   If one reads the story carefully, one will discover a symbolism that deepens it.

The rewritten sentences are leaner, stronger, more muscular; in concise prose, as in a well-trained body, every part is in prime working condition.

3. Overuse of the passive voice

Most of the time we speak and write in the active voice.

She wrote the book.

He read and reviewed the book.

The critics praised it.

A verb is in the **active voice** when the grammatical subject of the sentence is the one who does the action of the predicate. *Who* wrote the book? (*she* did); who read and reviewed it? (*he* did). Occasionally, we want to emphasize that which is acted upon, so we place the complement in the subject position:

Her book was nominated for the Pulitzer Prize.

Only exceptional books are chosen.

In these sentences the doer of the action—nominating, choosing—is unknown or irrelevant to the statement being made. To write *A jury nominated her book for the Pulitzer Prize* is to place undue emphasis upon an anonymous group of people to the detriment of *her book,* which the sense of the sentence seems to insist is more important and, therefore, should occupy the important subject position. The thrust of the statement, of course, could make *jury* of more interest than *her book: A hastily selected jury, which later was accused of favoritism, nominated her book for the Pulitzer Prize.* Here the sense of the sentence puts the emphasis firmly on *jury,* so it is in the subject position and the verb is in the active voice. Note that in the subordinate clause (*which . . . favoritism*), where the fact that the committee was charged is more consequential than who made the charge, the verb is in the **passive voice.**

14b

There is no right or wrong use of the passive or the active voice. The conventions of scientific and technical writing dictate frequent use of the passive voice, since it is the experiment and not the performer of the experiment that is significant:

> A cubic centimeter of water was added to the solution, and the test tube was heated. The experiment was conducted under adverse conditions, and the results were considered worthless.

But in most writing the doer of the action is important, and the sentence should declare who she or he is. Because passive constructions are formed by the past participle and a form of the verb *to be,* the predicate is more wordy than a predicate in the active voice. The performer of the action must be mentioned in a prepositional phrase—*by me, by the committee*—which also adds to the number of words in the sentence. Overuse of the passive voice can lead to wordy, flabby assertions:

14b

> **Weak**   Classics like *Middlemarch* will always be appreciated by readers.
>
> **Weak**   The question "Who ever reads an American book?" was asked by an English critic in the nineteenth century.

Translated into the active voice, these sentences are concise and forceful:

> **Strong**   Readers will always appreciate classics like *Middlemarch.*
>
> **Strong**   "Who ever reads an American book?" an English critic asked in the nineteenth century.

Overuse of the passive voice often leads to a false subject, which can make the sentence confusing as well as wordy.

> **Confusing**   The changes that *had been made* in the conservation bill by the Committee *were accepted* by the Senate, which voted to pass the bill.

One can hardly tell what happened here. Who did what? The real subject is *the Senate;* what it did was to pass a bill, and the sentence should be written accordingly.

> **Clear**   The Senate passed the conservation bill as amended in committee.

A good style is a blend of the active and passive voices, with the active voice predominating. Be alert during revisions for the inadvertent, vague passive— the voice that is shirking the responsibility of judging and making, often on the basis of little evidence, some rather grand assumptions. *It has been decided that, it is known, agreement has been reached, it was thought* are constructions that should be challenged with the question, *by whom?* The introduction of the agent of the action into the sentence may result in sharper thinking and more exact phrasing:

> **Vague**   It was thought that the world's natural resources were inexhaustible.
>
> **Clear**   Only a handful of the relatively few people who considered the question thought that the world's natural resources were inexhaustible.

4. *There is* and *It is* constructions

Beginning a sentence with *There is . . .* or *It is . . .* is a common idiomatic construction.

Correct There is no reason to doubt his honesty.
[*There* is an introductory word; the grammatical subject is *reason.*]

Correct It is true that he had been drinking at the time.
[In this idiomatic construction, *it* anticipates the actual grammatical subject, the clause *that he had been drinking.* The writer uses this construction to imply that a concession is being made.]

Used unnecessarily or simply as a means of filling up the page, however, this idiom can lead to awkward, weak, and repetitious sentences.

14b

Weak It was to no avail that I made an effort.

Weak It was in the year 1927 that Virginia Woolf's novel *To the Lighthouse* was published

Weak There are a large number of readers who consider this her finest work.

Emphasizing the subject of the sentence results in these brisk versions:

Strong My effort was useless

Strong In 1927 Virginia Woolf's novel *To the Lighthouse* was published.

Strong Many readers consider this her finest work.

Exercise 5

One way to alert yourself to wordy sentences is to write them deliberately. For each sentence in the following exercises, give yourself 5 points if you succeed in making it wordier without adding anything to the meaning. Perfect score 100.

1. Pad out each of the following sentences by using the passive.
    a. The women's volleyball team won all of its home games last season.
    b. Lock all doors and leave the keys at the desk.
    c. The Valley String Quartet decided to hold extra rehearsals during the week and agreed to postpone other activities.
    d. He cut the wood with his ax.
    e. Some college students choose medicine as a career as early as the beginning of their sophomore year.
2. Pad out each of the following sentences by adding dead phrases or clauses.
    a. Many writers dislike personal publicity because the lionizing keeps them from their work.
    b. The apartment rooms were small, boxlike, and painted in a hideous green.
    c. The City Council agreed to work with the Board of Education to determine the principles for zoning schools and homes.

   d. In 1960, Kennedy won by a very small plurality.
   e. Sometimes I study from 8 P.M. to 2 A.M.
3. Pad out each of the following sentences by using the verb *to be* and a clumsy complement to replace the precise verb.
   a. I like musical comedies and I collect record albums of them.
   b. David Riesman, author of *The Lonely Crowd,* thinks many Americans lack a firm sense of individuality.
   c. Ms. Spaulder lives in Cincinnati but teaches in the suburbs.
   d. Distance bicycling requires stamina and ten gears.
   e. He has given up cigarettes and now he feels better.
4. Pad out each of the following sentences by expanding the modifiers into phrases and clauses.
   a. A *mano* is a hand stone for grinding corn in a large hollowed stone metate.
   b. A biographer lacks the artistic freedom of a novelist because the biographer cannot invent her characters or move them about as she pleases.
   c. Since Paul was tired when he took the Civil Service examination, he missed several easy questions and did poorly on familiar topics.
   d. A number of educational theories and practices still regarded as dangerously "modern" and "progressive" date back to Rousseau.
   e. If my mother, born in the Kentucky backwoods, had stayed there and spoken only with her childhood friends, she would never have had to change her speech habits; only when she moved north and began associating with teachers and business people did she realize how much people scorned her grammar and pronunciation.

14b

Exercise 6

Reduce the wordiness in the following sentences. Be prepared to explain your changes.

1. It is my intention to be affiliated with some large automobile manufacturer in connection with sales of cars and accessories.
2. There are all too many instances of condemnation of a person by other human beings before "sufficient knowledge" has been found.
3. I was especially interested in going to the University of Southern California because of the fact that it was near home.
4. Respect is the individual's personal ability to be aware of another person's unique individuality.
5. Owing to the fact that quick action was taken by this employer, a major crisis was averted.
6. He is often thought to have a lack of responsibility; hence, he is not trusted to any great extent by those who know him.
7. I am now very sorry that I didn't find reading a meaningful and worthwhile experience when I was younger.
8. The reason that Lincoln kept in close contact with his generals by writing them letters was that he felt that he was responsible as commander-in-chief for the running of the war.

14c Pronoun reference

A pronoun is a substitute for a noun. The noun it stands for is called the **antecedent** because it usually goes (*cedere*) before (*ante*) the pronoun.

  antecedent   pronoun

Rita Martinez lives in Boulder, but *she* has relatives in San Diego.

    antecedent   pronoun

When the *plane* left O'Hare, *it* was already behind schedule.

Note, though, that the antecedent—despite its literal meaning—may *follow* the pronoun in some constructions.

  pronoun   antecedent

Although *it* was behind schedule, the *plane* finally took off.

As you read over your sentences with an eye to revising them, examine every pronoun to make sure its antecedent is clear.

1. Ambiguous reference

When persons of the same sex are mentioned in the sentence, confusion may occur about which person the pronoun refers to:

Unclear The novelist Virginia Woolf assured her sister Vanessa, who was a painter, that *she* was a great artist.
[We cannot be sure whether Woolf was assuring her sister that she (Woolf) or Vanessa was a great artist.]

Correct The novelist Virginia Woolf told her sister Vanessa, who was a painter, "You are a great artist."

Do not use a pronoun in such a way that it might refer to either of two antecedents. If there is any possiblity of doubt, revise the sentence to remove the ambiguity.

Unclear In *Nostromo* Conrad's style is ironic and his setting is highly symbolic, so that *it* sometimes confuses the reader.
[Does *it* refer loosley to *Nostromo*, Conrad's style, his setting, or to a combination of these? Banishing the pronoun from the sentence, the writer is forced to say exactly what he means.]

Correct Conrad's ironic style and highly symbolic setting in *Nostromo* sometimes confuse the reader.

Correct In *Nostromo*, Conrad's style is ironic, and his highly symbolic setting sometimes confuses the reader.

Each of the sentences is now clear and each is saying something different from the other.

2. Remote reference

A pronoun too far away from its antecedent may cause misreading. Either repeat the antecedent or revise the sentence.

Unclear The two major highways converging at the sign are lined with huge billboards that rise above the corn stalks and obscure the gently rolling hills. *It* is a convenient location for hitching rides.
[The pronoun *it* is too far removed from its antecedent, *sign.*]

Clear The two major highways converging at the sign are lined. . . . The *sign* is a convenient location for hitching rides.
[The antecedent has been repeated.]

Clear The two major highways converge at the sign, a convenient location for hitching rides. Each highway is lined. . . .
[The sentences have been recast.]

14c

Sometimes the noun to which a pronoun refers cannot logically be its antecedent.

Incorrect The Tzotzil Indians are only nominal Catholics, using *its* symbols and adapting them to the traditional Mayan religion.
[The antecedent of *its* has to be inferred from the noun *Catholics,* which means people who belong to a church and not the institution itself with its symbols and names.]

Correct The Tzotzil Indians are only nominal Catholics, using the symbols and the names *of the Church* and adapting them to the traditional Mayan religion.

Make sure the pronoun is not placed next to a word that cannot possibly be its antecedent.

Incorrect The botanist told us the plants' names that were all around us.
[Clearly, names were not sprouting out of the ground, as the sentence says.]

Correct The botanist told us the names of the *plants that* were all around us.

3. Broad pronoun reference: *this, that, which*

In speech we often use the relative pronouns, *this, that,* or *which* to refer broadly to the idea of the preceding clause or sentence. In writing, however, such loose pronoun reference can be misleading or confusing. If the preceding clause contains a noun that might also be mistaken for the antecedent, the reference may be ambiguous as well. If there is any doubt in your mind about whether or not the reader may wonder what is the word or phrase to which a *this,* or *that,* or a *which* refers, revise the sentence to eliminate the pronoun or to give the pronoun a definite antecedent.

Unclear   The beginning of the book is more interesting than the conclusion,
               which is unfortunate.
               [On first reading, the pronoun *which* seems to refer to *conclusion,* even though
               conclusions are not usually described as fortunate or unfortunate. The writer wants
               the *which* to refer to the whole idea of the main clause, but the noun at the end
               gets in the way.]

Revised, the sentence might read:

Correct   Unfortunately, the beginning of the book is more interesting than the
               conclusion.
               [The pronoun has been eliminated and the sentence is crisper.]

In the following sentence, the *which* is being made to stand for more than it can
clearly express.

Unclear   In the eighteenth century, more and more land was converted into
               pasture, *which* had been going on to some extent for several centuries.

The inclusion of a noun (*a process*) in the revised version both defines and
reiterates the idea.

Correct   In the eighteenth century, more and more land was converted into
               pasture, *a process which* had been going on to some extent for several
               centuries.
               [The vague pronoun reference has been cleared up by adding *process,* a noun that
               summarizes the idea of the main clause and gives the pronoun *which* an
               antecedent.]

The pronoun *this* should not be used as the beginning word in a sentence that
follows another sentence of great length and complication.

Unclear   The Japanese fugu, or puffer, is one of the most lethal fishes in the
               world, its poison 275 times deadlier than cyanide, yet it is considered a
               choice dish in Tokyo, Kyoto, and other cities, where it sells for more
               than $200 a plate. *This* means that its preparation must be controlled
               and supervised.

To revise the sentence, the writer must ask: this *what?* That the fish is so
deadly? That the fish is so expensive? The idea serving as the antecedent for
This is unclear. The revision depends on what the writer means.

Correct   This *toxicity* means that its preparation must be controlled and
               supervised.

Correct   This *costliness* means that its preparation must be controlled and
               supervised.

4. Indefinite use of *it, they, you*

English contains a number of idiomatic expressions using the impersonal
pronoun *it: It is hot, It rained all day, It is late.* The pronoun *it* is also used clearly
in sentences like "It seems best to go home at once," in which *it* anticipates the

real subject, *to go home at once.* Avoid, however, the unexplained *it,* the *it* that needs a clear antecedent and has none.

> **Unclear**   Lewis Thomas, author of *Lives of the Cell,* is a physician and writer who spends his spare hours practicing *it.*
>
> **Correct**   Lewis Thomas, author of *Lives of the Cell,* is a physician who spends his spare hours practicing writing.

The indefinite use of *they* is always vague; it can sound childish or paranoid.

> **Unclear**   If intercollegiate sports were banned, *they* would have to develop an elaborate intramural program.

Who, the writer should rigorously ask, are *they?* And answer by revising the sentence:

> **Correct**   If intercollegiate sports were banned, *each college* would have to develop an elaborate intramural program.

14c

Watch out for the vague, accusatory *they,* which can swell to dark proportions.

> **Unclear**   At registration *they* made us line up on the outside of the gymnasium and wait until *they* called the first letter of our last names; *they* made some of us stand in the rain for hours.

Be exact in describing the event and in assigning responsibility:

> **Correct**   At registration *we* had to line up on the outside of the gymnasium and wait until *a monitor* called the first letter of our last names; *some of us* had to stand in the rain for hours.

The indefinite use of the pronoun *you* to refer to people in general is widespread in conversation and frequent in informal writing: *Around here, you never know what the neighbors will say.* Formal usage, however, still prefers to limit *you* to mean *you, the reader,* as in *You can use these review questions to enhance your understanding of the poems,* and to substitute the pronoun *one* or a general noun for people in general.

> **Informal**   Small classes give *you* a chance to take part in discussions.
>
> **Formal**   Small classes give *one* a chance to take part in discussions.
>
> **Formal**   Small classes give *the student* a chance to take part in discussions.

While the impersonal or general use of *you* is both natural and appropriate in certain informal contexts, it is clearly inappropriate in other contexts:

> **Inappropriate**   During the American Revolution *you* were forced to choose sides.
> [The pronoun *you* cannot mean *you, the reader* in this context.]
>
> **Revised**   During the American Revolution *colonists* were forced to choose sides.

If the pronoun *one* seems stilted, try recasting the sentence.

> **Awkward**   In proofreading, *one* should catch all of *one's* careless errors.
>
> **Better**   In proofreading, *writers* should catch all of *their* careless errors.

Exercise 7

Revise the following sentences to correct the ambiguous reference of pronouns.

1. The runner lunged toward the tape, threw out his chest, and snapped it.
2. In the course of the argument, Jack told his father that he needed a new car.
3. It wouldn't hurt people to read about addicts because they live in a different kind of world and they don't have to follow their example.
4. Both parents were there when the twin brothers graduated together, and we couldn't help noticing how happy they were.
5. Under Roosevelt's leadership, the Democratic party, which had not really been united under one president for some years, came together effectively for a time. Historians tend to agree that this was a case of the right man at the right moment.
6. The hives buzzed with activity, and the beekeeper covered himself with netting before going after the honey and then motioned for us to follow at a distance. It was about fifty feet away.
7. In Updike's novel, he delights in complex allusions and in playing with words.
8. The spider gently shook the strands of his web as he scurried toward the fly and the moth. Although they were barely visible, they were obviously strong.
9. Engineering is the profession that applies scientific knowledge to the building of such things as bridges, harbors, and communication systems. This is my ambition.
10. Ethics must not be understood to be the same thing as honor because this is not the case.
11. When there is no harmony in the home, the child is the first to feel it.
12. Most of the students at the work camp were inexperienced, and many of them had never seen raw poverty before, but on the whole they were up to it.
13. It says in the brochure that in Japan they drink sake instead of wine.
14. Malamud's *A New Life* successfully used farcical incident and character development as tools for his satire in the novel.
15. Since the white settlers held the Indians to be of no significant value, they regarded their rights as equally nonexistent. This is exemplified by several incidents in Kroeber's account.

14d Dangling modifiers

A **modifier,** you will recall, is a word or phrase that functions in the sentence to modify, that is, to limit, qualify, or restrict another word or group of words. If there is no word or group of words in the sentence for the modifier to qualify or limit, the modifier is said to dangle, as in the following sentence.

Dangling   *Having eaten our lunch and waited an hour to digest our food,* the lake felt cool and pungent on that first hot afternoon of summer.

The literal syntax of this sentence states that the lake, well fed and well digested, felt cool on a summer afternoon. Of course, that is not what the writer meant, but the subject the modifying phrase is intended to limit—*we* or *the picnickers* or *the class of eighty-four?* (there is no way of knowing)—is not in the

14d

sentence. *Lake,* then, is the only possible body, even if it is of water, for the participial phrase *having eaten our lunch and waited an hour to digest our food* to modify.

Almost all dangling modifiers occur at the beginning of the sentence, and almost all result from carelessness or oversight. Once detected, they can be mended in either of two ways.

1. By supplying the noun or pronoun that the phrase logically modifies:

> modifier
> **Correct**   *Having eaten our lunch and waited an hour to digest our food,*
>
> word modified
> *we* plunged into the lake, which was cool and pungent that first hot afternoon of summer.

2. Or by changing the dangling construction into a complete clause:

> **Correct**   *After we had eaten our lunch and waited an hour to digest our food,* we swam, that first hot afternoon of summer, in the cool and pungent lake.

14d

1. Dangling participial phrases

Participial phrases are verbal modifiers that function in the sentence as adjectives do. Like adjectives, they should be placed next to the words they modify.

> **Dangling**   *Analyzing Joan Didion's style, her essay* seemed to me to be cool, detached, and uncommitted to purpose or point of view.
> [It is unlikely that an essay will analyze the style of the author who wrote it, but that, in effect, is what this sentence says. The writer has tossed off the participial phrase without examining its function in the sentence.]
>
> **Correct**   *Analyzing Joan Didion's style, I discovered* that the writing, especially in this essay, was cool, detached, and uncommitted to purpose or point of view.

Dangling modifiers at the end of a sentence are less frequent than those at the beginning, but they are often confusing and always awkward.

> **Dangling**   The mountains were snow-covered and cloudless, *flying over the Rockies.*
>
> **Correct**   *Flying over the Rockies, we saw* snow-covered, cloudless mountains.
>
> **Correct**   *When I flew over the Rockies,* the mountains were snow-covered and cloudless.

2. Dangling gerunds

A **gerund** is a verb form ending in *-ing* that is used as a noun. A gerund phrase dangles when the subject of the gerund is not apparent to the reader.

Dangling	*After explaining my errand to the guard,* an automatic gate swung open to let me in. [Obviously, a gate cannot explain an errand to a guard, or to anyone else. There is nothing in the sentence to indicate who is doing the explaining.]
Correct	*After explaining my errand to the guard, I drove* through the automatic gate, which had opened to let me in.
Correct	*After I had explained my errand to the guard,* an automatic gate swung open to let me in.

Often dangling gerunds result when the gerund functions as the object of a preposition, and the grammatical subject of the main verb would not be the subject of the gerund were the gerund to take a subject.

Dangling	*In writing a term paper,* notes should be carefully entered on 3 x 5 cards. [The subject of the main verb *should be entered* is *notes*, which could not possibly be the subject of *writing*.]
Correct	*In writing a term paper, one* (or *we* or *the writer*) should carefully enter notes on 3 x 5 cards.

3. Dangling infinitives

An **infinitive** is a verb preceded by the word *to,* and is said to dangle when the subject of its action is not expressed.

Dangling	*To be considered for law school,* the aptitude test must be taken.
Correct	*To be considered for law school, a student* must take the aptitude test.

This faulty construction is similar to the dangling gerund. Its revision is equally simple.

Always look carefully at an infinitive phrase to make certain that *who* is doing the action is clearly expressed.

Dangling	*To develop a lively writing style,* all kinds of sentence structures should be used.
Correct	*To develop a lively writing style, the writer* should use all kinds of sentence structures. [*Sentence structures* are not going to develop *lively writing styles* as the faulty sentence claims, but writers are, and the sentence should make that agency clear.]

4. Dangling elliptical clauses

Sometimes we omit the subject and main verb from a dependent clause and write *while going* instead of *while I was going,* or *when a child* instead of *when he was a child.* Such shorthand phrasing results in an **elliptical clause** which is perfectly acceptable as long as its subject is made clear in the rest of the sentence. If the subject of an elliptical clause is not stated, the construction may dangle.

14d

Dangling	*When six years old,* my grandmother died.
Dangling	*At the age of six,* my grandmother died.
Correct	*When I was six years old,* my grandmother died.
	[In both faulty sentences, the implied subject of the elliptical clause, *I*, is omitted. The addition of the subject and verb eliminates the dangling modifier and, unlike the other two, makes sense.]

The implied subject of the elliptical clause can be the subject of the main clause. If so, that subject status should be made clear.

| **Dangling** | *While hitting high E,* a wine glass was shattered by the tenor. |
| **Correct** | *While hitting high E, the tenor* shattered a wine glass. |

| **Dangling** | Do not add the beans *until thoroughly soaked.* |
| **Correct** | Do not add the beans *until they have been thoroughly soaked.* |

14d

5. Permissible introductory expressions

Some verbal phrases, such as *to begin with, judging from past experience, considering the situation, granted the results,* or *to sum up,* have become well established and need not be attached to any particular noun.

Judging from past experience, he is not to be trusted.

Granted the results, what do they prove?

To sum up, all evidence suggests that the decision was a fair one.

An **absolute phrase** should not be confused with a dangling modifier. Such a phrase consists of a participle with a subject (and sometimes a complement) grammatically unconnected with the rest of the sentence and usually telling when, why, or how something happened.

His mind preoccupied with his marital problems, William forgot his lunch date with the chancellor.

The dinner for the new athletic director started late, *the guest of honor having been caught in the five-o'clock traffic.*

Exercise 8

Revise the following sentences to eliminate the dangling modifiers.

1. When waiting for the dentist, every sound from the office is nerve-wracking.
2. After correcting my original calculations, the problem was finally solved.
3. Having seen Tharp's *Sue's Leg,* my attitude toward modern dance has changed completely.
4. The directions were clear, and my trouble could have been prevented, if followed correctly.
5. After hurrying to buy the rug, the clerk told the customer it had been sold.
6. In order to see the comet in detail, a small telescope was set up in the backyard.

7. The zoning petition was widely supported, after having canvassed many people in the neighborhood and stirred up concern about the proposed high-rise apartment building.
8. Being covered with plastic, I did not expect the car seats would be cool, having sat in the hot parking lot for several hours.
9. At last able to earn my car insurance, my parents allowed me to buy my own car.
10. Although tired and out of practice, the last set of the tennis match was too much of a personal challenge for me to resist.

14e Misplaced modifiers

Modifiers dangle when there is no word or group of words within the sentence for them to modify. A modifier is **misplaced** if it is not close to the word it is intended to modify. In English, word order is crucial to meaning. Adjectives, adverbs, and phrases or clauses that function as modifiers are placed close to the words they are intended to limit or define:

> She *hurriedly* read the printed notice that came in the mail.

The difference that the placement of a modifier makes in a sentence becomes clear if we observe what happens in the following sentence when the adverb *only* is moved about:

> The notice said *only* [said *merely*] that clients were invited to see the exhibit on the third floor.

> The notice said that *only* clients [clients *alone*] were invited to see the exhibit on the third floor.

> The notice said that clients were invited *only* [invited for the *one* purpose] to see the exhibit on the third floor.

> The notice said that clients were invited to see the exhibit on the third floor *only* [the third floor *alone*].

Many modifying phrases and clauses can be moved around to various positions in the sentence. An introductory clause, for example, can be shifted from the beginning of a sentence to the middle or the end.

> *Whatever the public may think,* I am sure that Picasso will be remembered as one of the greatest artists of our times.

> I am sure, *whatever the public may think,* that Picasso will be remembered as one of the greatest artists of our times.

> I am sure that Picasso will be remembered as one of the greatest artists of our times, *whatever the public may think.*

This freedom, however, has its dangers. Movable modifiers may be placed so as to produce misreadings or real ambiguities. Unlike the dangling modifier, which cannot logically modify any word in the sentence, the misplaced modifier may seem to modify the wrong word or phrase in the sentence:

Misplaced   She wrote the full story of her harrowing escape *from memory.*

Unless the writer meant the rather unlikely statement that the author was freed from her own memory, the sentence should read:

Correct   She wrote *from memory* the full story of her harrowing escape.

Be especially careful that adverbs are placed exactly where they belong in the sentence.

Misplaced   He scolded the student for cheating *severely.*

Correct   He *severely* scolded the student for cheating.

Misplaced   I have followed the advice *faithfully* given by the manual.

Correct   I have *faithfully* followed the advice given by the manual.

14e

1. Squinting modifiers

Modifiers are said to squint or to look two ways at once when they are placed so that they might refer to either a preceding word or a following word in the sentence.

Squinting   The child who lies *in nine cases out of ten* is frightened.

Correct   *In nine cases out of ten,* the child who lies is frightened.

Squinting   The tailback who injured his knee *recently* returned to practice.

Correct   The tailback who *recently* injured his knee returned to practice.

Correct   The tailback who injured his knee returned *recently* to practice.

2. Split constructions and infinitives

It is best to keep the parts of tight grammatical constructions together. The insertion of a modifier between the parts of a verb phrase or an infinitive can jolt the reader.

Split   *I have,* more than the rest of the class, *been* in a panic since the term paper was assigned.

Correct   More than the rest of the class, *I have been* in a panic since the term paper was assigned.

Split infinitives—that is, infinitives with a modifier between the *to* and the verb (*to personally supervise*)—may be awkward, especially if the modifier is long.

Awkward   I should like *to,* if I ever get the chance, *take* a trip to Spain.

Correct   I should like, if I ever get the chance, *to take* a trip to Spain.

Frequently, however, an adverb fits naturally between the two parts of an infinitive:

Correct   Some young couples regard children as a nuisance, but as they grow older they begin *to actually look* forward to having a family.
[If the modifier is moved and the sentence reads . . . *but as they grow older they actually begin to look forward . . .* , the emphasis is slightly changed and the stress the adverb receives in the original sentence is lost.]

Exercise 9

Revise the following sentences to correct misplaced words, phrases, and clauses.

1. He wore a ring on his right finger which was made of topaz.
2. The film about the life of the white shark that I saw downtown was very interesting.
3. She wrote her book on surfing in New York.
4. We camped in a small shelter near the edge of the cliff that had not been used for months.
5. Bread that rises rapidly too often will have a coarse texture.
6. The dean told me I could return to school in a high rage.
7. He was hit by a rotten egg walking back to his condominium one night.
8. Wild and primitive, with hidden snags and rapids on one side, jungle and savage natives on the other, danger is ever present.
9. I promised during the evening to call her.
10. Often she would spend hours on the edge of the beach watching her small son build a sand castle with half-closed eyes.

Exercise 10

Revise the following sentences to correct the split constructions.

1. At the end of the period we were told to promptly hand in our bluebooks.
2. The pharmacist told her she should, since she needed the medicine in such a hurry, have the doctor phone in the prescription.
3. The term *reactionary* can be applied to political, social, or economic (or a combination of the three) beliefs.
4. After nicking a submerged rock, the canoe began to slowly but steadily leak and to gradually settle deeper in the water.
5. She told him to for heaven's sake shut up.

14f Confusing shifts

Shifts in sentence structure lead to confusion. If the first clause of a sentence is in the active voice, the second clause should not be in the passive voice unless there is a good reason for the change. Similarly, a sentence that begins in the present tense should not lapse into the past tense halfway through, and one that starts with the first person *I* point of view should not shift to *you*. Sharp revision should ensure consistency in mood, tense, voice, and person. Watch out for shifty sentences.

1. Confusing shifts of voice or subject

A shift from the active to the passive voice almost always involves a change in subject. Such a shift in voice makes a sentence doubly awkward.

Awkward After *I* finally *discovered* an unsoldered wire, the *dismantling* of the motor *was begun.*

Correct After *I* finally *discovered* an unsoldered wire, *I dismantled* the motor. [The subject of this sentence shifts from the *I* of the dependent clause to the *dismantling* of the independent one; the voice shifts from active in the first clause to passive in the second. The sentence would be logically consistent if both verbs were in the passive voice: *After an unsoldered wire was found, the motor was dismantled.* But the passive voice is not required by the sense of the sentence. Reinstating *I* as the subject of the independent clause produces subject and voice consistency.]

14f

Confusing shifts from the active to the passive voice can also lead to questions of agency.

Awkward He *left* the examination after his answer *had been proofread.*

Correct He *left* the examination after he *had proofread* his answer. [The passive second clause of the faulty sentence leaves us with the puzzling question of who proofread the answer. The translation into the active voice of the correct sentence reinstates the subject and tells who performed the action.]

2. Confusing shifts of person or number

A common—and, to the reader, annoying—shift in unskillful writing is from the third person (*he, she, they, one*) to the second person (*you*). Another common shift is from a singular number (*a person, one, he*) to a plural (*they*). The inconsistencies usually occur when the writer has little or no sense of audience. Having no particular individual in mind as a listener, such a writer speaks in vague platitudes to an even vaguer anybody or everybody. The result is fuzzy, vapid writing with no focus.

Awkward When *one* tries hard enough, *you* can do almost anything.

Correct When *you* try hard enough, *you* can do almost anything.

Correct When *a person* tries hard enough, *he or she* can do almost anything.

Correct When *we* try hard enough, *we* can do almost anything.

Correct When *people* try hard enough, *they* can do almost anything.

A shift in number from singular to plural confuses the reader and results in faulty pronoun agreement.

Shift   If *a customer* is ignored or kept waiting, *they* should complain to the management.

Correct   If a *customer* is ignored or kept waiting, *he or she* should complain to the management.

Correct   If *customers* are ignored or kept waiting, *they* should complain to the management.

3. Confusing shifts of mood or tense

14f

A sentence should end in the same mood with which it begins. If the opening mood is an order or a command, the sentence is imperative and should not shift without good reason to the indicative mood.

Shift   First, *locate* the library on the campus map; then *you should find* the card catalog and the reference section.

Correct   First, *locate* the library on the campus map; then *find* the card catalog and the reference section.
[The first clause is an order, a command addressed in the imperative mood to an understood *you*. The second clause, which is a statement giving advice, is in the indicative mood. The revision puts both clauses in the imperative mood.]

A sentence that begins in the past tense should not change to the present tense.

Shift   *I stood* on the starting block and *looked* tensely at the water below; for the first time in my life *I am* about to swim the fifty-yard freestyle in competition.

Correct   *I stood* on the starting block and *looked* tensely at the water below; for the first time in my life *I was* about to swim the fifty-yard freestyle in competition.

Correct   *I stand* on the starting block and *look* tensely at the water below; for the first time in my life *I am* about to swim the fifty-yard freestyle in competition.

Remember that it is a convention to use the historical present in writing about literature: *Hamlet stabs Laertes, Isak Dinesen writes about South Africa.* Be careful not to lapse by habit into the past tense; keep the historical present consistent.

Shift   At the beginning of the *Divine Comedy,* Dante *finds* that he has strayed from the True Way into the Dark Wood of Error. As soon as he *realized* this, Dante *lifted* his eyes in hope to the rising sun.

Correct   At the beginning of the *Divine Comedy,* Dante *finds* that he has strayed from the True Way into the Dark Wood of Error. As soon as he *has realized* this, Dante *lifts* his eyes in hope to the rising sun.

Exercise 11

Correct the shifts in voice, person, number, mood, or tense in the following sentences.

1. After I finished planting my garden, the seeds were watered daily.
2. The matinee was enjoyed by all the children because they saw two monster films.
3. A person can always find something to criticize if they look hard enough.
4. In the school I attended, you had just five minutes between classes, and that was not enough time for most of us.
5. Don't ride the clutch; you should keep your left foot off the pedal.
6. Parson Adams went to London to try to sell his sermons and finds out that people are neither kind nor generous; he does not worry about taking money with him because he thought that people would be hospitable to him.
7. Thus, in *Daniel Martin,* Fowles is telling his readers to look ahead; he tells them not to be caught without knowing what is going on around you.
8. Of course, knowing how to use one's leisure is also important, but I do not think that it is up to the college to more or less arrange your social life, as many colleges do.
9. Fifty years ago, your house was the center of your everyday life; today, we Americans practically live in our cars.

14g   Mixed constructions

We designate as **mixed constructions** these sentences that begin in one way and end in another. For example, we may start a sentence with a modifying phrase, leading the reader to expect a substantive that it will modify. But instead of a noun the reader finds a verb, so that the modifying phrase becomes the subject of the sentence.

Mixed   *By requiring* drivers to have their cars periodically inspected *is one way* to cut down on accidents.

Correct   *By requiring* drivers to have their cars periodically inspected, *we can* cut down on accidents.

Correct   *Requiring* drivers to have their cars periodically inspected *is one way* to cut down on accidents.
[In the first revision, the prepositional phrase at the beginning of the sentence is given a subject, *we,* to modify. In the second revision the preposition *by* is dropped and the construction becomes a gerund phrase, subject of the verb *is.*]

1. Dependent clauses used as subjects and complements

A **dependent clause,** by definition, stands beside an independent clause for support. Using a dependent clause as the subject or the complement of a verb can produce a badly mixed construction.

Mixed   Because they installed solar heating when they remodeled their house made their fuel bills lower.

Correct   Because they installed solar heating when they remodeled their house, their fuel bills were lower.

Correct   Installing solar heating when they remodeled their house made their fuel bills lower.
[The first revision subordinates dependent to independent clause by means of the complex sentence construction. In the second revision the gerund phrase is the subject of the verb *made*.]

Common to speech, *the reason . . . is because . . .* construction is redundant. *Reason* means *because*.

Mixed   *The reason* their fuel bills were lower *is because* they installed solar heating when they remodeled their house.

Correct   Their fuel bills were lower *because* they installed solar heating when they remodeled their house.

Correct   *The reason* their fuel bills were lower *is that* they installed solar heating when they remodeled their house.

14g

2. Adverbial clauses used as nouns

A frequent cause of mixed constructions is the illogical use of *when* or *where* as part of the complement of *is*—the "is when" or "is where" habit.

Incorrect   One *thing* that keeps me from driving to the city *is when* I think of the traffic jams.

Correct   One *thing* that keeps me from driving to the city *is the thought* of the traffic jams.

Correct   I won't drive to the city because of the traffic jams.

Incorrect   *Symbiosis is where* dissimilar organisms live together in a mutually advantageous partnership.

Correct   *Symbiosis is a state where* dissimilar organisms live together in a mutually advantageous partnership.

Correct   *Symbiosis is the* mutually advantageous *partnership* of dissimilar organisms living together.
[The faulty sentences are mixed constructions that link a noun with an adverbial clause. They are revised by retaining the *is* verb and linking the noun with a noun or an adjective (or with groups of words that function like nouns and adjectives) or by dropping the *is* and subordinating dependent to independent clause.]

3. Idiomatic comparisons

In making comparisons, use the same idiom throughout the sentence.

Incorrect   The amateur typist will find erasable paper easier *to type on than on bond.*

Correct   The amateur typist will find erasable paper easier *to type on than bond is.*

Correct   The amateur typist will find it easier *to type on* erasable paper *than* [to type] *on* bond.

Exercise 12

In the following sentences, analyze the constructions that have been mixed and revise the sentences.

1. Because Porter's stories are written with the greatest skill makes each and every character come alive before the reader's eyes.
2. In the container is where the experiment takes place.
3. For college students, I feel that teaching assistants who read papers for the professors are really a disadvantage to the student.
4. It would be hard for me to say what the outlook on life a person with this disease would have.
5. In choosing the class play, we found small reading groups much easier to work with than with the whole committee together.
6. In my high school, which is rated as one of the best in the state, it is my opinion that it was much too easy.
7. As the volume of sound increases in the earphones, the nearer the submarine is approaching.
8. Of course, if I decide to become an education major doesn't mean that it is too late to change later on.
9. By defining the term "socialism" accurately will save us argument.
10. When waiting for the mail on the day a check from home is expected is very frustrating.

14h Incomplete constructions

14h

Do not omit words and expressions necessary for grammatical completeness.

Incorrect	The very sound of the poem gives the *feeling fleeting* light and life.
Correct	The very sound of the poem gives the *feeling of fleeting* light and life.

Incorrect	Like Hamlet, he pondered the question *being or not being.*
Correct	Like Hamlet, he pondered the question of *to be or not to be.*

1. Incomplete verb forms

When the two parts of a compound construction are in different tenses, the auxiliary verbs should usually be fully written in so that their meanings will be clear.

Incorrect	Language *has* and always *will be* a profitable subject in a college curriculum.
Correct	Language *has been* and always *will be* a profitable subject in a college curriculum.

When there is no change in tense, part of a compound verb can be omitted:

Correct	Information will be sent to all students who *have signed* up for the Education Abroad program and [who have] *paid* the fee.

In sentences where the predicate is the linking verb *to be*, the verb must agree with its subject in number.

Incorrect	He *was lecturing* and the students *taking* notes.
Correct	He *was lecturing* and the students *were taking* notes.
	[The plural *students* requires the plural auxiliary *were.*]

2. Idiomatic prepositions

English idiom requires that certain prepositions be used with certain adjectives and verbs; we say, for example, "interested in," "aware of," "devoted to." We expect others "to agree with," or "to object to," or even "to protest against" our plans. Use the proper idiomatic preposition with each part of a compound construction. Your dictionary will help you decide which is the right preposition.

Incorrect	He was *oblivious* and *undisturbed by* the noise around him.
Correct	He was *oblivious to* and *undisturbed by* the noise around him.
Incorrect	No one could have been more *interested* or *devoted to* her constituents than Senator Chong.
Correct	No one could have been more *interested in* or *devoted to* her constituents than Senator Chong.

3. Incomplete and inexact comparisons

In comparisons, do not omit words necessary to make a complete idiomatic statement.

Incorrect	She is as witty, if not wittier, than her brother.
Correct	She is as witty as, if not wittier than, her brother.
Correct	She is as witty as her brother, if not wittier.
	[If we delete the *if not wittier* interjection in the faulty sentence, it becomes apparent that the statement says *She is as witty than her brother,* which makes no sense.]
Incorrect	Leonardo da Vinci had one of the greatest, if not the greatest, minds of all time.
Correct	Leonardo da Vinci had one of the greatest minds, if not the greatest mind, of all time.
	[No one, not even Leonardo, can have *the greatest minds.* Comparisons should be complete, logical, and unambiguous.]
Incorrect	His expectations were more modest than *his brother.*
Correct	His expectations were more modest than *those of his brother.*
Correct	His expectations were more modest than *his brother's.*
	[A brother may be modest, but it is unlikely that the comparison was intended by the writer. That his brother had expectations, too, is made clear in each of the revisions.]

14h

Incorrect	The food here costs no more than any other restaurant in town.
Correct	The food here costs no more than [it does] at any other restaurant in town.

Avoid the illogical use of *than* or *any*.

Incorrect	For many years the Empire State Building was taller than *any* building in New York.
Correct	For many years the Empire State Building was taller than *any other* building in New York. [*Any building in New York* includes the Empire State Building, and a building cannot be taller than itself.]

Make sure the reader can tell what is being compared with what.

Incorrect	Claremont is farther from Los Angeles *than* Pomona.
Correct	Claremont is farther from Los Angeles *than* Pomona *is.*
Correct	Claremont is farther from Los Angeles *than it is* from Pomona. [In the two revisions, both terms of the comparison are completely filled in, and there is no ambiguity about what is being compared.]

14h

Many commercials and advertisements make claims that rest on incomplete comparisons. Both the student of language and the consumer should challenge ungrammatical and empty statements.

Incorrect	Philsoc Gas gives more and better mileage for the dollar. [We should ask, more and better than what? Than a team of mules? Than another kind of gasoline? If so, which one?]
Incorrect	Buy the bigger, crunchier, crisper, better-tasting breakfast cereal. [Again: than what?]

If clearly indicated by the context, the standard of comparison need not be specified:

Correct	Boulder Dam is big, but the Grand Coulee Dam is bigger.

Note that the words *so, such,* and *too* when used as comparatives are completed by a phrase or clause indicating the standard of comparison.

Correct	I am *so* tired *that I could drop.* I had *such* a small breakfast *that* I was starving by noon, and when we stopped for lunch, I was *too* tired *to eat.*

Exercise 13

Revise the following sentences by filling out the incomplete or illogical constructions.

1. The reasons for leaving are at least as good as staying.
2. Disneyland is as large, if not larger, than any other amusement park in the country.
3. The Hondas and Yamahas weigh less and are cheaper.
4. My father complained that his income tax was higher than last year.
5. The distributor was cleaned and the points adjusted.

6. Vale did some of her best work and learned a great deal from her high school history teacher.
7. Because of their climate and soil, Florida and Texas raise more citrus than all the states put together.
8. According to our map of Arkansas, Fort Smith is farther from Little Rock than Pine Bluff.
9. As your Class Secretary, I have and will continue to send you all the news that I receive about the class of '85.
10. Trying to analyze my good points and weaknesses made me a happier and secure person.

Exercise 14

The following sentences contain faults discussed in the preceding chapter on coherence—faulty reference of pronouns, dangling and misplaced modifiers, confusing shifts, and mixed and incomplete constructions. Identify the causes of incoherence in each sentence, and then revise the sentence.

1. Entering the door, after walking up several steps made of concrete, there is a police officer sitting behind the desk, who will gladly give you any needed information.
2. The politician has dinners given, ads filmed, and attends rallies.
3. If someone knows that a certain person is a "cheat," they wouldn't want to be around them and they wouldn't trust him.
4. By the way she tells the story is indication enough of how Mansfield feels.
5. I found Charlie Macklin to be the closest thing to perfection, but at the same time still being human, than any other I have either read about or known in real life.
6. Pulled through a broken window with pieces of glass scattered about, a passing motorist rescued a woman in her home early this morning, which was blazing.
7. One advertisement shows a washing machine "growing" before our eyes to be ten feet tall, and in a different commercial for soap portrays a giant in your washer who labors to clean your clothes.
8. While personally finding nothing to recommend Marx's system, it is fitting to examine him in order to see how and why so many people have believed in it.
9. He certainly didn't look like a man of my father's age and he certainly didn't have a particle of dignity that I so commonly associated with my father of having.
10. Just because our campus radio station plays so much popular music is no reason for the college to cut its funds.
11. The Lilliputians are much more like the human race than the giants.
12. After being locked in the cabin about two hours, our first roll call of the evening took place.

14h

15 Revising Diction

The great archetypal activities of human society are all permeated with play from the start. Take language for instance—the first and supreme instrument which man shapes in order to communicate, to teach, to command. Language allows him to distinguish, to establish, to state things; in short, to name them and by naming them to raise them into the domain of the spirit.

—Johan Huizinga

Language is a link between self and other: in playing with language, we experience the world; in sharpening our words, we make the world manageable. Our discovery of these powers begins early and unselfconsciously. If, for example, we move back to our childhood games (or perhaps the games of our parents and friends), we may rediscover these powers. We may live once again in the child's jeering or shame of "Tattle-tale, tattle-tale,/ Stick your head in the garbage pail"; the ritual oath of "Cross my heart and hope to die/ Drop down dead if I tell a lie"; or the gleeful celebration of "Made you look, you dirty crook,/ Stole your mother's pocketbook!" We distinguish the "tattle-tale" (what naming could be more specific?); we establish our laws ("Cross my heart"); we state the victory of "Made you look." We communicate, teach, command.

But, looking back, it appears that we did more. We twisted our tongues with "She sells seashells by the seashore"; mocked authority with "Teacher, teacher, I declare/ I spy a hole in your underwear"; and counted off with "One potato, two potato, three potato, four." We *tested* words for their sounds, their shock value, their rhythmic combinations. In playing (often very intently) with language, we did not merely master the different ways of naming and therefore of making the world inhabitable; we learned that the emotional colors, the sounds, and the contexts of particular words belong to their meaning as much as a deep, insistent voice belongs to the Siamese cat or the horny rings of warning belong to the rattlesnake. We learned a fundamental lesson about **diction,** or word choice: that different words not only name different realities but that the ways they name are as curious and as complicated as the reality itself.

We may even have sensed dimly that each word has a long history behind it, a fascinating ancestry of origins, of slowly changing meanings, of curious and forgotten uses as well as current, living ones—in short, an etymology. For instance, the word *diction* is derived from the Latin *dicere,* to say, and ultimately from the Indo-European root *deik,* to show or to point out, as its kinship with the Latin word for finger, *digitus,* and the English *digit* reveals. We point forward to things we don't know the names for. Words point backward to their roots and growth, if only we choose to look. Whether it is hybrid or pure stock, domestic or foreign, plant, flower, or weed, part of a word and its essence lies in its ancestry. To know the root or roots of a word is to know something valuable about its heredity.

One of the complex ways by which words gain their power to name is through their past. Some of the other ways will be discussed in this chapter: *the more you become sensitized to and experiment with these various ways,* the greater the precision in your *naming.* ("Sharpening words" may suggest the imagery of grinding an axe, a fitting picture if meaning were only logs to be split by forceful blows and keen steel; the image might just as well refer to more delicate wood carvings. Or, to discover another meaning, the image might suggest the sharpening of taste, learning to discriminate among and to savor words as if they were wines.)

Granted, no word can ever duplicate the reality of the thorn that pierces our thumb, the sunset that moves us to silent joy, or the turbulence of first infatuation. Recognizing this limitation of language, however, writers who are attentive to diction achieve precision and depth by selecting words that most nearly approximate their thoughts and feelings. For it is only through words on the printed pages—not the blank spaces above or below them—that one is understood in writing. Too often the complaint "You know what I meant" or "You know what I'm saying" is really the hurry of someone who cannot be bothered— someone in too much of a rush to learn about words.

The first, most elementary principle is the following: we draw on the names of those things and events that are the most important to us. The Eskimos have a rich vocabulary to discriminate among the colors, degrees of wetness, and textures of different kinds of snow. Americans have a similar vocabulary for cars. (How many types and makes can you name? What beyond the Mustang, Camaro, Reliant, Chevette, Rabbit, each a current, separate model, not to mention the Edsel, Pierce-Arrow, Hupmobile, and others of the past? Each model named is another reality.) The corollary of this principle is that the more we develop our ability to name, the greater is our ability to discover and specify meanings. To do this, we need a large, active vocabulary that we can use confidently in writing as well as in reading; good writers own, paw through, and wear out their dictionaries.

Begin, then, by looking up both the meanings and pronunciation of the unfamiliar words you come across in reading and those that seem familiar but which you cannot define. Jot them down on a slip of paper, a matchbook cover, or a paper napkin, if necessary. Keep a vocabulary notebook and try these words out in conversation and writing. You may falter or blunder, just as you might in learning a new dance step with a new partner. Becoming acquainted with a new word, like learning a new dance, demands the willingness to stumble at first as we learn its expressive possibilities and the appropriate occasions for its use. But taking the risk is the only way of learning, and the confidence gained with practice soon wipes out the memory of an occasional word circled in red pencil on a returned manuscript.

15a Denotation and connotation

The first of the complex ways that words name is by their denotations and connotations. Their **denotations** are their most literal meanings. For instance, to take a stark example, *body, corpse,* and *cadaver* can all have the same denotation—a dead human being. **Connotations,** on the other hand, are a word's overtones, echoes, emotional colorings, and associations. Thus we would hardly speak of going to a funeral home to view the *corpse* of a friend, let alone the *cadaver. Body* is the most intimate in its connotations, expressing the sad acknowledgment that someone we care for is no longer there and that those familiar features will soon be gone forever: the word, in this context, connotes a commonly shared grief over an irrevocable reality. By contrast, *corpse* and *cadaver* connote the coldly impersonal, the anonymous, the institutional, as when police officially speak of finding an unknown corpse in a field or when medical students speak of dissecting a cadaver.

The connotation of each word must be appropriate to the context. For instance, *to compliment* and *to flatter* may denote the same action—giving praise to another person—but note the differences in their connotations. Usually, *to compliment* (or *compliments*) is used in the context of generous, justified praise given publicly or freely: "I'd like to compliment you on (or pass on a compliment about) your performance." Occasionally, it may suggest doubts—"I'm not sure he deserved all the compliments," or "I don't want to compliment her for simply doing her job"—but in these cases the *context* ("not sure," "don't want to," "simply doing her job") makes our uncertainty clear. We are not sure the connotations apply.

To flatter (or *flattery*) connotes excess, even deception. Sometimes it may be harmless enough, as when we speak of "a photographer who flatters his subjects," or innocent, self-admitted smugness as when we say, "I flatter myself that. . . ." More often, though, it connotes gratifying vanity, favor-seeking, blandishments. Still, if forced to choose between being called a *flatterer* and an *apple-polisher,* most of us would probably elect the former. The context in which *apple-polishing* is used is unmistakable: blatant insincerity and favor-seeking which are obvious to everyone, except perhaps the recipient. Such slang is always powerfully connotative.

Not all connotations are pejorative, of course, not by any means. *Kindness, compassion, thoughtfulness; strength, fortitude, guts; witty, amusing, funny;*

15a

vitality, liveliness, vigor; to comfort, to console, to solace; religious, devout, reverent—in each of these groupings, the words denote more or less the same thing but have different connotations. (Would you speak of Lincoln's "strength" or his "guts" in issuing the Emancipation Proclamation?) Even with these and similar words, however, context determines appropriateness.

In short, context—the relevant environment of speaker, audience, and subject—is all. Consider the shifting contexts in the following: "I am slender; you are thin; he is skinny." To determine appropriateness, try testing words *aloud.* Good abridged desk dictionaries (see Chapter 11) will also help; they frequently discuss the differences in connotations among terms that have similar denotations. Pocket dictionaries and thesauruses, insofar as they merely list rough synonyms without distinction, can be quite misleading. A heightened sensitivity to connotation and denotation is essential for all effective speaking and writing.

One final word: many connotations stem from deep, often unconscious associations that we have. When, for example, the poet Phyllis Thompson concludes a poem "When I die, I will turn to bone/like these. And dust of bone. And then, like God,/to stone," she draws on these associations in rhyming "bone" and "stone": hardness, dryness, gray-whiteness, inertness. Drawing on equally deep but different associations, Andrew Marvell three centuries ago praised "a green thought in a green shade." He knew very well that readers of English after his lifetime would bring to the phrase associations of grass, trees, growth, life, tranquility. These associations often reveal our most elementary hopes, desires, experiences, and fears. For instance, the campaign of American blacks to replace certain negative connotations of *black* with positive ones of power and beauty has been a conscious one by users of the language to alter the ways in which we respond to words. The history of linguistic change is, among other things, the history of oppressed peoples striving to change the associations—and often the words—we live by in order to make their world more inhabitable.

15b Abstract and concrete

If you can describe clearly without a diagram the proper way of making this or that knot, then you are a master of the English tongue

—H. Belloc

The second of the complex ways that words name is by their abstractness and their concreteness. Words that name specific, tangible things are **concrete;** words that designate general qualities, categories, or relationships are **abstract.** A general term like *food* is a name for a whole group of specific things: tomato soup, fried chicken legs, chilled lettuce and alfalfa sprouts, sliced apples, cheesecake, and so forth. Note that *abstract* and *concrete* are relative, not absolute terms. Using S. I. Hayakawa's well-known model, we may speak of going up the "ladder of abstraction":

1. The tree *Charter Oak* which exists at the atomic and subatomic level, incredibly complex and changing;
2. The tree *Charter Oak* that we experience, not the word but only the limited number of features our nervous system selects from the complex reality;
3. The word *Charter Oak* itself, which is the name we give the particular perceived object but which is not the object itself, already tremendously simplified;
4. The word *oak,* which stands for what $Charter\ Oak_1$ and oak_2, oak_3, etc. share in common—in short, thousands of oaks of different ages, sizes, conditions, etc.;
5. The word *tree,* which stands for the traits we have abstracted that oaks, palms, pines, etc. share in common and which, of course, omits much, much more;
6. The word *plant,* which includes any living organism that cannot move voluntarily and usually makes its own food by photosynthesis—trees, flowers, bushes, etc.;
7. The word *organism,* which includes any living thing;
8. And so on up the ladder, as far as we choose to go.

15b

The point, then, is not just that "abstractness: and "concreteness" are relative as terms, but also that general words as well as specific ones are necessary. For certain subjects or in certain contexts, we have to generalize, abstract, deal in whole categories. And at its own level of generality such prose can have great precision. The English philosopher John Stuart Mill, writing on "The Subjection of Women" in the late 1860s, is as intelligible to us now as he was to his contemporaries because of such precision:

> For what is the peculiar character of the modern world—the difference which chiefly distinguishes modern institutions, modern social ideas, modern life itself, from those of times long past? It is that human beings are no longer born to their place in life, and chained down by an inexorable bond to the place they are born to, but are free to employ their faculties, and such favorable chances as offer, to achieve the lot which may appear to them most desirable. Human society of old was constituted on a very different principle. All were born to a fixed social position, and were mostly kept in it by law, or interdicted from any means by which they could emerge from it.

He continues, with the same forceful generalities, to argue that what is becoming true for the men of Western Europe and America should also be true for women. Discussing the slaveries that have vanished and "The Subjection of Women," which still remains, he is necessarily well up "the ladder of abstraction": long historical periods and change, abuses of one half of humanity, and the huge social costs are all part of his argument.

But even writers as skillful as Mill is at this "rung" come down the ladder because abstract terms at some point (preferably sooner rather than later) have to be given the substance of concreteness by comparisons or examples. In the following passage, for instance, Jonathan Swift makes us see and feel what the term *war* meant in the eighteenth century:

> And being no stranger to the art of war, I gave him a description of cannons, culverins, muskets, carabines, pistols, bullets, powder, swords, bayonets, battles, sieges, retreats, attacks, undermines, countermines, bombardments, sea-fights; ships sunk with a thousand men, twenty thousand killed on each side; dying groans, limbs flying in the air, smoke, noise, confusion, trampling to death under horses' feet; flight, pursuit, victory; fields strewed with carcases left for food to dogs, and wolves, and birds of prey; plundering, stripping, ravishing, burning and destroying. I assured him that I had seen them blow up a hundred enemies at once in a siege, and as many in a ship, and beheld the dead bodies drop down in pieces from the clouds, to the great diversion of all the spectators.

15b

The abstract term *war* is translated into the realities it too often obscures: massive cruelty, pain, and dying—pieces of human bodies dropping "from the clouds, to the great diversion of all the spectators."

This passage from Swift should suggest why teachers of writing urge their students to be specific, to be concrete. Too often beginning writers use vague generalities that seem to have no reference to the world of anyone's experience. Yet when we are learning a language we begin with that world; we ask for the names of what we see, hear, smell, touch, taste: *red, thunder, burning, smooth, salty.* While the best writing moves gracefully from abstract to concrete and back from particular to general, most of use are prone to sacrifice the sharp and concrete for the colorless abstraction. Consider the following:

Vague and general	For dinner we had some really good food.
Specific	For dinner we had barbecued steaks and sweet corn.
Vague and general	She liked to argue about controversial subjects.
Specific	She liked to argue about politics and religion.
More specific	She liked to argue about God's existence and the merits of socialism.

Paragraphs—even entire papers—that settle for "really good food" and "controversial subjects" are dull to read and thin in content because only the most shallow of broad surfaces is being glanced at; no real thought is taking place because, like an unfocused camera, the writer is not registering anything in particular.

Chapter **13** discussed several of the ways by which you can revise vague paragraphs and suggests means of noting the details to be used in giving depth to generalities. In reworking sentences, remember that a specific statement often requires no more space than a vague one, yet it can communicate much more information:

Vague	One member of my family has recently begun his professional career.
Concrete	Last week my brother Ken joined the law firm of Bailey, Harney, and Johnson.

To sum up, you will achieve only as much reality in your papers as your words actually name; you may find that the effort to think concretely takes time and imagination, but it's the only way you have of discovering your meaning.

15c Idiom

Still another of the complex ways that words name is by **idiom,** an expression peculiar to the language, not explainable by the principles of logic or the ordinary meaning of individual words. Idioms, in short, are arbitrary, as when we say *make out* (succeed), *make up* (reconcile), and *make do* (be satisfied with). They are as fixed as the Spanish "Hace frio" ("It's cold"), which literally and unaccountably to one learning the language translates as "It makes cold."

15c

In English, we rely on prepositions to indicate subtle but essential relationships. To take a stand *on* an issue, to be *in* a quandary, *out* of luck, *off* your rocker—these idiomatic expressions make a kind of spatial sense as figures of speech: we can, if we stop to visualize it, imagine standing on an issue, defending our point of view, planting our feet firmly on an ideological turf we call our own. Some verbs require prepositions that are arbitrary and unexplainable. How can persons who are learning English and know the words *take, in, up, down,* and *over* deduce the meaning of the following: *take in* (comprehend), *taken in* (fooled), *take up* (begin to do something), *take down* (humiliate), *take over,* and *overtake?* They can't, any more than they could figure out the differences among *put up with* (tolerate), *put on* (assume), *put away* (deposit, renounce), and *put down* (suppress), Each of these idioms has to be learned separately. Here are some idiomatic uses of prepositions:

abide *by* a decision

agree *with* a person; *to* a proposal; *on* a procedure

argue *with* a person; *for* or *about* a measure

angry *at* or *about* something; *with* a person

compatible *with*

correspond *to* or *with* a thing; *with* a person

differ *from* one another in appearance; differ *with* a person in opinion

independent *of*

interfere *with* a performance; *in* someone else's affairs

listen *to* a person, argument, or sound; listen *at* the door

with regard *to*

stand *by* a friend; *for* a cause; *on* an issue

superior *to*

wait *on* a customer; *for* a person; *at* a place; *in* the rain; *by* the hour

Idiom demands that certain words be followed by infinitives, others by gerunds. For instance:

Infinitive	Gerund
able to go	capable of going
like to go	enjoy going
eager to go	cannot help going

If two idioms are used in a compound construction, each idiom must be complete.

Incomplete	He had no love or confidence in his employer.
Complete but awkward	He had no *love for,* or *confidence in,* his employer.
Improved	He had no love for his employer and no confidence in him.
Incomplete	I shall always remember the town because of the good times and the friends I made there.
Complete	I shall always remember the town because of the *good times I had* and the *friends I made* there.

15d Figurative language

The last broad category to be discussed is that of **figurative language**. When we speak figuratively, we speak nonliterally: we compare one quite distinct thing with another for some quality we think they have in common, or identify one thing by another in terms of a common quality. Figurative language is a complex and powerful means of creating, showing, or limiting relationships. Thus, when we speak of costs being "cut," of price "gouging," or of a state "draining" its taxpayers, we are using metaphors; so, too, when we speak of a "head" on the beer, the "hands" of a clock, or the "heart" of the subject; so also when we speak of "losing our shirt," "covering" a subject, or "building up" expectations. Of course, a merchant charged with price "gouging" has not, in fact, taken a chisel and scooped grooves on his customers any more than we have made a chest incision and inspected the right auricle and right ventricle when we speak of "getting to the heart of the subject." These metaphors, dead metaphors, are economical and precise: price "gouging" says how we feel when we think we have been defrauded (we speak of the "chiseler"); "getting to the heart of the subject" names our intent to discover the source of its life, the vital center.

A **metaphor** is, then, a direct comparison of two things on the basis of a shared quality. The word *metaphor* is itself a buried metaphor since it means *to transfer* or *carry across:* when we compare, we are carrying a trait from one thing to another as if over a bridge or road. Metaphor says that one thing is another: "All the world's a stage"; "Snow blanketed the ground"; "The road of excess leads to the palace of wisdom." A *dead metaphor* has, so to speak, become so common in usage that it has lost its life, its capacity to startle us with the appositeness of the comparison; but it is not really "dead," only moribund, and can be brought back to life, as when we complain: "The beer was all head and no body."

Metaphor is one of the most powerful causes of linguistic growth, change, and vitality. To speak of large, expensive, inefficient automobiles as "gas-guzzlers," a sharp decline in the value of currency and a sharp rise in prices as "runaway inflation," or citizens receiving inadequate services for their money as "the public's being shortchanged"—to employ these and other metaphors that have come into general use is to be conveniently brief, exact, and vivid. In fact, whether we realize it or not, we organize whole categories of our experience through certain metaphoric structures. For example, we systematize our concepts of vitality and power through metaphors of upwardness, our concepts of debility and weakness through metaphors of downwardness: She is at the *peak* of her fame, or she *fell* from the public's favor. He is *on top of* the situation, or he is *under* the control of others. The stock market *rose,* or the stock market is *declining.* Language is always vitally metaphoric because our realities—our hopes, desires, circumstances, and fears—change. The relevant issue is not whether metaphors are employed but whether they pinpoint accurate relationships, or whether they are forced, mixed, or trite. We will return to these abuses later.

One final, positive word about metaphors, and some advice: begin to feel their presence; make a practice of discovering them not only in nouns (the *heart* of the subject) but also in verbs. Such verbs (and nouns) give nourishment in ways that the junk food of needlessly abstract phrasing never can—the difference between saying *"Cut* out the *deadwood"* and "Avoid repetitious or unnecessary phrasing." American English has been wonderfully rich fare for our writers, as the following passage from *Huck Finn* may suggest:

> Once or twice of a night we would see a steamboat slipping along in the dark, and now and then she would *belch* a whole world of sparks up out of her chimbleys, and they would *rain* down in the river and look awfully pretty; then she would turn a corner and her lights would *wink* out.

Granted, Twain's prose is in a dialect that only a gifted writer could imitate; but the presence of metaphor here is clear enough. In more standard English, F. Scott Fitzgerald's metaphors deepen the vision of Long Island and America as a lost Eden at the end of *The Great Gatsby:*

> Most of the big shore places were closed now and there were hardly any lights except the shadowy, moving glow of a ferryboat across the Sound. And as the moon rose higher the inessential houses *began to melt away* until gradually I became aware of the old island here that *flowered* once for Dutch sailors' eyes—a fresh, green *breast* of the new world. Its vanished trees, the trees that had *made way for* Gatsby's house, had once *pandered in whispers* to the last and greatest of all human dreams; for a transitory enchanted moment man must have *held his breath* in the presence of this

15d

continent, compelled to an aesthetic contemplation he neither understood nor desired, face to face for the last time in history with something commensurate to his capacity for wonder.

Other types of figurative speech—techniques for making an image—include simile, analogy, and allusion. As comparisons, these sometimes tend to be more self-conscious and formal than metaphors, though they also can be forced or become trite. A **simile** uses the words *like* or *as* to state a comparison:

Simile   "I sensed a wrongness around me, *like* an alarm clock that has gone off without being set."

—Maya Angelou

Simile   ". . . her tepid, sluggish nature, really *like* something eating its way through a leaf."

—Katerine Anne Porter

Simile   [a muddy sow that would] "stretch out and shut her eyes and wave her ears whilst the pigs was milking her, and look as happy *as if* she was on salary."

—Mark Twain

A comparison can be extended into an **analogy,** which not only illustrates a point but also suggests an argument or point of view (Chapter **8** discusses the use of analogy in building paragraphs; Chapter **17,** their uses and abuses in reasoning). Consider, for instance, Mary Ellman's startling analogy between astronauts and pregnant women:

The astronaut's body is awkward and encumbered in the space suit as the body of a pregnant woman. It moves about with even more graceless difficulty. And being shot up into the air suggests submission too, rather than enterprise. Like a woman being carted to a delivery room, the astronaut must sit (or lie) still, and go where he is sent. Even the nerve, the genuine courage it takes simply not to run away, is much the same in both situations—to say nothing of the shared sense of having gone too far to be able to change one's mind.

In an **allusion** the comparison is made between some present event, situation, or person and an event or person from history or literature. Usually, the allusion is a brief reference to something the reader is assumed to know, as when journalists allude to a recent scandal as "another possible Watergate." Sometimes the writer may employ several allusions, as when Adrienne Rich says of a woman who reads about women in books written by men:

She finds a terror and a dream, she finds a beautiful face, she finds La Belle Dame Sans Merci, she finds Juliet or Tess or Salome, but precisely what she does not find is that absorbed, drudging, puzzled, sometimes inspired creature, herself, who sits at a desk trying to put words together.

A sense of audience should determine what allusions, if any, are appropriate. There is no point in throwing away allusions or in alienating your readers by appearing to be more knowledgeable than they. An allusion can deepen the meaning of a statement for those who recognize the comparison, but the statement should still make perfectly clear sense without it.

And what of the abuses of figurative language, especially metaphors and similes? In "Politics and the English Language," George Orwell writes: "Modern writing at its worst does not consist in picking out words for the sake of their meaning and inventing images in order to make the meaning clearer. It consists in gumming together long strips of words which have already been set in order by someone else, and making the results presentable by sheer humbug." Much of the time these "long strips of words" are the tritest of metaphors and similes. No thought is involved, no feeling evoked; thus we get *the man in the street,* whose *home is his castle,* whose wife is *the little woman,* along with the son who is a *chip off the old block;* this is the *All-American family* lucky to live in the *land of opportunity, working like the devil to* keep *the cancer of communism from our shores,* and generally preventing others from *undermining the foundations.* Ludicrous? Yes, it is, but only when the plastic phrasing is strung out this way. Here is a typical list of such clichés:

15d

acid test	more than meets the eye
agony of suspense	moving experience
all boils down to	other side of the coin
as luck would have it	out in the cold
beat a hasty retreat	poor but honest
bitter end	proud possessor of
bolt from the blue	quick as a flash
breathless silence	rotten to the core
checkered career	slow but sure
cool as a cucumber	straight from the shoulder
deep, dark secret	tempest in a teapot
depths of despair	trials and tribulations
doomed to disappointment	undercurrent of excitement
few and far between	uphill battle
gone off the track	walking on air
green with envy	water under the bridge
growing by leaps and bounds	wave of optimism
heave a sigh of relief	work hand in hand
hit the nail on the head	worth its weight in gold
in this day and age	young in spirit
jumping on the bandwagon	youthful glee

Forced figures of speech often begin in dead metaphors and end in clichés.

> **Forced**   I was so eager for people to like me that I would take any position they
> wanted and bend over backward to please them.
> [Here, the dead metaphor *take any position* has led the writer to the cliché of *bend
> over backward* and into an image that strains visual and conceptual belief.]

Mixed figures usually occur when writers have stopped thinking about the logical and visual sense of what they're saying. Used deliberately, they make their point by comic incongruity; for example:

"Whenever he saw a spark of genius, he watered it."

"The early bird gets the worm—but who wants the worm?"

Most of the time they are confused, bizarre, or both:

> **Mixed**   I know it sounds like sour grapes, but that's the whole kettle of fish in a
> nutshell.

> **Mixed**   The southern states, being completely argicultural, hinged around the
> barn.

> **Mixed**   He was saddled with a sea of grass-roots opinion that his campaigners had
> ferreted out for him.

> **Mixed**   She penetrated the impervious gaze of her challenger.
> [One can no more *penetrate an impervious gaze* than *be saddled with a sea of grass-
> roots opinion* that others have *ferreted out*—except, perhaps, in the world of Monty
> Python.]

15e Other pitfalls to avoid

For the most part, we have been emphasizing the complex ways that words name in order to improve your prose. Writing that is puffy with abstractions, flabby with clichés, or thin and undeveloped requires new exercises: more climbing down the ladder of abstractions, as well as up, more agile play with connotations, more striving for concreteness. We have concentrated primarily on nouns and verbs because they are the best conditioners; they do the most basic naming.

Words also have complex ways of confusing, obscuring, and deceiving. Misleading connotations, unidiomatic expressions, and mixed metaphors exemplify some of the means by which we can go awry; there are others. In illustrating these other ways, we will necessarily be saying, "Don't, don't." What we intend to affirm continually is the fact that the disciplined writer, the one who truly loves and considers words, will not want to use them carelessly. As you read, try to recall where we began—with that childlike delight, awe, and mastery that increase as we learn to communicate, teach, and command. Recalling something of that playfulness is about as close as we will ever come to the "naming day in Eden."

1. Weak verbs

One way in which writing goes awry—never really even gets started—stems from the needless use of weak verbs. Anemic writing results when, rather than using a vigorous verb, we connect subject and complement with the verb *to be*. Such verbs, called **linking** (or **copulative**) **verbs,** also include *become, seen, appear, remain,* and others. We cannot, of course, write without linking verbs, especially when indicating logical equivalents:

> Yoruk doctors, with extremely rare exceptions, were women—all their great doctors were women.
>
> —Theodore Kroeber
>
> [The linking verb *were* functions as an equal sign in mathematics and is appropriate to Kroeber's sentence.]

15e

Used excessively, however, linking verbs make for bland and predictable prose.

Make your verbs work. Good writers enliven their observations by selecting sharp verbs and by using verbals as modifiers. Consider these sentences from an essay by the naturalist Edward Hoagland:

> Mountain lions spirit themselves away in saw-toothed canyons and on escarpments, and when conversing with their mates, they coo like pigeons, sob like women, emit a flat slight shriek, a popping bubbling growl, or mew, or yowl. They growl and suddenly caterwaul into falsetto—the famous scarifying scream functioning as a kind of hunting cry close up, to terrorize the game. They ramble as much as twenty-five miles in a night, maintaining a large loop of territory which they cover every week or two.

The verbs that assert, *spirit away, coo, sob, emit, growl, caterwaul, ramble,* and *maintain,* and the infinitive *to terrorize* are reinforced by the action of the verbals, *conversing, popping, bubbling, scarifying, functioning, hunting,* and *maintaining.* Even the nouns *shriek, growl, mew, yowl, scream,* and *loop* contribute to the energy of the passage, since in other contexts they function as verbs and carry these active connotations with them. Action verbs and verbals make us feel, see, hear, smell; they appeal to our senses and body knowledge, our primary ways of knowing and understanding.

Occur, take place, prevail, exist, happen, and other verbs expressing a state of affairs have legitimate uses, but they are often colorless, tossed in merely to complete a sentence.

Weak	In the afternoon a sharp drop in the temperature *occurred.*
Stronger	The temperature *dropped* sharply in the afternoon.
Weak	Throughout the meeting an atmosphere of increasing tension *existed.*
Stronger	As the meeting progressed, the tension *increased.*

Linking verbs completed by an adjective or participle are usually weaker than concrete verbs.

Weak   He *was* occasionally *inclined to talk* too much.

Stronger   Occasionally he *talked* too much.

Weak   In some high schools *there is a very definite lack of emphasis on the development* of a program in remedial English.

Stronger   Some high schools *have failed to develop* programs in remedial English.

2. Wordiness and euphemisms

Wordiness and euphemisms blur the horizon of clear meaning. Writing that is needlessly repetitive has a strained, awkward effect. If handled carefully, repetition can be effective:

> The really important question is: "What does the *composer* start with; where does he begin?" The answer to that is, "Every *composer* begins with *a musical idea—a musical idea,* you understand, not a mental, literary, or *extramusical idea.*"
>
> —Aaron Copland
>
> [Copland emphasizes his declaration by repetitions intended to make his meaning unmistakable.]

Often, however, repetition is cumbersome:

Awkward   *Probably* the next *problem* that confronts parents is the *problem* of adequate schooling for their children.
[There is no reason for emphasizing *problem* and no excuse for clumsily echoing its sound in the cautious *probably.*]

Improved   Parents next *must find* adequate schooling for their children.

Read you writing aloud to catch offenses to the ear which are elusive to the eye. Alliteration and other repetition of sounds, functional in poetry, are rarely suited to expository prose.

Unsuitable   Henderson *set some* kind of record by *sliding* farther on the *slippery slope* than anyone else had *slid.*

Intensives, such as *really, very, so, much,* which may give emphasis to conversation, weaken written language. They are often coverups for the fact that the writer lacks a vocabulary with a wide range of emphatic words. Why settle for *really angry* when there are *enraged* and *furious,* for *so happy* when there are *joyful, delighted, cheerful,* for *very bad* when there are *wicked, detestable, rotten, vile?* Every time you are tempted to dump a "really" before a word, look that word up in a good college dictionary and try to discover a word that will convey the meaning you want in all its intensity.

Often when we want to avoid harsh facts we resort to a particular kind of circumlocution, the **euphemism.** The Greek word means "good speech," but euphemisms seldom are good for writers. Too often they are cosmetics to cover up painful realities. To avoid facing the finality of death people have always used euphemisms: *passed on* or *passed, gone west, met his Maker, gone to her reward.* The *dear departed* rests in his casket in the *slumber room,* often having been *prepared* by the *funeral director,* who today is likely to preside at a *memorial service* instead of a funeral. Ultimately, the *loved one* is not buried but *laid to rest,* not in a graveyard but in *The Valley of Memories.* Such sentimental wordiness is intended to comfort the bereaved by pretending that death is sleep, but its effect is one of stilted insincerity. There is no need, however, to go to the opposite extreme and speak ill of the subject. *Croak* and *kick the bucket,* while brisk and salty, are no closer to the fact of dying than *wrestled with the Angel of Death and was vanquished.*

3. Jargon and pretentious diction

15e

Once again, Orwell: "The great enemy of clear language is insincerity." Sincerity implies candor, trust, unaffectedness. Jargon and pretentious diction mislead and boast. They are the most morally objectionable ways of using language, short of outright lying.

There are two kinds of jargon: the technical language used by certain professionals and the empty generalities that are the bluff of the insincere or incompetent writer. Here, we are not concerned with the inevitabilities of technical language: even handbook writers and readers need terms like *dangling modifier, comma splice,* and *faulty subordination* to name specialties of the trade. We are concerned, rather, with the ponderous, wordy, inflated prose that obscures the obvious. This is the jargon we object to; this is the language of bureaucrats, publicists, politicians, college professors, and students when they hope the inflation of their prose will raise the commonplace to the significant.

Our minds are befogged every day by phrases like *capability factor, career potential, divergent lifestyles, socio-personal development, decision-making process, social interaction, holistic learning procedures, methodologies, technical implementations, fundamental value structures.* We cannot easily escape from this publicized network of confused language, but if we learn to recognize the stylistic flavor of jargon, we may avoid it in our own writing. Jargon words are, by and large, abstract rather than concrete, and contain more than one syllable (as if the jargon writer assumed that the addition of a syllable would add weight to the word). Jargon words are often nouns masquerading as verbs: *concretize, finalize, interiorize.* Sometimes nouns are turned into adverbs or adjectives by the addition of the suffix *-wise: languagewise, subjectwise, moneywise, weatherwise.* Jargon is best deflated by a translation into clear English:

> The leader-follower relationship must be looked upon as a field situation and such a field will be structured and sustain its structure only when the views of the leader are acceptable to the followers. The leader-follower field will be extended to the degree that the leader is seen to have authority to assume the leader role.

> As the relation of the leader's apparent right to authority is moved progressively away from the problem area confronting the group, there will be an increasing tendency for the leader-follower field to disintegrate.

This specimen, while not the worst, typifies the habits of jargon—inflated prose and overuse of the passive voice. Thus *leader* and *group* become *the leader-follower relationship* in a *field situation,* and the leader's meddling becomes a movement *away from the problem area confronting the group.* Stripped of their jargon, these sentences mean no more than:

> A group will fall apart when its members no longer agree with the views of their leader. Whatever degree of authority leaders have, they gain from the group's willingness to grant it. The more the group feels its leaders is meddling, the less likely it is to follow.

15e   In addition to being obscure and tiresome, jargon, when it conceals or distorts the reality it describes, can be dangerous, even deadly. The phrase *anti-personnel detonating devices* obscures the chilling reality of bombs that kill men, women, and children. Similarly, the deviousness of official statements like "The U.S. cannot foreclose any option for retaliation" distracts us from the protest we might register had the writer said what he meant: "The U.S. will use nuclear weapons if necessary."

Pretentious diction, like the pretentious person, is stiff and phony—in short, a bore. Our diction becomes pretentious if we always choose the poly-syllabic word over the word of one syllable, a Latinate word when an Anglo-Saxon one will do, flowery phrases in place of common nouns and verbs. Writing should be as honest and forthright as plain speech. And since we have the opportunity to revise and edit what we write, it should be even more economical, direct, and to the point.

Sometimes, ordinary words seem inadequate to carry the weight we want our thoughts to have, so we decorate statements with ornate language:

> His charismatic appeal profoundly influences the personal lifestyles of all those fortunate enough to call themselves his friends.
> [The sentence says little more than *His popularity influences the way his friends live,* but the fancy language is out of proportion to the statement it makes.]

To guard yourself against this sort of thing, read your papers aloud to a classmate. If he or she looks uncomfortable or laughs at the wrong places, examine the diction of your paper for phony phrases, for words that don't sound like you. Be wary of words that dress up simple facts: *charisma* for *popularity, interface* for *meet, utilize* for *use, profitable enterprise* for *money-maker, purchase* for *buy, decision-making process* for *leadership.* As you consult your college dictionary to develop your vocabulary, note the fine distinctions among synonyms and listen to thousands of words to judge whether they will strike your reader as counterfeit or genuine. Keep in mind Samuel Johnson's advice: "Read over your compositions and, when you meet a passage which you think is particularly fine, strike it out."

Exercise 1

Pick one or two words that interest you (nouns, verbs, adjectives, and adverbs are your best bet) and consult the *Oxford English Dictionary* in your library. The OED (its familiar title) is the indispensable reference for anyone curious about our language: it gives a word's first known appearance in print, its changing uses (with historical examples), and the fullest record we have of its connotations and denotations. Write a full paragraph in which you (1) note the word's primary shifts in meaning, (2) analyze these shifts for some common principle, logic of associations, or consistency in figurative use that runs throughout, and (3) indicate what you take to be its primary connotations and denotations now.

Exercise 2

15e

With the help of a dictionary (and perhaps a dictionary of Roman and Greek mythology) discover the concrete particular in which each of these words originated. Write a brief explanation of why and how you think some of these words came to mean what they mean today.

cereal	cupidity	hackneyed	panic
chapter	erotic	infant	paradise
comma	genius	language	surgery

Exercise 3

Choose three words that have similar denotations: for example, *to please, to gratify, to delight; concerned, involved, committed; fame, celebrity, stardom.* Then write a paragraph on the differing connotations of each word, and compose a sentence or two to show how the word is used in context.

Exercise 4

Choose three concrete nouns and take them up three or four rungs on "the ladder of abstraction," beginning above the atomic and subatomic rung.

Exercise 5

Choose three abstract nouns (for example, *wealth, humanity, art*) and take them down four or five rungs on "the ladder of abstraction."

Exercise 6

Analyze the following paragraphs for jargon, pretentious diction, and clichés. Translate the paragraphs into Standard English if you can, and if not, be prepared to say why.

1. A corollary of reinforcement is that the consequences of responding may be represented exhaustively along a continuum ranging from those that substantially raise response likelihood, through those that have little or no effect on response

likelihood, to those that substantially reduce response likelihood. An event is a positive reinforcer if its occurrence or presentation after a response strengthens the response. Sometimes good grades, words or praise, or salary checks act as positive reinforcers. An object or event is a negative reinforcer if its withdrawal or termination after a response strengthens the response. Often bad grades, shame, or worthless payments act as negative reinforcers. The above notion sounds complex and difficult to apply but is indeed extremely simple.

2. All courses (process or outcome) in the University system that are judged to contain written or oral communication goal statements should constitute a set of courses from which a student must select some number. This client-oriented marketplace approach to core requirements is a solution. Enrollment determines which courses will survive and which will not. However, academic tradition is rife with distrust of student judgment; and it can result in a self-fulfilling prophecy where faculty compete in playing to the "house" because they are convinced that ultimately only those who do will survive. This solution is usually condemned without trial.

15e

Exercise 7

Analyze the following paragraphs for clichés, pretentious diction, jargon, and so on. Translate the paragraphs into Standard English if you can, and if not, be prepared to say why.

Henry

As human beings, each of us grows and benefits in some way from ordinary experience each day. For the past five years I have sought a higher understanding of human attitudes, especially those of a positive nature, and of the mental processes which underlie and reinforce them. By listening to people, I have gained much wisdom; by seeking out those who have much to share, I have grown. I have begun the arduous but satisfying search for maturity.

One individual who has given me special insights is Henry. A married, older person who has had much experience in diverse walks of life, he is a special person. One day he joined a group of us after classes while we were sitting on the grass. I immediately felt his desire to communicate some special aspect of his life—something that was preoccupying him very deeply.

Henry began to relate the experience of his recent separation from his wife. It bothered me at the time that someone with such an understanding nature as his would have such a deep personal problem, and I questioned him regarding the reasons for his trouble. At the time I was involved in a personal relationship and wanted our communications to be open. What Henry told me became one of the most valuable teachings of my life. He told how he and his wife had stopped making a conscious effort to work at their relationship. Their life had become a burden and a sorrow.

My own relationship has grown into a beautiful experience, but it is one I have to work at and strive to improve. Henry made me realize that we have to lose our selfishness. I feel that I have matured, and we have grown together, and I am a better person for it. Today is the first day of the rest of my life.

Exercise 8

Analyze several of your themes and, for each theme, list all the clichés, weak verbs, and examples of jargon you find. Review these lists with the following questions in mind: Are there significant differences among the lists in the frequency of clichés, weak verbs, examples of jargon? Can you see some connection between the topic and the frequency of your ineffective diction? If so, what seems to be the connection? Are there any particular clichés, weak verbs, or jargon words you use often?

Exercise 9

Select one of the papers used for Exercise 8 and rewrite it, or at least the offending passages. Revise the diction by making it as concrete and fresh as you can.

Exercise 10

Analyze the diction of the following sentences for exactness, connotation, figures of speech. Be prepared to say what words or figures of speech would more effectively express the writer's meaning.

15e

1. Our balloons of egotism filled with the air of freshman knowledge were soon to be pricked by the pinpoints of self-awakening.
2. As the town grew, the theater obtained a foothold in the hearts of the citizens.
3. Drinking seems to have its claw in the economy of San Francisco.
4. Poring through *Paradise Lost* was like wading in deep water.
5. A good education is the trunk for a good life for it is the origin of all the branches which are your later accomplishments.
6. His immaturity may improve with age.
7. The basic objective of the indoctrination program is to build strong class spirit and to weed out those who are leaders in the class.
8. Darwin's *Origin of Species* began an epic of materialism.
9. Margaret Mead's book had a great success because Americans are grossly interested in sex.
10. Jefferson and Madison were two of the most prolific characters our nation produced at that time in history.
11. Because he did not follow the code, he was blandished from society.
12. He was a male shogunist pig.
13. She succeeded in deleting her flaw and, in doing so, became a stronger, ursine being.
14. In Tillie Olsen's story "I Stand Here Ironing," the mother paradoxically loves her child but has to farm it out to a day-care center.
15. Sarty does not realize that his father is the noose around his neck until Sarty gets his feet planted firmly on the ground to stop his mutation into a passive being.
16. He reflects on the way Sarah has been ostersized.
17. O'Neill seems to be saying that alcohol and narcotics are not helpful devices in problem solving.
18. He has a vicarious relationship through his son.
19. His trip around the world is a soul search.
20. She is still young and arouses bodily disturbances in Robert.

Part IV

Critical

Reading and

Thinking

16 *Thinking Critically*

Any expository writing that is more than just a summary of dates and events involves critical reading and thinking: interpreting evidence, making generalizations, arriving at conclusions. You may be discussing a book that you find persuasive or unpersuasive; you may be arguing for or against some new policy; you may be explaining your actions or beliefs. In each case, you are trying to convince your readers, and if you credit them with intelligence, you will want to convince them by logic.

As used in this section, the terms "critical reading and thinking" apply in the broad sense of sound and adequate reasoning. Our treatment is necessarily brief, ignoring many technicalities more suitably taken up in a full course in logic. It also omits discussion of certain specific expository techniques that aid clear reasoning but are more properly taken up elsewhere. These techniques include the *definition and restriction of terms,* the ways of achieving *paragraph coherence,* and the ways of achieving *sentence unity.* You may wish to review these techniques in conjunction with this section, or your instructor may assign you to do so (see the index for the relevant chapters).

We start with a principle that underlies all that follows in these chapters. It is this: *unsound reasoning is often the result of ignorance rather than intentional deception or incurable bigotry; the person has not known enough, and perhaps has not cared enough, about the subject and has generalized hastily.* Consider a commonplace, daily example—the difference between an uninformed driver and the skilled mechanic. The car suddenly stalls and won't start. What does this driver frequently do? He or she checks the gas, finds the tank half full, opens the hood, and pokes around. With luck, he happens upon the fan belt and finds it intact. Now stuck, he concludes the battery must be dead because that's what happened last time. While looking for a phone and hoping that someone will stop, he again vows to himself to take a course in auto maintenance offered at the community college and to read through the manufacturer's manual, lying unopened these last months.

With skilled mechanics, it is quite otherwise. Taking their time, they proceed systematically, checking various possibilities until they find the source of trouble. Drawing on their knowledge about cars in general and this model in particular, they reason from known effect to probable cause until they solve the problem or realize the car will have to be towed to the garage for further inspection. Because they are informed, they do not generalize rashly; because they care, they are not hasty.

The point of this rather ordinary example is, first of all, our need to recognize what we don't know and to do whatever is necessary to become knowledgeable. When our information is scanty, our awareness is probably dim. We cannot see complexity, nuance, or difference. We do not know how to proceed and we risk the impulsive conclusion. (The skilled mechanic can be as foolish as anyone else on subjects he or she is ignorant about.) But most college subjects do demand that we recognize complexity, nuance, difference—as, indeed, do many of the things we study outside of the academy. Presently, we will discuss some guidelines for evaluating and shaping complex data into complex arguments and for judging among authorities in particular fields. Here, before looking at some more specific principles of critical reading and thinking, we simply wish to reiterate in slightly different terms the principle we began with: *to enhance sound reasoning, take the time necessary to do research and to be informed about your subject.*

16a The structure of an argument

The preliminaries of an argument are usually definitions. Having defined capital punishment as "execution, the death penalty for a crime," you can then argue for or against it. One "argument," or "reason," you might give for capital punishment is that it deters murder. A "reason" or "argument" against it might be that it does not deter murder. Note that the words "argument" and "reason" are interchangeable and that they imply an identical process of thinking.

In most discussions of logical analysis, the word *argument* signifies any two statements connected in such a way that one is drawn from the other. The argument has two parts: a premise (or evidence) and an inference (or immediate conclusion):

premise or evidence	inference or immediate conclusion
Capital punishment deters murder.	It should be continued.
Because capital punishment does not deter murder,	it should be abolished.

We use arguments constantly in writing and in speaking, and we recognize them by the actual or implied presence of connectives such as *because, so,* and *since,* and by auxiliaries such as *ought, should,* and *must.* The structure of an argument, then, is an observed fact or set of facts, or else a generalization presumably based on facts (the premise), leading to a conclusion (the inference). And usually we intend, though we may not always state explicitly, a final conclusion or point of the argument:

premise ————————▶ inference

I'm tired out *because* I've been studying too hard.

final conclusion

So I'll take a break now.

final conclusion ◀—— inference ————————▶ premise

She wasn't angry. She didn't mean it *since* she was joking about it later.

Usually, a final conclusion has several arguments, not simply one, to support it. The inference of one argument may be the premise for the next, and so on in a chainlike pattern to the final conclusion, the clasp:

premise 1 and . . .   premise 2

National prestige is fostered by   Successful countries
success in the Olympic games.   use professional athletes.

(inference from premises 1 and 2 becomes premise 3)

Since we wish to be successful in maintaining our prestige,

(inference from premise 3 becomes premise 4)

we cannot afford to field amateurs.

16a

final conclusion

Consequently, we should begin a program of national recruiting and full-time support for our Olympic athletes.

Several distinct strands of argument may be knotted into the one final conclusion, itself often the beginning of a paper or conversation:

final conclusion

There is no good reason for our starting a program of national recruiting and full-time support for our Olympic athletes.

first argument introduced   premise 1

To begin with, the modern games were not founded to foster nationalism. Professionalism is contrary to the intent of the games (inference from premise 1).

second argument introduced   premise 1

In the second place, nationalistic rivalries have made the protection of the athletes difficult and costly. This politicizing has made the games a great burden for the host country (inference from premise 1).

third argument introduced   premise 1 and so on to the end

Moreover, if one looks at the remarkable record of success that amateurs have had . . .

Just as a paragraph can develop several arguments to support one conclusion, so several paragraphs can each develop one or more arguments to support a thesis, itself a final conclusion.

If you are required to identify the premises and inferences of an argument— your own or someone else's—try an outline. Outlining assists critical reading by isolating the major issues and evidence; and it assists critical writing by systematically pinpointing areas of disagreement. So far, however, we have considered an argument's structure, not its truthfulness. An argument's structure may be quite consistent, yet its premises and conclusions may be unsound. One of the commonest causes of unsound arguments is the writer's failure to examine the key assumptions.

16b Key assumptions

A key assumption is a connection between the premise and the inference which is *taken for granted before* the argument is advanced; and it is a *presupposed* relationship between the argument and the final conclusion. Consider the following:

premise 1 and . . .   premise 2
Hayes has an A – average   Brookes has a B – average
(inference from premises 1 and 2 becomes premise 3)
Since Hayes is obviously a better student
(inference from premise 3 becomes premise 4)
he should do better work in a restricted creative writing course.

final conclusion
Consequently, he certainly should be given preference over Brookes.

Clearly, unless you *took for granted* that high school grades and creativity are related, you couldn't very well argue that Hayes's superior average was proof that he would do better work in the writing course than Brookes. The argument assumes *beforehand* that grades and creativity are connected. Nor could you *conclude* that Hayes ought to be given priority unless you had *presupposed* this relationship. Key assumptions are essentially a form of deductive logic, in which one moves from the general to the particular:

If   Academic success and success in creative writing are connected   **Premise**
If   Hayes has a better grade average than Brookes   **Premise**
Then   Hayes will be more successful as a creative writer.   **Conclusion**

Like the premises in deductive logic, the key assumptions underlying an argument must be sound before they are built on. If the assumptions are false or only partly true, the whole thing collapses. If the assumptions are unjustified, writers risk overlooking troublesome details that do not support them, and they may find unreal evidence that does. For example, if you were to assume that academic success and creativity are related (the key assumption), you would have to overlook the students with mediocre or even poor averages who are gifted painters, dancers, or poets, and you would have to ignore the intelligent honor students who seem to lack imagination, or at least seldom do more than safe, thorough work.

Key assumptions occur all the time, in all kinds of arguments and contexts—letters to the editor, talk show controversies, reviews of films and books, political campaigns. Consider each of the following arguments. Each (in one variation or another) is popular; each has one or more key assumptions. We need to ask two questions about each of these arguments: (1) What are the key assumptions? (2) Do these assumptions require explaining or defending? The first argument:

Argument: A great many of the movies that Hollywood makes give an unfair picture of American life because they show mainly its violence and its obsession with sex.

Assumptions:
1. That movies should give a "fair" picture of whatever they are picturing.
2. That there is such a thing as a "fair picture."
3. That violence and obsession with sex are not "typical" of American life.

Question: Are these self-evident assumptions?

The second argument:

Argument: Enriched courses for gifted students are a valuable addition to the high school curriculum because such courses offer these students a chance to fulfill college requirements and to begin specializing earlier.

Assumptions:
1. That college students should choose their major and specialize as soon as possible.
2. That the purpose of enriched high school courses is to satisfy college requirements, not to master a subject for its own sake.
3. That gifted students are particularly deserving of special attention.

Question: Are these self-evident assumptions?

16b

Because we *do* take key assumptions for granted not only in what we read and hear but also in what we write, we need to be especially conscious of our own. With a little attentiveness, it is relatively easy to detect the key assumptions others make. It is less easy to detect the ones we ourselves make. For example, when students write about short stories narrated by a first person "I," they sometimes *assume* that there must be a one-to-one correspondence between the narrator and the author in real life—that what happens to the narrator of the story is exactly what happened to the author. By failing to distinguish between the "I" as a device for telling the story and the writer's personal history and identity, the reader turns the story into autobiographical self-confession and distorts fact and fiction alike.

There are at least a couple of things you can do to help protect yourself against unsound assumptions and arguments built on them. These practices are essential to critical reading and writing. First, *make it a habit* to ask what other people are taking for granted in their arguments. If their key assumptions need challenging, challenge them. Second, *make it a habit* to ask yourself what you have taken for granted in your argument. If these assumptions need explaining, explain them; if they need defending, defend them. The exercises that follow are designed to give you this kind of practice.

Exercise 1

Consider each of the following arguments. Each (in one form or another) is wide-spread; each has one or more key assumptions. Analyze the argument to determine the key assumptions it makes and which of these, if any, would need to be explained or defended. If you find the assumptions shaky or untenable, specify your reasons for challenging them.

1. Politicians who take an unpopular stand during an election are foolish because they simply increase their chances of losing.
2. Civil rights laws are useless because morality can't be legislated.
3. Arguments about artistic merit or performance are pointless because all such judgments are based merely on personal likes and dislikes.
4. Nuclear policy should be left to the experts because the average person doesn't have enough information to know what's best.
5. It's a mistake to argue with teachers because they'll only mark you down; just give them what they want and take a good grade.

Exercise 2

Choose one of the topics below (or one of the arguments in Exercise 1) and write one paragraph of two hundred words or so, as rapidly as you can, and take a firm stand. Then analyze your paragraph with the following questions in mind: (1) What are the key assumptions? (2) Do they need defending? (3) What kinds of arguments or evidence would support them? Then *rewrite* the paragraph in the light of your analysis and compare it to your original. Have you made significant changes in your case?

1. Colleges should (should not) have required courses for all freshmen.
2. The major television networks should (should not) be left to themselves in matters of programming and censorship.
3. Public universities should (should not) impose fixed quotas on the number of out-of-state students they will admit.
4. Ticket scalping at popular events should (should not) be prohibited.
5. Drunk drivers should (should not) automatically be deprived of their licenses for a fixed period of time on their first arrest.

16b

Exercise 3

> Analyze a recent paper that you or your instructor found unsatisfactory as an argument with these questions in mind: (1) What are the key assumptions? (2) Should they have been questioned? (3) If so, how would you modify or defend them?

Exercise 4

> Ask the questions in Exercise 3 about an argument from a book or an essay you found unpersuasive.

16c The differences between fact and judgment

As the preceding exercises may have suggested, what can be proved and what one approves of do not always coincide. The differences between fact and judgment, though not always easy to determine in a given case, are important. A **fact** may be defined as any statement, any declarative sentence, that can be proved true. The definition says nothing about who does the proving, what their qualifications are, or how they prove it. It merely stipulates the possibility of verifying the statement, the central idea intended here. It rules out commands, questions, and exclamations as provable assertions—no one will try to prove or disprove utterances like "Shut the door!" "How old is she?" "Wow!"

The definition eliminates more than these obvious examples. "Water is wet"; "A yard has 3 feet"; "New York has more people than Chicago"; "Shakespeare was born in 1564"—most people would agree that such statements are all "facts." But saying "Water is wet" isn't the same as saying "The paint on the door is wet." The first sentence is either a *tautology*, a needless repetition of an idea to anyone familiar with the qualities of "waterness," or else instructions to a very young child on how to identify the feeling of liquid on his fingers. To say "A yard has 3 feet" is also to state a truth-by-definition—quite different from saying "The track was only 99 yards long." We can touch the paint and measure the track and thereby answer "Yes, it is" or "No, it isn't" to the assertion. But what point is there in responding "Yes, it is" or "No, it isn't" to statements like "Water is wet" or "A yard has 3 feet" except to agree with definition?

Some statements are verifiable facts because they are stated in quantifiable terms, that is, in such a way that what is asserted can be weighed, measured, or counted: "Jean weights 80 pounds," "The last discus throw was 147 feet," "There are two bluebooks apiece for the thirty-five of you." Even in these cases, of course, you assume that the scale or the tape measure is accurate, that neither has been jiggled, and that your index finger has not missed a cover or pointed at the same head twice. Other facts presuppose greater faith: If you believe that "New York has more people than Chicago" and "Shakespeare was born in 1564" are factual statements, you are not simply accepting the authority of an almanac and an encyclopedia. You are trusting the accuracy and conscientiousness of every census taker hired in these cities by the Bureau of the Census in 1980 and the reliability of scholars who have inspected the parish records of baptism in Stratford-on-Avon.

Admittedly, life is too short for anyone to verify personally more than a fraction of the "facts" he or she learns, and many things have to be taken on authority. Still, you ought to cultivate the habit of skeptical analysis in reading and writing. It can help you detect those judgments that are unverifiable—that are often "proved" in writing by heavy underlining and double exclamation marks and in conversation by rising voices and tempers. How, for instance, can one prove (or disprove) such statements as "You can't change human nature" or "Materialism is the greatest threat to our way of life"?

A **judgment** is a conclusion expressing some form of approval or disapproval. The term should not be dismissed because it is taken to connote "mere opinion." There are, after all, reasonable grounds and confirming facts for "good judgment" as well as the arbitrary assumptions and disregarded facts in "poor judgment." Sometimes the judgment is a fairly simple, safe inference from the facts, as in the judgment "Helen Wills Moody was one of the finest tennis players in the game's history," which is based on her winning the Women's National Singles seven times, the Women's National Doubles three times, and the Women's Singles at Wimbledon eight times. The phrase "one of the finest" is a judgment of her record. Sometimes, a judgment is a complicated inference from many facts, none of which is immediately clear. Consider three propositions, in which the judgments are italicized:

1. In 1940, there were 131,669,275 Americans, averaging 44.2 people per square mile; by 1980, *the population was larger and denser,* 226,545,805 people averaging 64 per square mile.

   This first statement contains the terms "larger" and "denser," which denote a factual inference. The statement is clearly factual and the inference results from a simple computation.

2. Between 1940 and 1980, as the *country became more urbanized and heavily populated, the American farm became more efficient through improved mechanization and specialization; it is now able to cultivate more land and feed an expanding population.*

   This second statement, a judgment, not only presupposes the first statement's facts but others as well. It presupposes the first statement in the judgment "more urbanized and heavily populated." But it assumes much more. To prove "efficient through increased mechanization," the writer would need figures showing the increased use of electricity and various kinds of power machinery. To prove "specialization," the writer would need

16c

data showing the increased percentage of farms that raise only crops of livestock, or produce only dairy goods. The evidence exists, of course, to defend the judgment that "the American farm has become more efficient."

3. *Profit-seeking specialization and mechanization are destroying the small, self-sufficient family farm in America and the deep attachment to the land and tradition that are so much a part of the family farm.*

In this third statement, the judgment is far more conspicuous than in the first two, and the facts are less immediately evident. To prove, for example, the existence of "the small, self-sufficient farm" with its "deep attachment to the land and tradition" would require detailed information. This information would have to include data about income, expenses, size of family, acreage worked, period of ownership without tenancy, length of political and religious affiliations, and a study of attitudes toward marriage, education, and the like. Such information might take the form of statistics or the extensive observations of qualified observers, or both. It would have to include the New York family raising some sheep and a few cows, some acres of wheat and garden tomatoes; the North Carolina family raising a hillside of tobacco and corn, supplemented by hogs and hunting; the Illinois family running a small dairy and orchard; the Colorado family raising grain and beef near the foothills of the Rockies; and the California family raising grapefruit and oranges near the desert's edge. Then the information about all of these families would have to be analyzed to see whether there is such a type as "the small self-sufficient family farm" with distinct values or whether there are sharply different regional variations.

16c

You can no more help making judgments about human actions and goals than the writer of the third statement could help feeling strongly about the changes taking place in the American farm. In fact, the writer might say that information about income and attitudes toward marriage had little to do with her judgment, that she was talking about qualities that could only be experienced personally. The grounds for this judgment might be her own life on a small Iowa farm or New Mexico ranch; novels like Willa Cather's *O Pioneers!,* Steinbeck's *The Red Pony,* or Harriette Arnow's *The Dollmaker;* short stories like those in Hamlin Garland's *Main-Travelled Roads;* movies like *Hud;* or the memories of a country doctor. The question would then be what other qualities are slighted. Do the films, fiction, and memoirs show only loyalty, belief, the close-knit family, and hard work? What of the fatigue and boredom, the bigotry and blighted vision, the drudgery and failure they reveal? Fiction, films, and memoirs are images of possibility, not mathematical probability: they can make us see, feel, and share the intensity and variety of human life in a particular time and place rather than convince us of statistical likelihood. If the writer argues that their details and experiences are "factually typical," she or he then assumes as true what only statistics or the extensive testimony of many qualified observers could confirm.

When you make judgments, then, express your facts clearly and accurately and show clearly the way in which the facts warrant your judgment; when you don't know the facts or have reason to suspect their authority, suspend judgment. And don't be reluctant to ask others to do the same. Try to distinguish between those judgments that involve personal preference and are not provable and those that may be supported by evidence and arguments. For your college writing, this advice implies your willingness to do research; to distinguish among facts, statements that may be factual, and judgments; and to tolerate uncertainty. The last is especially hard to do: often the experts in specialized fields are so much at odds that you either are tempted to give the matter up entirely or else arbitrarily decide "one side *must* be right, the other wrong, so I will choose." If, for example, you were to look up the statistics and analyses on capital punishment, you would find no clear-cut agreement among the criminologists, psychologists, and various law officials as to what the figures prove— and no agreement among the statisticians, either. But lives—the victim's, the accused murderer's, and their families'—are too important to be ignored simply because you cannot prove conclusively that capital punishment is or is not a deterrent. There are other factual grounds that may help you form a judgment: How many innocent men or women have been executed, or how many saved at the last minute? Do the poor and the uneducated receive the death sentence more frequently than others convicted of murder? How often are murderers declared insane, later to be released to commit another murder?

16c

As has been pointed out, we cannot verify personally more than a fraction of the "facts" we learn, and necessarily we have to take many things on authority. Still, when experts disagree about their facts and their judgments, there are a few helpful guides.

The first guide is to be sure that a supposed expert is an authority on the subject at hand. If a famous physicist and a chemist differ about disarmament, you may have to suspend judgment as far as their argument about the technical difficulties is concerned, but you don't have to feel that either of them is an expert on the Soviet Union and Soviet foreign policy. Other writers and scholars have made the study of Soviet aims and behavior their life's work, and you should turn to them.

A second guide is to consider the experts' probable motives in relation to their testimony. An executive for a major car manufacturer who testifies that "all reasonable efforts have been taken to make economical, unpolluting cars" may well not be as reliable an authority as a writer for an independent trade magazine or engineering firm.

A third guide is to see whether others in the field agree about the strengths or weaknesses in an expert's research. Suppose that you are doing a project on the attitudes of high school students toward their teachers. If book reviewers generally praise a husband-and-wife team for their studies of suburban students but criticize their failure to study inner-city students as thoroughly, you would want to confine yourself to the couple's discussion of suburban students only, and look elsewhere for evidence about the feelings of inner-city students.

Exercise 5

For practice, consider the following statements. Determine which parts of each are facts and which parts are judgments. For each judgment, decide what kind(s) of facts or evidence, if any, could be cited to support the judgment.

1. Smoke Cigarmellos! They last longer, burn cooler, and are easier on you than cigarettes. They are cleaner and cheaper than pipes.
2. Julius Caesar, Rome's greatest general and ruler, was asassinated in 44 B.C. by Cassius, Brutus, and other personal enemies.
3. A meter equals 39.37 inches.
4. A kilometer contains 1,000 meters.
5. Kareem Abdul-Jabbar is one of the finest offensive players of all time in professional basketball.
6. If one compares the number of talented women now entering law schools with the number twenty years ago, one sees how wasteful of abilities those sexist admissions policies were.
7. The concern over "computer literacy" is just another educational fad, largely promoted by manufacturers rather than by genuine demand.
8. Real mastery of a foreign language means the ability to think in the language, not simply to translate headlines and signs, word by word.
9. There is no clear evidence one way or another about the effectiveness of strict gun laws in preventing crime.
10. The early bird catches the worm—but who wants the worm?

16c

Exercise 6

Pick a controversial issue you feel strongly about and summarize your views in two or three sentences. Then analyze your sentences with the following questions in mind: What evidence can you cite to support your judgments? Do you make judgments that are difficult to support?

Exercise 7

Choose two of your papers—preferably a good one and a weaker one—and analyze each to determine how well the judgments were supported by evidence. Is the weaker paper characterized by unsupported judgments or unsupportable judgments? Try revising a paragraph or two to make the judgments more convincing.

Exercise 8

Choose a paper to be revised (either a rough draft for a paper due or an essay that has been returned for rewriting) and go over it carefully, marking every judgment. If you find judgments that are unsupported, try revising them to make them more convincing.

Exercise 9

Choose a piece from the editorial page—a signed opinion column, a letter, an editorial—and underline its judgments. Are they supported? If not, draft an answer in which you show how or why they are unreasonable or unconvincing.

16d Believability and tone

From one viewpoint, the aim of most writers is believability. Novelists usually strive to make their stories realistic. Dramatists usually contrive to make their plots and characters credible. Even authors who play with the fantastic and the imaginary want to gain the reader's consent. A satirist like Swift in *Gulliver's Travels,* a fabulist like Tolkien in *Lord of the Rings,* or a science fiction writer like Ursula K. Le Guin in *The Left Hand of Darkness* tries to make a fictional world that is internally consistent and that obliquely refers to our world. Here, as the term applies to argumentation, we will use "believability" in a more limited sense. By it, we mean the reader's belief that the writer's reasoning can be trusted.

Several factors contribute to your reader's trust in your case. These include the orderliness of your argument, the plausibility of your assumptions, the persuasiveness of your evidence, and the accuracy of your logic. But these factors may not be enough to earn the reader's confidence. Even if the assumptions are defended, the conclusions supported by detail, and the arguments free of obvious errors, the tone may offend. Quite rightly, readers become skeptical when they feel the writer is trying to crowd them or compel their assent by vehement or dogmatic insistence. Consider the following paragraph:

> Lurking behind the walls of trailers and apartments, concealed by the privacy of homes, suppressed by the terror of its helpless victims, domestic violence is destroying the integrity of the American family! It shatters children and marriages; it releases the most hideous emotions and feelings humans are capable of. It is the most sordid display of depravity one can imagine. No social evil is more vicious! Domestic violence threatens the very foundations of our society.

What offends here is not the writer's choice of subject (the destructiveness and prevalence of domestic violence can be documented) but his choice of tactics. He assaults his topic and reader with exclamation marks, unqualified statements, and highly charged words like *hideous, sordid,* and *vicious.* He leaves no room for honest differences of opinion and judgment; for example, readers who might feel that drug addiction or alcoholism poses as great a social problem as domestic violence does. However reasonable the rest of his case, he has risked losing the reader's trust by a lack of moderation. Now consider the same paragraph rewritten to earn credibility:

> One of the serious social problems in America is domestic violence. Because its victims, usually women and young children, are often frightened and silent, the magnitude of this problem is not always recognized. The privacy of the home—whether trailer, apartment, or house—too frequently conceals its consequences. But the bruised child, the battered wife or lover, and the angry, confused male all find themselves trapped, the law and social agencies unable to intervene until violence has already occurred, and not always easily even then.

The revision solicits concern, not unquestioning acceptance or submission.

A believable tone is a moderate one. It allows for other viewpoints and alternatives without compromising the writer's basic conviction. For instance:

> For many Americans, domestic violence may seem a deplorable but less acute social disorder than alcoholism. The effects of domestic violence are not, perhaps, as visibly publicized and dramatic as certain effects of alcoholism—the televised image of the totaled car and the paramedics arriving, and the escalating rates of injury and death. But its long-term results are, far too often, the battered child who becomes the battering adult. Although it receives less attention and less research funding than alcoholism, its consequences are not less tragic.

A moderate tone also recognizes connections where connections exist and concedes what is unknown:

16d

> In reality, domestic violence and alcoholism are not wholly separate social disorders. Each frequently contributes to the other, and neither is fully understood in its causes.

In short, a moderate tone trusts its evidence and the reader's intelligence. The argument is believable because the writer invites belief.

To summarize, the basic ingredients in persuasion include the elements we have discussed so far. We now turn to more specific problems in reasoning, instances where the logic is faulty and needs correcting.

Exercise 10

Choose one of the following topics and write a paragraph in which you make the tone as dogmatic and as vehement as you can. Then rewrite the paragraph to make the tone moderate and believable.

1. A case for or against athletic scholarships.
2. A case for or against a minimum legal drinking age.
3. A case for or against prayer in public schools.
4. A case for or against police roadblocks to catch drunken drivers.
5. A case for or against the use of animals in medical research.

17 Avoiding Errors in Reasoning

The failure to examine key assumptions and the confusion of fact with judgments are not the only causes of faulty reasoning. Of the other causes, hasty generalizing is one of the most common. And, as with other causes of unsound logic, hasty generalizations often result from the writer's not knowing enough about the subject. Faulty reasoning can also result from mistaken causal relationships and bad analogies, both to be discussed later in this chapter.

17a Hasty generalizations

To generalize is to *draw conclusions* about a *whole class* or *group* after studying some members of the group. A **hasty generalization** is one drawn from too few members or from nontypical members. Suppose, for instance, that after meeting two bright, articulate, and friendly freshman counselors who are also English teachers, you are convinced that the English department must be outstanding for its teaching. Do you have reasons to question this generalization? Yes, because your sampling may be quite unrepresentative and in any case is quite small. The counselors were probably chosen for this job because they are so effective. But even so, suppose you still have a hunch that the English department is outstanding for its teaching. How would you establish such a generalization?

Establishing an accurate generalization usually requires several steps. First, you would have to identify the group *outstanding department* by defining it as, say, the one whose members consistently receive the highest ratings on student evaluations. Otherwise, the generalization is no more than a vague judgment. You would then have to show that there was a higher percentage of the English department rated at the top of the evaluations than other departments. Otherwise, the outstanding department is no more likely to be the English department than any other.

To establish an effective generalization, you have to identify clearly the group or groups about which you are generalizing, and you must study enough individual members of the group to ensure that they represent the group as a whole. Failure to observe these principles usually results in hasty generalizations.

Not all generalizations can be as easily established as the one above. In cases where all the relevant facts about a limited group are available, one may indeed generalize by simply counting or checking accurately—a parking attendant inspects each car on the lot and generalizes that all headlights are off; a dean reviews all the high school transcripts and generalizes that every freshman has had at least a year of foreign language before entering the college. But much of the time it is not possible to do a complete check. Necessarily, one also generalizes by **induction,** that is, by observing a number of specific examples of the group and then concluding that other examples will *probably* be like those observed. Young children use induction when, after grabbing at two or three cats, they conclude that all cats scratch. Later, when they understand what grabbing is and when they have seen more cats, they learn to generalize that most cats will not scratch unless they are grabbed. Pollsters use induction when they question a representative sample of the voters to determine how all voters feel or will probably vote. If their cross section is not representative, they will be embarrassed. A consumers' research organization uses induction when it purchases all the different brands of a mass-produced item, tests several samples of each brand carefully, and then generalizes about which brands are likely to be the best buys and in what ways.

The **stereotype** is one form of hasty generalizing—the trite, unchanging picture of an ethnic group, a profession, or social role. "He's the typical macho male—a sexist and a bully." "She's the typical feminist—loud and aggressive." Other stereotypes are the bossy mother-in-law, the dumb athlete, the crooked politician, the happy, singing Italian, the stoned Californian, and so forth. Stereotypes are crude caricatures that deny the variety and diversity of actual life.

17a

Oversimplification is another form of hasty generalizing. Usually, it entails making a question seem easier than it is. Statistics, especially, can lead to oversimplifying. For example, if two groups have a markedly different class average on a reading comprehension test, you could not generalize that every member of the first class was better than every member of the second class. Since a few very high scores might have pulled up some mediocre ones in the averaging, you would have to compare all the individual scores to reach such a conclusion. Still less would you be entitled to simplify the results by generalizing that one group was "innately" better than the other. You would have to know a great deal about the income and the education of the parents, the reading matter (if any) in the homes, each child's previous training, the hours spent watching TV, and other crucial factors before drawing any conclusions.

The **unqualified generalization** makes a third form of hasty generalizing, the exaggerated claim made from insufficient evidence. Some years ago, on the basis of a peace petition signed by a few thousand college students, a commentator generalized that all undergraduates were becoming pacifists. His sampling was highly inadequate. He ignored not only those who refused to sign but also those who were being drafted. The unqualified generalization is a rather frequent weakness in college writing: for example, "All the freshmen think 'Orientation Week' is a waste of time" or "Not one woman student in the whole college trusts the Dean." To the question "How do you know? Have you talked with every freshman or every woman?" the writer usually answers: "Of course not, but I know several [or some] people who feel. . . ." The least the writer can do is to rephrase the generalization more accurately and responsibly by identifying the approximate numbers involved and the source of the real evidence: "Several of us who are freshmen and attended 'Orientation Week' with high hopes have decided that . . ." or "After the women on our corridor had met with the Dean, we agreed that. . . ."

In order to generalize effectively, you need to know some criteria of generalizations. Since generalizations are made about classes or groups, *the first criterion of generalizations is that the evidence be typical of the class or group.* An assignment using freshmen on the debate team as the basis for generalizing about the speaking abilities of all members of the freshman class would be as unconvincing as an essay that used the followers of the Ayatollah Khomeini to generalize about the beliefs of all Moslems.

Often, though, the untypicality is less crude, more a question of interpretation than of outright error. Are Hemingway's heroes and heroines in *A Farewell to Arms* and *The Sun Also Rises* "typical" of the period in their disillusionment with World War I and its aftermath? If you read Hemingway's novels you will agree on some conclusions: Hemingway's heroes and heroines do distrust "causes" and conventional moralities—they say so and ignore them. Many of your most interesting writing assignments will be ones like this, or at least ones in which you use complex facts for complex judgments. When you have to evaluate typicality, define what features you believe typical and show how these features are found in the evidence. If you had read only the two Hemingway novels, but none of F. Scott Fitzgerald, John Dos Passos, or Ford Madox Ford about this period, you would want to confine your discussion of typicality to Hemingway's novels.

The second criterion of generalizations is that the evidence be adequate. Americans spending a few days in London or Madrid, Europeans touring the United States for two weeks, or students visiting Washington, D.C., for a weekend have many superficial impressions, some of them probably accurate. But if they generalize "The English are reserved" or "Americans are friendly but ignorant," they reveal more about themselves than about the English or Americans. Other examples of inadequate evidence are the essay citing the two police officers who were reprimanded for roughness as proof that the city's thousands of police officers are brutal, or a term paper citing the suicide of one rock star to show that all rock stars are deeply unhappy, tormented people. Like typicality, adequacy is sometimes difficult to judge—anthropologists finding only a jaw fragment and a few bones or archeologists finding only a faded temple painting may have to infer what they can and hope for more evidence. But you can assist yourself and your reader by saying why you think your evidence is adequate and for what, if there is likely to be doubt. If only one half of the 250 freshmen vote for class officers, you have adequate evidence that "something" is wrong with morale, but you would have to talk with many of the nonvoters to find out what it is.

The third criterion of generalizations is that the evidence be relevant. Figures showing that all fraternities on campus have a "C" average or better would not be proof that fraternities produce outstanding students. The figures would be more pertinent to the generalization that fraternities care enough about their eligibility to satisfy academic requirements. In a different fashion, the fact that an artist or musician was once a communist or a fascist is irrelevant evidence to prove his work incompetent, if you define incompetence as a lack of artistic ability or skill. The only way he can be shown to be incompetent is by musical or artistic standards of performance. You might find it personally distasteful to attend his exhibit or recital, but if you condemn his present work because of his past associations, you adopt the propaganda view of art and the illogic used by the Nazis in persecuting "non-Aryan" writers and writing, and by the Soviets in their harassment of Pasternak, Solzhenitsyn, and others.

The fourth criterion of generalizations is that the evidence be accurate. This standard seems self-evident, yet if you were to read through the long, careful book reviews in such publications as *Scientific American,* the *American Historical Review,* or the *Journal of American Folklore,* you would find two common criticisms: that the writer has been careless about checking facts, and indiscriminate about sources. In cases of extreme carelessness, the reviewer legitimately questions the author's right to be trusted, regardless of how original the ideas are. The most helpful guides you have are the ones for expert testimony: Does the information come from a recognized source? What are the person's announced motives or position in relation to the evidence? What agreement is there among others in the field about strengths or weaknesses in the researcher's work? Like an editor or reviewer, your teacher has greater confidence and pleasure in conclusions based on accurate evidence.

17b Mistaken causal relationships

Mistaken causal relationships are errors in reasoning about cause and effect. Perhaps the two most frequent kinds are the *post hoc, ergo propter hoc* fallacy and the *reductive fallacy.*

The **post hoc, ergo propter hoc** fallacy is the error of arguing that because B follows A, A is the cause of B. (In Latin, *post hoc, ergo propter hoc* means "after this, therefore because of this.") Sequence is not proof of a causal relationship. The fact that B follows A is not proof that B was caused by A. Primitive beliefs like a full moon "causing" pregnancy and their modern equivalent in the television commercial connecting marriage with a change in deodorant are easy enough to laugh at. But clear thinking on serious social problems can be obscured by this fallacy. For example, the assertion that heroin addiction is the result of smoking marijuana not only ignores the fact that most people who try or use pot never touch heroin but it also may divert attention from the real need—the understanding of the psychological and physiological factors that do contribute to addiction. And what of the unqualified generalization that makes the loss of religious belief the cause of crime? Crimes are also committed by people who profess religious belief; and not every person who loses his or her faith commits a crime.

The **reductive fallacy** occurs when simple or single causes are given for complex effects, creating a generalization based on insufficient evidence. In history, when motives and events are enormously complicated and cannot be exactly duplicated, such generalizations as "Athens fell because of mob rule," "Luther caused the Reformation," or "The need to rebel caused the campus demonstrations of the 1960s" are reductive. That is, instead of specifying the mob or Luther as one important condition, these assertions make Luther or the mob the single agent of causation. Such generalizations tend to reduce history to caricature. Strictly speaking, historians rarely uncover the cause or causes of events. Rather, they try to decide which conditions were important and were more probably necessary for the event to take place. In scientific studies when a sequence cannot be directly observed and controlled and the investigators cannot know whether Y is the result of X only or W and X together, or whether X and Y are both the result of W, they speak of a correlation. In 1964, when the Surgeon General announced a high correlation between cigarette smoking and lung cancer, he indicated that one was probably a contributory cause of the other. But since not all heavy smokers die of lung cancer and since there is evidence that industrial fumes and car exhaust are injurious in this regard, one cannot say that smoking is the only cause of lung cancer. Insofar as they cannot directly isolate, identify, and control each factor in a sequence, scientists, like historians, usually observe the test of sufficiency; only if A alone is sufficient to produce B can it be called the cause of B.

Except for laboratory reports in physics or chemistry and perhaps a research project in psychology or education, you will seldom have space or occasion in college writing to prove a strictly causal relationship. Usually, so far as causal relations are concerned, you will be judging or reporting on research done by others, or else trying to determine what the probable connections are between an effect you have observed or experienced and events preceding it.

To let your readers judge the *sufficiency* of your argument, define its conditions and limitations as clearly as you can. With complex relationships, it is

17b

often helpful to know that there is a significant difference between saying "It is due to" and "It has been helped by," just as there is between saying "Luther caused" and "Luther contributed to" or "The reason for the Revolution" and "One reason for the Revolution." The limited statement can be more exact because it is more tentative: It implies that other conditions, other contributing factors, may be as important as the one singled out for discussion. This kind of exact tentativeness requires careful, analytical thinking. When you analyze complex historical events and personalities, complex social issues, and complex motives, avoid the reductive fallacy.

17c Reasoning by analogy

An **analogy** is a comparison between two different things or events showing the way or ways in which they are similar. To illustrate, for example, how the novelist works, one could draw the analogy between the writer and the potter: both begin with a rough idea or image, but discover the particular shape of the plot or vase as they work with their materials, often modifying the outlines several times before they are satisfied.

Analogies can vividly illustrate and clarify difficult ideas. In the following student paragraph, for example, the writer has used her analogy skillfully to describe the complex techniques of a satirist:

17c

> The sight of a monkey pushing through the jungle, leaping from tree to tree, seems "natural" and, perhaps, graceful. However, when a monkey is placed in a small cage or zoo, his boundings from side to floor to side to ceiling seem antic and "unnatural." The satirist employs the same techniques of limitation. He confines his subject, as it were, to a small cage, or at least one tree, for purposes of close observation. The setting in which he moves his object is limited and its barriers are precisely drawn. The satirist, in effect, traps the victim in his most ridiculous positions and does not allow him to wander off or in any way escape an intensely mocking portrayal.
> [The writer recognizes that her analogy, however vivid, is an illustration, not proof, when she says, "He confines his subject, *as it were*. . . ."]

Analogies have been fruitful in science because they have suggested new lines of research and testing. Franklin saw a similarity between lighting and electric sparks; the similarity between X rays and the rays emitted by uranium salts raised questions about the source and nature of this energy, and eventually led to Marie Curie's discovery of radium; mathematicians such as John von Neumann, instrumental during the early development of computers, saw an analogy between the way the human nervous system works and the way a relay of vacuum tubes can be made to work. In science, an analogy only sets up a hypothesis to be proved or disproved. Although it suggests a possibility, it is not proof by itself.

An analogy can be illustrative or suggestive, but it cannot be conclusive. You do well to suspect any conclusions that are supported only by an analogy. Sometimes, a false analogy offered as proof is relatively easy to detect. The student who argued that the new African countries should have federated into a United States of Africa to solve their political and economic problems ignored some obvious dissimilarities with the American colonies. The latter, unified by language and a common foe, had in most cases a long tradition of local self-government. African countries are separated from each other by deep linguistic and cultural differences and in several cases are inwardly divided by tribal rivalries. This analogy also ignores the difficulties we had—the failure of the Articles of Confederation and the opposition to the Constitution.

Often, however, false analogies may be even more deceiving. Two principles will help you cope with them:

1. The more concrete similarities there are and the more instances that can be cited, the higher is the possibility that the conclusion is true.
2. The greater the magnitude of the differences and the more irrelevant the similarities that do exist, the less is the chance the conclusion is true.

False analogies obscure the real issues of and prevent clear thinking about serious and difficult questions. To detect analogies used as proof, examine the argument to see if any evidence is offered other than a comparison between two different things or events. In your own writing, if you think an analogy is essential to your argument, rethink your entire case: don't allow yourself to be taken in by shallow or deceiving similarities.

17d Avoiding the question

When writers fail to give relevant evidence for their arguments or fail to draw relevant inferences, they are **avoiding the question.**

Begging the question is one such common failure. A question is begged when writers use as a proven argument the very point they are trying to prove. For example, columnists who argue that the poor are lazy and cite families on welfare as "evidence" are assuming without proof that only lazy opportunists take relief—the very point to be demonstrated.

The **ad hominem** argument—the argument "to the man"—is a second common form. Here, the tactic is to condemn the morals, motives, friends, or family of one's opponent and to divert attention from the substance of the opponent's argument. For instance: "How could you possibly agree with Berloff about the school bond? I hear from some people he's a real snob." The issue is the school bond, not Berloff's alleged snobbery. The evaluation of expert testimony should not be confused with the *ad hominem* argument: in the former, you ask what a person's professional credentials are and the reasons for his or her position—that is, you attempt to distinguish between fact and judgment; in the latter, you insinuate by sarcasm or similar means that a case is unsound because there is something wrong with the person making it.

The **straw man** is another device commonly used for avoiding the question. As the label implies, the technique is to stuff and set up a dummy issue that is substituted for the real issue. If the question is whether or not Shylock deserves his punishment and the writer goes to great lengths to prove that bitterness can make a man lonely, the writer is erecting a straw man. The issue is whether Shylock is treated too severely, by either his own standards or Christian ones. No one argues the fact that bitterness can isolate people.

17e False alternatives

The false **either/or** deduction is a common but easily avoided error. The error lies in assuming that there are only two alternatives and that if one of them is true, the other must be false. If parents tell a child, "You must be lazy because the only reasons for poor school work are laziness or stupidity, and I know you aren't dumb," the parents commit this error. They ignore other alternatives: the child may be bored with easy work, or he may lack adequate training, or he may be unhappy for a variety of reasons. Ideological slogans often make this kind of phony simplification—"Communism versus Capitalism," "The Free World versus Tyranny," "Education versus Indoctrination," and the like. The careful writer will rethink the false alternatives in order to discover what the more complex possibilities really are.

17f

17f Non sequiturs

In Latin, *non sequitur* means "It does not follow." A **non sequitur** occurs when there is no connection between the premise and the conclusion, as in the following: "Carolyn likes algebra so she ought to be a good treasurer." The connection between liking algebra and taking care of money is entirely unclear.

Exercise 1

To sharpen your eye for others' fallacies, take a newspaper and turn to the editorial and opinion section. Go through it carefully, isolating and analyzing any errors you find. Better still, if there's an issue you feel strongly about or a column you find particularly objectionable, write a letter to the editor pointing out how the reasoning is unsound.

Exercise 2

To sharpen your eye for fallacies in your own writing, go over some of your back papers as if they had been written by a stranger. What kinds of logical errors do you find? Now, try revising the material logically, as if you were doing a favor for a good friend.

Exercise 3

Analyze each of the following generalizations by the four criteria suggested in **17a**. Be prepared to explain *which* generalizations are defective and in what ways.

1. From a recent faculty committee meeting: "Students are making a farce out of the government's low-interest loan program for college financing. The percentage of students who deliberately default is steadily rising, and there's no reason to think it will drop or that students will begin to feel responsible for paying the money they owe. The whole program is just a waste of the taxpayer's money."
2. From a recent "Letters to the Editor" column: "How can your editorial writer deny that Americans are the most wasteful, extravagant consumers of gas in the world! Drive along any expressway or freeway at rush hours and count all the cars with only one passenger and look at the miles of bumper-to-bumper traffic."
3. From a recent college newspaper: "This school has the worst meals of all the state colleges. Any athlete or debater can tell you the meals you get at other colleges make the ones we get look awful."
4. From the *Guinness Book of World Records:* "The only admissible evidence upon the true height of giants is that of recent date made under impartial medical supervision. Biblical claims, such as that for Og, King of Bashan, at 9 Assyrian cubits (16 feet 2½ inches) are probably due to a confusion of units. Extreme mediaeval data from bone measurements refer invariably to mastodons or other nonhuman remains. Claims of exhibitionists, normally under contract not to be measured, are usually distorted for the financial considerations of promoters. There is an example of a recent 'World's Tallest Man' of 9 feet 6 inches being in fact an acromegalic of 7 feet 3½ inches."

Exercise 4

Analyze each of the following statements of causal relationship to determine which ones are guilty of the *post hoc, ergo propter hoc* fallacy or the reductive fallacy.

1. More than two thirds of the people in our state voted for the limitation on the state property tax and deliberately deprived local communities of all kinds of services. The only explanation is sheer selfishness; they were afraid of higher taxes.
2. All the children in the remedial reading class watch at least twenty hours of television a week. With all that passive sitting, no wonder they can't read.
3. It is not surprising that the divorce rate is climbing; all those young couples splitting up now grew up during the chaos of the 1960s; they never had a chance at a stable environment.
4. Since 1940, the government has gotten bigger and bigger, and taxes have gone higher and higher. The conclusion is obvious.

Exercise 5

Analyze each of the following analogies to determine whether it is used as an illustration, a hypothesis suggesting further investigation, or proof.

1. From a pamphlet: "Pornographic literature is arsenic that poisons the system. It's not enough to label it and put it on the shelf. Just as some children can't read the

label on the bottle and others want to experiment, some juveniles and adults can't discriminate and others are tempted by the warning. Such books should be locked up in libraries where only scholars with reason for using them can get at them, in the same way druggists only sell arsenic from behind the counter by special permission."

2. From a composition handbook: "Many of the rules in this book, making no mention of exceptions or permissible alternatives, are dogmatic—purposely so. If a stranger is lost in a maze of city streets and asks for directions, one doesn't give him the several possible routes, with comments and cautions about each. He will simply become more confused and lost. One sends him arbitrarily on one route without mentioning equally good alternative ways. Likewise, the unskilled writer can best be set right by simple, concise, stringent rules."

3. From a student editorial: "The administration never gets tired of telling us that the state college is part of society as a whole. It harps on student responsibility for 'good taste' in plays and publications, student responsibility to obey state laws about drinking and driving, and student responsibility for property. By the same line of reasoning, then, how can the administration claim it has the final right to approve of campus organizations and their speakers? If the state university is part of 'society as a whole,' it ought to recognize our rights as well as our obligations. We aren't asking for the privilege of being subversive; we are asking for the civil rights we have in 'society as a whole'—the rights to hear whom we wish and join the groups we wish."

4. From a student theme: "The college has the same obligation to satisfy the student that a store does to satisfy the customer. Students and their parents pay the bills, and they ought to have a much freer say about what courses they take. No clerk would think of telling a customer he had to buy several things he didn't want before he could buy the item he came for. And no store would keep as clerks some of the men the college keeps as professors. They can't even sell their product."

5. From a medical journal: "If you place a number of mice together in fairly close quarters and then systematically introduce an increasing variety of distractions— small noises, objects, movements—you increase the probability of neurotic behavior. Cannot something like this process help explain the growth of neurotic behavior in our ever more crowded, complex society? The possibility is worth considering."

17f

Exercise 6

Pick one of the following analogies and write a paragraph using the analogy as proof. Then, in a second paragraph, show precisely how the analogy is false or misleading, as you have developed it.

1. The family budget and the federal budget
2. The referee in boxing and the arbiter in labor disputes
3. The captain of a ship and the president of a democracy
4. Packaging the goods well and giving a lecture well
5. Determining the warnings on chemicals and determining the ratings of films

Exercise 7

The following statements contain unsound reasoning. Identify the different kinds of fallacies and specify what change, if any, would improve the argument.

1. Either you trust a person or you don't. And you don't do business with someone you don't trust. The same principle ought to be observed in foreign affairs; you don't do business with countries you can't trust.

2. Anyone with a grain of sense would have known that the county didn't need to buy land for a park. But those officials don't learn easily. It wasn't proof enough for them that a majority voted against the purchase in the election. They had to go to the state legislature and get voted down, too.

3. Freshman "Hell Week" is one of the oldest and dearest traditions of the college. Many of us alumni can remember having our heads shaved and getting up at midnight for roll calls and jogs around the track. Those of us on the Alumni Board oppose the abolition of the custom. We find the arguments for doing away with "Hell Week" childish and tiresome. We were good enough sports to go along with the sophomores in our time.

4. I don't see why I received such a low grade on this term paper. I put in hours of work on it and did several rough drafts. And I followed the format you asked for. It doesn't seem fair.

5. Any man who supports the Equal Rights Amendment has either been brainwashed by feminists or else has no guts.

6. To be an actor, you have to be on a real ego trip. That's why people become actors. All you have to do is look at any famous star and you'll see the living proof.

7. Laws against smoking on trains, in restaurants and theaters, and in other public places discriminate against my right of free choice. If I want to take the risks with my health because of the pleasure I get, that's my business. I'm not trying to tell others how to live their lives.

8. "Reflection on Ice-Breaking"
   Candy
   Is dandy
   But liquor
   Is quicker

   —Ogden Nash

Exercise 8

The following is a satire, written by a student, of the arbitrary assumptions, unexamined generalizations, and misleading analogies, which all too often are found in print. In analyzing the argument, see how many of these logical errors you can find.

Why Have Teachers?

In the early days of America, before the establishment of compulsory schooling, moral standards were high. People were contented with the simpler virtues. Girls learned to sew, cook, and keep house; men, to farm or work at some trade. Marriages were stable and happy; there was no such thing as divorce. Today this happy scene has changed—the morals of modern America

17f

are corrupted. Every newspaper carries stories of murder, embezzlement, adultery, and divorce. What has caused this shocking situation? Is it possible to regain the happy state of early America?

The most influential institution during the formative years of each American is the school, governed and dominated by the teachers. From these teachers children learn the human faults of blind obedience, prejudice, and the betrayal of one's kind in the form of tattling. These early sown seeds bear the bitter fruit of low morality. Clearly, teachers do much to undermine the morality of American children, and through them, that of society.

The obvious solution is to eliminate the teacher as much as possible. The modern child is increasingly capable of educating himself. There are more college students today than ever before, a fact which proves that youth today possess superior intelligence. By educating themselves, they would not be subjugated to the influence of teachers. They would share their knowledge willingly, each gaining from the other, with no one person dominating the others.

Cynics will sneer that this system is impractical, that students need guidance and even indoctrination in fundamentals before they can think on their own. Nothing could be further from the truth! One of the most clear-thinking, intelligent men in this nation's history, Abraham Lincoln, was almost entirely self-educated. Think of the effect on our society of an entire generation with the training and characteristics of Lincoln. The present immorality would disappear; a high moral standard would be developed. The group that is undermining morality would be minimized in its influence, and the education of American youth placed where it belongs—in the hands of these same youth.

17f

18 Writing about Literature

I know noble accents
And lucid, inescapable rhythms;
But I know, too,
That the blackbird is involved
In what I know.

From "Thirteen Ways of Looking at a Blackbird,"
by Wallace Stevens

Like the speaker in Stevens's poem, as readers we have known "noble accents" and "lucid, inescapable rhythms" in the poems, plays, and stories we have read. And, like the speaker reflecting on the blackbird, perhaps we have reflected on our involvement with the work. Stevens's lines suggest several major challenges in writing about literature. How to understand our relationship to the work? How to share our experience of it most effectively with other readers? How to convince others that ours is a valid way of looking at the work?

Obviously, in this short chapter we can only offer a few guidelines to thinking and writing about literature. These are complex subjects, certainly not to be reduced to rules such as those for the uses of the apostrophe. Nevertheless, we can say some things about the questions posed above that will make your writing about literature more effective and more pleasurable. For convenience, we will divide our discussion into three broad categories: Inhibiting Assumptions, Productive Questions, and Useful Strategies.

18a Inhibiting assumptions

By "inhibiting assumptions," we mean those preconceptions and attitudes students often bring to the academic study of literature that block clear thinking and writing. Such assumptions make students distrust their abilities, or make them defensive and dogmatic, or both. You are probably familiar with one of these inhibiting assumptions: the notion that writing about literature requires some esoteric technique or special logic, mastered only by the gifted few. You may have heard friends say (and felt yourself) something like the following:

"What does she want me to say? I don't know how to write about poetry." "How am I supposed to put this essay together? I don't know what to do with the novel."

These and similar remarks frequently assume that reasoning about literature is different from, say, reasoning about history, psychology, or biology. Clearly the materials being reasoned *about* do differ. Literary characters and events are not the same as actual persons and historical events, or the theories of perception and personality studied in psychology. But a little reflection should suggest that the principles of clear exposition—defining and developing a topic, observing and describing evidence accurately, supporting generalities by detail—do *not* change. Consider your own experience of discussing a film or novel with friends outside of class. You agree or disagree that a character or event was or was not significant and say why (stating a topic and its implications). You recall your impressions of the character or event as fully as you can; sometimes you are corrected by your friends, sometimes you correct them (observing and describing evidence). And you connect the details you remember to the judgment you are defending (supporting generalizations).

In short, we question the assumption that thinking and writing about literature require a special logic because we often do make sense about it to each other. Usually, such discussions occur naturally and spontaneously, without our worrying self-consciously about method. The belief that there must be some arcane technique for discussing literature probably results, in part at least, from the way subjects are divided by the curriculum—literature in one room, history in another, and biology in a third, each subject with its own procedures and terminology, none apparently related to the other. But this division of labor (and that is mainly what a curriculum is) can unduly inhibit us. It can make us question our ability to communicate effectively in the academic setting, even though we have talked intelligibly about a variety of works in more informal settings.

18a

This, then, is one inhibiting asumption. Another assumption—a pair of assumptions, actually—concerns the authority of interpretations. At one extreme is the belief that there must be a single, unambiguous, "correct" interpretation of a given work. At the other extreme is the belief that since all interpretations are wholly subjective and individual, none is better than another. You recognize these contrary views in the simple ways they are often stated. In effect, the first says, "Well, what *is* the right interpretation of the poem? There must be one." The second says, "I don't see what's wrong with my interpretation. After all, it's just a matter of personal opinion."

Now these assumptions are not entirely unwarranted. We have been taught that right answers exist. We have also learned that people's tastes differ, sometimes irreconcilably. But, again, if we turn to our experience outside of the classroom, we probably find that we are more discriminating. Experience has very likely taught us that right answers may be found in some areas but not in others. In matters that involve simple calculation or measurement—arithmetic, chemistry labs, and the like—we reasonably expect to find the correct solution. In matters of human choice, motive, and action (the substance of literature), however, we have to master the demanding discipline of tolerating ambiguity and perplexity. The poet John Keats called this discipline "Negative Capability" and described it as one's ability to accept "uncertainties, mysteries, doubts, without any irritable reaching after fact and reason." However strongly we may wish otherwise, we learn that adulthood involves the recognition that certain situations and differences have to be accepted and lived with. So, too, with plays, poems, and stories: because they so often are complex explorations of human motive and actions, they cannot be reduced to a single "correct" statement of the author's "message." In simple terms, what is *the* meaning or "message" of *Hamlet, Pride and Prejudice,* or the *Iliad?* If you sometimes find yourself irritably wanting to simplify the meaning of a work, resist the temptation. The assumption that such a single, correct statement of its meaning exists can inhibit your response to the work's depth and power, transforming it into a formula, a slogan, at best a ten-word telegram.

18a

The other inhibiting assumption is that all interpretations are equally valid because all are equally subjective. Once again, it is an assumption that is frequently contradicted by our behavior outside the classroom. If, for instance, we are discussing the history of science fiction or the achievements of its major writers, we are unlikely to accept all views equally. We know that some friends have read widely and deeply, while others have narrow views based on limited exposure and knowledge. The same holds true in dozens of other interests we may have—gymnastics, interior decorating, chess, country music, whatever. We don't usually insist that others share our interests, only that they not make snap judgments and offer facile interpretations out of ignorance while claiming the right to do so because "it's just a matter of opinion." By contrast, we often give heed to those we know to be sensitive and informed. While not compelled to treat them as experts, we have learned that they see, feel, and grasp more, that they can make more connections, that they make us understand more fully than we can by ourselves. We don't necessarily assume that their judgments and interpretations are always right but rather that their views are probably more inclusive and penetrating than other opinions—in short, better.

What does all of this imply about the study of literature? Most immediately, it implies your need to prepare and to be informed—to use dictionaries for unfamiliar words and allusions, to consult a glossary of literary terms for the meanings of such terms as *irony* and *dramatic monologue,* to reread shorter works several times and at least parts of the longer ones. Beyond such preparation, it implies an open attitude, a readiness to consider varying interpretations (including your own) as rough approximations. Consider them as hypotheses about a work's meaning. In the natural sciences, hypotheses are tested against all the facts and, other things being equal, those with the greatest explanatory power are judged better. That is, those hypotheses uniting the most features into a coherent pattern with the least complication are considered the more probably true. Admittedly, the analogy between literary interpretations and scientific hypotheses is only partial because literature often depends on the kinds of irreducible paradoxes and ambiguities that science tries to avoid. Nevertheless, the analogy points out certain shared characteristics. Hypotheses are subject to frequent review in the light of new data, just as interpretations may be reviewed in the light of new evidence found in the text. Hypotheses are provisional and sometimes modified, just as interpretations may be tentative and sometimes revised. We urge you to think of interpretations as resembling hypotheses because such an attitude increases the likelihood of greater understanding of the work. This attitude can shift the reader's attention away from defensiveness about an entrenched view and toward what he or she shares in common with other readers—the evidence of the text. Consider the following example.

Two students in a class discussion take different viewpoints on *The Adventures of Huckleberry Finn*. One interprets the novel as essentially the story of Huck's coming of age and learning he cannot trust the adult world. As evidence, the student points to Pap's abusiveness and selfishness, the unthinking violence of feuds and mobs, the barbarity of the small towns, and the duplicity of the King and the Duke. The other student interprets the novel as essentially Twain's attack on slavery. As evidence, the student points to Huck's experiences with Jim, their growing friendship, and Huck's crisis of choice when he decides he would rather go to hell by helping Jim escape than return him to slavery. If the two students construe the different interpretations primarily as differences of opinion or as mutually exclusive alternatives, they risk becoming locked into their positions and ignoring what they might learn from each other. If, however, they construe their interpretations as tentative explanations—as hypotheses— they enhance their chances of improving their understanding. They can rethink their analyses to include what they have omitted. Thus, they might find they can synthesize their separate arguments into a more comprehensive one. They might conclude that as Huck comes of age he learns he cannot trust the adult world but only his personal feelings, especially in his relations with Jim. This revised interpretation is richer than the two originals because it incorporates the evidence of *both*. But it is only provisional, not final. Interpretations, like hypotheses, are approximations, not absolute and unchanging truths.

So far, we have been questioning a few assumptions that impede full responses to and clear thinking about literature. You might call these the "negative factors" and still wonder about some positive ones. What are the kinds of questions and strategies that will sharpen your focus in thinking about poetry, drama, and fiction?

18a

18b Productive questions

In one of her poems, Emily Dickinson says,

Tell all the Truth but tell it slant—
Success in Circuit lies
Too bright for our infirm Delight
The Truth's superb surprise

We may read her lines to identify three major kinds of questions to be asked. The first concerns the "slantness" and the "circuit" the writer has chosen. How is the work put together? What are the resulting effects and meanings? Why this particular direction or slant? These we will call questions of **interpretation.** The second kind of question concerns our "Delight," infirm or otherwise. How well do we judge the work to have succeeded? By what standard? For what sort of audience? These we will call questions of **evaluation.** The third kind of question concerns the "Truth," all or partial, surprising or familiar. How can the individual work or writer be related to some larger context or perspective? What religious, social, or artistic ideas does the work contain? What aspects of human experience in general? These we will call questions of **integration.**

Now clearly a given essay may address all three kinds of questions, though it will usually emphasize one kind more than the others. Normally, writers don't ask themselves whether they are interpreting, evaluating, or integrating, any more than they worry about which method of paragraph development they are using. Nevertheless, good criticism in the arts is primarily the act of pointing— of singling out important details or features, specifying how a particular effect is achieved, noticing resemblances among works. And effective pointing depends on asking the relevant questions to *focus* attention. We begin with questions that focus attention on interpretation.

1. Interpretive questions

To ask *what* a work means, you will find it helpful to begin with a prior question: *How* does it mean? How is it constructed? How are the parts—the stanzas, the chapters, the scenes and acts—related to each other? Through whose eyes is the story told? Why? Is there a dominant image throughout? How is it developed or modified? Any or several of these questions will help answer the fundamental question interpretation tries to answer: How are we to understand the work?

Consider the question of who tells the story and why. What does Twain gain by having Huck tell his own story in his own words? Surely one major result is that we come to know Huck's sweetness and shrewdness, his untutored decency and wit, better than we know most people's qualities in actual life. We realize that Huck *is* his word in every sense. His arguments with and caring for Jim, the inventive lies he tells to save the two of them, his acute perceptions about the fraudulence of others, his ignorance of history and culture and his knowledge of immediate realities—all of these Twain renders in Huck's words, which reveal his essential character. And, on reflection, we may raise other questions: What else has Twain made us experience through the colloquial, seemingly spontaneous language of this largely natural boy? How have we been made to feel about Pap's drunken brutalilty and vulgarity? About the Widow Douglas's gentility? About Tom's zeal for adventure at Jim's expense? Eventually, we may conclude that Huck's words are the ones by which we measure all else in the novel—the characters; the events; what it means to be a slave, a piece of disposable property; the possible cost of civilization itself, a loss of a vision like Huck's.

The most important thing you know about a poem or a story is what you were thinking and feeling while reading the work. Begin by asking what elements in the work help account for whatever you felt and thought. (Even your boredom and irritability, your disbelief or disappointment, can be instructive, if you analyze them in relation to the work itself.) If you find your impressions are vivid but difficult to verbalize, begin with the work's title and its chapters or subtitles if it has any. Effective titles are frequently *governing images* of meaning. They are a condensed shorthand of the direction the writer intends to go—what Emily Dickinson means by the "slant" or "circuit." For instance, Joyce Carol Oates has written a fine novel set largely in mid-20th century American cities and mainly focused on women whose lives are for the most part shaped by suffering and pain they do not understand; she has entitled the novel *them* and its first section "Children of Silence." If you were to read the novel, you would soon discover how powerfully the title unifies aspects of the work: "them" are the powerless, anonymous, marginally poor not usually written about; "them" are the losers in the pursuit of the American dream; and "them" are those other faceless figures and forces the losers blame for their suffering. Similarly, if you were to read the first section, set in the depression and war years when older men were often broken by unemployment and younger men depressed and even violent, and when women endured as best they could, you would realize that these are indeed "Children of Silence." Their lives warped by historical forces they have no words for, the men turn inward and sullen, the women to the empty clichés of romance or domesticity, and to vague hopes for a better life they cannot precisely describe.

Exploring the implications of the title is one way of organizing your impressions. Another way is to identify, review, and analyze a repeated image or a recurrent pattern of action the author has charged with meaning. In the following passage, a student is discussing Doris Lessing's novel *The Golden Notebook* and its heroine, Anna Wulf, a writer whose personal and professional life is in shambles:

> During the time Anna is seeing Mother Sugar, a Jungian psychoanalyist, she has her first dream, a nightmare, about "the joy in spite." She tells Mother Sugar, "It

18b

mocked, and jibed and hurt, wished murder, wished death. And yet it was always vibrant with joy." In Anna's dreams, the embodiment of this principle progresses from a jug, to a grotesque dwarf, a deformed creature, a half-human, to a person: the progression of terror of an object, to terror of the dream as myth, to terror of Saul, her actual lover. Anna must work through her fears of the principle of destruction if she is to write again. Her fear of the cruelty that destruction brings helps cause her inertia, her writer's block. She must learn to turn that force into a creative one.

Here, the student has chosen to concentrate on an image. In this next example, another student has chosen a recurrent pattern of action in Ralph Ellison's novel *The Invisible Man*.

> *The Invisible Man* begins with a prologue which informs the reader that the black narrator is an invisible man who lives in a hole. He is invisible "simply because people refuse to see me." But he is also invisible because he has fled from seeing himself and has allowed others to manipulate him. Throughout most of the novel, the narrator is kept running by different authority-father figures or systems, submitting to each though he unconsciously rebels against them, repressing his own anger, tension, despair, and humiliation. What Ellison shows (to me, at least) is that the narrator flees not only because other people can't see beyond his blackness but also because the narrator can't accept his own humanity and his responsibility for himself.

18b

These two examples of student writing demonstrate the value of isolating a significant image or action and asking yourself *what it adds up to*. We have used novels as illustrations so far, but you can often do the same with poems, short stories, and plays. By questioning a part and teasing out its meanings and effects, you begin to see the larger pattern of the work. In fact, the resonant part may be no more than a line or two, a sentence that you marked while reading because it gave shape to your own impressions. Frequently, such lines occur near or at the end of the work as thematic summaries. The journey completed, the writer looks back to see *what* the direction has meant. For instance, at the end of Arthur Miller's play *Death of a Salesman*, Linda, the wife of Willy Loman the salesman, stands next to his grave and sobs, "I made the last payment on the house today. Today, dear. And there'll be nobody home. We're free and clear. We're free. We're free." Reading these lines, we may feel that Miller is a bit insistent but we also certainly perceive his dramatic intent: to make us realize how unfree Willy was, how trapped by a certain American ideal of success, and how damaging and difficult it may be to achieve freedom from this ideal, not only for Willy's family but for us, "we," the audience.

Still another question you can pose concerns the tone of the work. What *is* the tone, the speaker's emotional stance towards the subject? This question is especially appropriate for (though not confined to) lyric poetry, in which there is no story, or only a vaguely suggested situation. By recognizing the tone, you can locate the cluster of feelings and attitudes that has moved you, not by the plot and events but by the curve and motion of the speaker's voice. Reading aloud, you can retrace the rises and falls, the beckonings and the separations, the reaching outward and the drawing inward that affected you on silent reading. The poet and critic R. P. Blackmur has spoken of "Language as Gesture," and this is the essence of lyric poetry—language *as* gesture. The speaker's voice gestures by greeting, by rejecting, by embracing. And as you perceive the tone, you may recall other lines or poems that echo it, that make similar gestures. One might, for instance, begin with Edward Fitzgerald's translation of *The Rubaiyat of Omar Khayyam:*

> Come fill the Cup, and in the fire of Spring
> Your Winter-garment of Repentance fling:
> The Bird of Time has but a little way
> To flutter—and the Bird is on the wing.

In turn, these lines might bring to mind Christopher Marlowe's "The Passionate Shepherd to His Love" and his invitation:

> Come live with me and be my love,
> And we will all the pleasures prove
> That valleys, groves, hills, and fields,
> Woods, or steepy mountain yields.

Catching the tone of both poems, one would discover differences as well as similarity. Both passages are a call to life, to test the joy of living in the body and through the senses; they both gesture by imploring. But Fitzgerald's lines contain a reminder, almost a warning, not found in Marlowe's—that the moment is brief, that "The Bird of Time" is "on the wing." Marlowe's tone, by contrast, is seductive in its promise of timeless youth. In fact, Sir Walter Raleigh answers Marlowe in "The Nymph's Reply to the Shepherd" with the speaker's skepticism of the young man on the make. Raleigh begins,

18b

> If all the world and love were young,
> And truth in every shepherd's tongue,
> These pretty pleasures might me move
> To live with thee and be thy love.

and concludes,

> But could youth last and love still breed,
> Had joys no date nor age no need,
> Then these delights my mind might move
> To live with thee and be thy love.

As you may have decided by now, interpretive questions probe by comparison and contrast. They investigate the ways titles unify diversities, parts resemble or differ, images evolve or change, voices agree or disagree. Begin with your experience of the poem or novel; select a feature that has lingered with you; reason from effects to causes. As you move from particular to particular, you will necessarily compare and contrast. And as you find likeness and difference, you will integrate your feelings about and understanding of the work. You will become the interpreter of meaning, the negotiator between the work and your reader.

2. Evaluative questions

In a broad sense, anyone who writes about literature evaluates continually. The scenes, characters, and lines to be discussed or omitted, the themes and ideas to be stressed or minimized, the works themselves to be singled out for analysis—all of these represent choices about what is significant or insignificant. Similarly, readers have likes and dislikes, preferences for certain writers or kinds of literature, aversions to others. Different readers have different needs and expectations. For certain readers, the romance, detective story, or historical novel is a pleasant narcotic, used to kill time, escape, or doze off with. For others, fairy tales and fantasy offer a kind of substitute world where good and evil, high adventure and vivid conflict are found undiluted. And so on. The uses readers make of literature are varied and personal and often changeable. The stories that we loved as children sometimes disappoint us when we reread them as adults; the best-seller we enjoyed four years ago may bore us when we browse through it again.

We mention these familiar facts for several reasons. The first is that it makes no more sense to quarrel about the reality of different tastes in literature than it does in clothing or music. One may admire some tastes and deplore others, but that is another issue. The second reason is that people usually become better readers by exploring a variety of genres, works, and writers on their own and at their own rate. What is right for one person at a given age or stage of development may not be for another. Individual growth cannot be computer programmed. The third reason is that the academic study of literature differs in important ways from one's own leisure reading. Teachers hope that the works they have chosen will prove challenging, stimulating, pleasurable, but they cannot guarantee these rewards for any given student. Rather, what teachers can promise is a more systematic examination of certain significant works, techniques, ideas, and genres than most people are likely to undertake on their own. For these reasons, we have stressed interpretive questions. Interpretive questions are the ones the academic study of literature can most effectively ask students to think and write about. The evaluative questions we will look at are, therefore, limited to those that most frequently arise in class.

One of the most common questions you will be asked is "How successful do you think the work is?" This is *not* the same as asking "Did you like the work?" You can like or dislike a novel or poem for many reasons, some of which may have little to do with the work itself—wishing to please a respected teacher,

18b

having fixed ideas about what literature should be, being burdened with too much work for thoughtful reading, and so forth. The question "How successful do you think the work is?" usually is asked in relation to specific criteria or in a specific context—or should be. The most productive question *you* can ask is "Successful in relation to what?" Discussable judgments and evaluations require a framework, a stipulation of terms or assumptions. In this respect, evaluating literature is no different from evaluating paintings, films, or other works of art.

Assumptions are particularly important. If they are not clear, they should be clarified. If they seem questionable, they should be scrutinized. For instance, one popular assumption—not always explicitly stated as such—is that a play or novel should be well-made, with a decisive beginning, middle, and end. But what does one mean by a "decisive ending"? Is it in fact true that important novels and plays always have such endings? Some important works—especially modern ones—do not end decisively; they simply stop. Ralph Ellison's *The Invisible Man,* for instance, ends with the narrator finally understanding more about himself and the world but still living in a hole. In fact, many contemporary works close with the survivors disabused of illusions or pretenses but with their futures quite uncertain—Albee's *Who's Afraid of Virginia Woolf?* and Golding's *Lord of the Flies,* to mention but two. We simply don't know what the characters are going to do after the end of the text.

Be clear about standards and assumptions, including your own, and be willing to take chances with the unfamiliar. Like certain acquaintances, some poems, novels, and plays will seem difficult, strange, sometimes even threatening, when you first encounter them. They have to be lived with for a while. Here, for instance, is what one student found after living with Tillie Olsen's fiction long enough to be moved by it:

18b

> Raised in affluent, upperclass America, I have rarely come in contact with the poverty Tillie Olsen describes in her short stories. But her treatment of suffering powerfully conveys the despair, the broken lives, the caring, and sometimes even the hope that poverty entails. I found that Ms. Olsen develops an intensity of pain, resentment, love, and understanding that simply does not exist in more privileged communities. She made me realize the terrible destruction of human potential and personality that poverty can cause, but she also made me see how easily one can become hardened by comfort. At the end of *Tell Me a Riddle,* I had some hope that poverty can be overcome, but I found this hope tempered by the realization that as one gains affluence, one too easily loses intensity of emotion and the ability to understand.

Notice what the writer has done. Rather than hurrying to make up her mind about whether Olsen's stories are good or bad, she has taken the time to ask an entirely different kind of question, something like "What have I felt and understood that I had not before?" We suggest that this type of question is the most productive for works you find unfamiliar or unsettling.

We read texts, but texts also "read" us. Certain writers and works, that is, disturb our habitual ways of thinking and feeling and our conventional notions about what literature should be. If we remain open, they make us feel our own limitations. If, as happens occasionally, you find you are expected to write about such a work, try beginning with the following questions: Why do I find this book strange or discomforting? Is there something about myself or my beliefs I resist coming to terms with? After thinking about these questions as honestly as you can, you are always free to decide that what you have discovered was not worth the bother. It is also possible, however, that you will discover some things about yourself that take you on a far more interesting journey than safer, more familiar works have.

3. Integrative questions

By integrative questions, we mean those that ask about the individual writer's or work's relationship to some larger context. Such questions may concern the connections between the work and the writer's life or times; the work and philosophical, political, or religious ideas; the work and certain artistic movements or forms; the work and human experience in general. To be specific: What does the fiction of Toni Morrison, Alice Walker, and Toni Cade Bambara say about the lives of black women in America? What did T. S. Eliot learn from Ezra Pound about poetry? What political and social ideas was Swift satirizing in *Gulliver's Travels?* How does Virginia Woolf's criticism illuminate her major novels? What are the relationships between Shelley's interest in philosophy and his poetry? How does Dickens's humor differ from Fielding's? Why were the Beat poets called "Beat"?

Integrative questions are often the most exciting ones you can ask. They encourage wide reading, research, and concentrated thinking. They invite you to pursue a line of inquiry in depth and to sustain it until you have found the answers that make the most sense. Courses that center on a historical period, one or two authors, a movement or theme, or a genre quite naturally provoke such questions—the instructor's, your own, or both. Even introductory and broad survey courses lend themselves to such questions. The satisfaction of answering these questions is that they allow you to interpret individual works and then to connect what you have found to a larger argument or thesis—in short *to integrate.* Integrating is the discovering of significant relationships among things.

What is a good integrative question? To begin with, it should be one that is answerable. To ask "What did Salinger really have in mind when he wrote *Catcher in the Rye?"* is to ask a question that is probably unanswerable: nobody but Salinger could know, and he's not saying. A more manageable question is "What central themes of *Catcher in the Rye* are found in Salinger's other works?" It is answerable because the texts are available. Effective integrative questions are essentially the same as those you ask in preparing to write any paper involving research and critical thinking. (Also see Chapter **19** on the research process.)

Unless your instructor assigns the topic, your first question is the hardest: What more do I want to know about the work or writer? The period or society that shaped the work or writer? Some philosophical, religious, or artistic idea that permeates the work or influenced the writer? Other similar works or writers? Even if the topic is assigned, you can normally sharpen it by posing your own question and checking with the instructor to be sure it's relevant.

The second question is closely related to the first: Why do I want to know more about this? Of course it's because you are interested, but *why in terms of the topic?* For instance, suppose you wanted to know more about some recent feminist writers. Why? Because of their treatment of women? of men? of women and men? of women's sexuality? of mothers and daughters? Sometimes, especially at the beginning, it won't be easy to answer why, and often your interests will change as you get into the topic. But the more you can at least *tentatively* answer this question, the more you clarify your focus.

The third question is also crucial: What more do I need to know to answer my question? Here your primary and secondary reading and your conversations with the instructor are essential. Occasionally, you may find that you need to know too much, that the question is too vast or complicated to be manageable. For instance, if you were to ask seriously "What are the differences between the treatment of World War I and World War II in American fiction?" you would be committing yourself to a very long program of reading and research. More frequently, though, what you will need to know involves not only the extensive reading. It also will involve the relevant concepts. We stress the importance of concepts because they represent your larger intellectual stake in the question; they provide the boundary lines of your chosen turf. For example, if you wondered how Achilles in the *Iliad* differs from Odysseus in the *Odyssey* as an epic hero, you would have to master the concept of "epic hero" to answer your question.

18b

Like interpretive questions, integrative questions are usually answered by making significant comparisons and contrasts. In doing so, you should keep two more stock questions in mind. Both questions concern the danger of over-simplification. The first is "Have I tried to make the concept do too much work or expanded it too widely?" Be wary of broad, catch-all ideas such as "search for identity," "crisis of faith," "Renaissance man," "Romanticism," and the like. Clearly defined and given a specific context, they can be extremely useful, but they can easily become pigeonholes into which everything is shoved. In a loose sense, for example, most novels do probably dramatize "the search for identity," but how does that help one understand the differences between Huckleberry Finn's flight and Hester Prynne's remaining on the scene of her disgrace in

The Scarlet Letter as "searches"? The second question is "Have I looked at important differences as well as important similarities?" Difference is as vital as similarity. Writers sometimes do change their themes, subject matter, or techniques and style. History does affect and modify beliefs, artistic conventions, individual lives. To echo the philosopher William James, every difference that is a difference makes a difference.

Throughout this section, we have emphasized questions because they give momentum to thinking. They nudge you to move from effect to cause, impression to source, individual case to general principle. To close this discussion, we include a student essay that effectively blends interpretive and integrative questions into one unified argument. The essay concerns the function of Old Hilse, a character in Gerhart Hauptmann's play *The Weavers,* a dramatization of a revolt by impoverished Silesian weavers in central Europe during the 1840s. The writer's central question is "Why is Old Hilse even in the play?" His answer is a persuasive demonstration of *how* Old Hilse changes our understanding of the play, the effect he has upon us.

Why Old Hilse?

18b

What Old Hilse does *not* cause or influence

    If one were to examine the contribution of Old Hilse to the plot of The Weavers, one would be hard put to find any excuse for his being in the play. He neither alters the course of the main action nor initiates any new actions. His speeches to the main characters are unheeded. He does not join the rebel weavers nor does he come to the defense of the manufacturers. He remains neutral in the battle, in no way affecting its outcome. His only connection with the action of the play is to be an unintentional and all-but-unnoticed casualty.

Focusing question

    Then why are his unheeded lines ever spoken? Why is this character brought into the play at all?

    The play begins with a dispute between the younger weavers and the manufacturer's buyer, builds up the weavers' discontent with their poverty and fatigue, and reaches a climax with their open rebellion. It roars toward what we hope will be its triumphant conclusion. But it runs head on into Old Hilse. Here is a man whom we fully expect to jump on the bandwagon, or at least act as a dramatic counterpoint by siding with the manufacturers. But Old Hilse just states his contempt for this particular uprising, reiterates his belief in duty, and goes back to his daily weaving. For a moment the rapidly moving picture of a community in revolt is frozen. The logic that has been leading up to the great truth of why all the weavers must kill all the owners is stopped just short of a final conclusion. The almost cornily beautiful victory of good over evil, already foreshadowed in the impoverished mass's sacking of a manufacturer's estate, falters. Old Hilse, the most respected weaver, the one most representative of simple devotion to weaving, will not join the rebellion.

> Old Hilse's action—his refusal to join the rebellion—and its immediate effect on our involvement in the plot

18b

In a moment the machine starts to rumble again. The drunken and possessed leaders of the rebellion rush out of Hilse's house to battle the government troops. The plot starts up again. But the reader left behind begins to question the rebels. Why won't Old Hilse join? Why does his refusal, although not altering the plan of the rebellion one bit, alter the meaning of it so greatly? Hilse is certainly not afraid. He is a wounded veteran of a much greater war. As he starts to talk about that war, the rebellion raging outside begins to shrink. It is nothing to him. What's more, it is nothing to anyone

> Further effects on the reader—the meaning(s) of Old Hilse's choice

Initial statement of what Old Hilse does cause—our seeing the plot in a new perspective

except those who are inside of it. <u>Suddenly the story of the young weavers battling for their rights and the older ones gradually joining them becomes a pathetic example of the pattern we see in the papers almost daily, the local rebellion. This is Hilse's contribution.</u> He is the only character who stands far enough outside the battle to see it as the futile effort it is, not as the glorious rebellion that the other weavers think it is. He has seen it all before. He can even predict jail terms for the leaders. <u>Hilse takes us far enough from the story to see it clearly.</u> Hilse, who is nothing to the plot's outcome, is everything to its meaning: he makes the plot change from a story in which we are as personally wrapped up as the characters into a dismal pattern of the universality of revolt born by suffering and hunger, which is doomed to be led astray by its own excesses, and thus defeated.

For summary and strong restatement of Old Hilse's function—final answer to "Why Old Hilse?"

18c Useful strategies

Apart from the questions we have discussed, you have other ways to assist your thinking and writing about literature. The most important of these, of course, is your paying close attention to the terms, themes, and techniques of analysis that your instructor stresses. We know of no substitute for the student's class participation, asking questions, and keeping up with the reading. The more actively responsible you become for your own education, the more likely you are to get what *you* want from it. The strategies we will suggest should help you achieve this end.

1. Keeping a journal

A time-proven strategy for increasing one's pleasure in and understanding of literature is keeping a journal or reading log. Many students who have kept journals find they do best to set aside two or three periods a week for writing about their class reading. Length of entry and format also vary: some students write several hundred words on each novel, play, or poem; others jot down short notes, impressions, or references to specific pages they wish to return to. The subject matter can also take varying forms: some students pursue a theme or two from work to work; some explore their personal feelings and thoughts and connect the work to their own experience; some isolate key passages, images, or characters and reflect on these; others, depending on the work, may try a combination of these. Unless assigned and collected by the instructor, such journals are entirely private. Journals allow the student to write about any aspect of the reading in whatever way is most congenial. That is part of the journal's value: its freedom.

The advantages of keeping a journal are several. To begin with, it allows you to explore your own reactions to the works at greater length and in greater depth than class sessions always permit. By doing so, you make the poem or story more fully your own. Moreover, the journal encourages you to sort out your impressions while they are still fresh. Sometimes, a few weeks after reading a work, you may recall having had some wonderful insights but have no idea now what they were. Journals help you remember. Finally, journals can assist your reviewing in either of two ways. Looking over your journal, you may find some topic you have discussed several times; this topic may be a subject for a paper. Or, reviewing your journal for in-class tests or essays, you may rediscover evidence and ideas that you might otherwise overlook.

18c

If you have not kept a journal before, you may find yourself a bit self-conscious and awkward when you begin one. These feelings are entirely natural and usually diminish as you become more experienced. At the very least, we encourage you to try one for a few weeks: it's an excellent way of making the academic study of literature a more personal inquiry.

2. Summarizing

Another useful strategy is summarizing. While this can take a number of forms, the summarizing technique we especially recommend is best suited for scenes or acts of plays, the sections or chapters of prose fiction, and the divisions of longer poems. Briefly, such summaries consist of a few phrases or sentences that set down the *primary* events, themes, and images; the summary is a record of the dominant impressions the section has made. Here, for instance is the summary of a chapter called "Pastoral," from V. S. Naipaul's moving novel *A House for Mr. Biswas,* based on the life of Naipaul's father, an Indian journalist growing up in Trinidad:

```
Brief pastoral. Mr. B's birth curse, death of calf and
father: family dispersed; no home.
```

And here is the summarizing note for the next chapter, entitled "Before the Tulsis":

> Beyond childhood: school, beatings, work with Pundit (&
> disgrace), liquor store, sign painter. This novel goes in
> real stages; youth—adolescence, concluding with sex,
> hopes of love and romance, a la Samuel Smiles.

At first, you may wonder of what possible value these summaries are to anyone but the writer. That is their point: they are the *writer's* record of his key impressions on first reading. They are not intended as a total synopsis of the plot, still less as the novel's "message." Rather, *they organize the passages that have been marked throughout the chapter into significant units to be examined more fully later.* They are, so to speak, mile markers on the road of meaning.

The value of this kind of summarizing is most obvious for long, complex works when you are reading them for the first time. Summaries help you go back over what you have read and sort out the central developments and ideas from the lesser ones; they map the major features of the territory you have just explored. Reviewing the territory later, you can inspect the details more analytically because you already have a tentative framework into which they fit. In a somewhat different fashion, summarizing can help unravel the knotty strands of shorter but nevertheless complex pieces. Though only 204 lines, Browning's poem "Childe Roland to the Dark Tower Came" is one of his most mysterious works. Here is one reader's summary of the poem that at least served as a start toward understanding it:

> Strange poem in several ways: dreams, snatches of memory of
> picture and verse, not B's usual control; the wasteland
> where all effort is futile, things mysterious and point-
> less—world does not mean intensely and mean good. Note poem
> filled with images of failure, betrayed strength, weak-
> ness, ageing and decay without honor—memory no help.

The main use of this note for the writer was that it underlined several ways this poem differed from others by Browning and therefore highlighted what had to be thought about.

Rather like some journal entries, the summarizing note is your own record in your own words of your primary conclusions. And, like its journal equivalent, its best use is as an aid for further, more carefully detailed analysis. It is another means of engaging yourself more actively with the reading.

18c

3. Working with the words

Plays, poems, and fiction are made out of words, not clay or copper. When you are caught up in a short story or sonnet, you are enmeshed in the *effects* of words—their connotations and denotations, their plasticity and firmness, their freshness and familiarity. And when you think and write critically about the story or poem, you are partially disengaging yourself from the words in order to look at them. Themes, images, and events do not exist in the abstract; they are embedded in and realized through the words, the stuff of language. Whatever "happens" in literature happens because of the patterns that have been made out of words. Whatever "happens" in analysis and criticism happens usually because these patterns have been *explicated,* or at least considered.

To explicate is to unfold. To explicate a piece of literature is to unfold the ways the words have been shaped into larger units of meaning—couplets, lines, scenes, chapters, completed works. As we will see presently, even a short poem may include *layers* of suggestiveness and *strands* of imagery. Explication, the unfolding of these layers and strands, is essential to critical thinking about literature. And while critical thinking and writing do not end with explication, they usually begin with it. Before you can go on to larger questions—how does this writer differ from that writer? this epic compare to that epic?—you have to work with the words. Even if you do not write about the language as such, you at least have to think about it as such.

18c

How do you think about "language as such"? To begin with, you will need to look up unfamiliar words and allusions and see how they are used in context. Beyond that, you should, at least with shorter poems and sections of plays, try reading aloud to catch the sounds, rhythms, intonations, and other elements that compose the body language of words. These are essentially preliminaries, however. Your main activity is more easily illustrated than described. To give you an idea of what's involved, we suggest you first read the poem that follows, written in the last years of Walt Whitman's life. After you have read the poem aloud a couple of times and looked up words like "hawser'd," try answering these questions: (1) How is the picture of old age embedded in particular images? (2) Why is the unifying image "The Dismantled Ship" rather than, say, "The Forgotten Ship"? (3) How can the poem be read as a picture of human loss and decay, particularly Whitman's?

The Dismantled Ship

In some unused lagoon, some nameless bay,
On sluggish, lonesome waters, anchor'd near the shore,
An old, dismasted, gray and batter'd ship, disabled, done,
After free voyages to all the seas of earth, haul'd up at last and hawser'd tight,
Lies rusting, mouldering.

Now compare your analysis with the following, an extract from a student essay:

> Whitman views a perishing man as a model for suffering and loss: the victim loses his strength and abilities, is helpless, alone, neglected. His central image, a rotting ship, helps develop this theme because it is easily associated with a weakening body, an ageing man, or even, as the editors hint, the elderly Whitman himself. The image conveys not just the idea of a decaying object or thing, but a decaying person. It invites the reader to empathize, to imagine the analogy between ship and human being, both now impotent and forgotten.
>
> Whitman's diction develops his theme. It makes the reader feel the tragedy of a man or ship perishing, of an outcast weak and abandoned. Like a ship rotting in "some unused lagoon," mired in stagnant water and cut off from the "seas of earth," so an ageing man may be shut up in a nursing home or live alone, confined, separated from life. He is "anchor'd near the shore," cut off by time, space, and thought from the ships and men sailing the wide oceans. He is "dismasted . . . disabled, done"; like a "mouldering" ship which has lost its source of power, his age has cost him his Freudian source of energy—his libido. He is "dismantled," unmanned. He is unable to make "voyages" of life and love from person to person and country to country, "free" to choose and "free" from cost or worry. The ship is no longer freshly painted and intact; the old man's skin is weathered, his body weakened. The "good gray poet" has become a "gray and batter'd ship."
>
> Nor is there any returning to the days of old, for time has him "hauled up at last and hawser'd tight." The inevitable price of the years of "free voyages to all the seas of the earth" is to become worn out, an empty hull to be dragged aside and secured to prevent drifting. Yet what is perhaps still worse about his decay is the lack of concern by others, for while his person cries out to be cared for—to stop the "rusting" and "mouldering"—he is alone. He is lonely but no one comes; he is feeble, but no one helps. The sluggish waters lapping against the hull are all that is heard.

18c

Notice *how* the student's explication proceeds. It finds three possible layers of meaning in the words—the image of the ship, of an ageing man, and of the poet Whitman. It does not say the poem "is" one layer only or has one "message," but instead tries to find correspondences and similarities among these layers. And it argues for such correspondences by finding them embedded *in* the words. To put it in different terms, the explication unfolds each image to see *how* it may be read in relation to the ship, an ageing man, and, on occasion, the poet Whitman. Still, the explication does not claim to be the complete or only interpretation of the poem. Explications are rarely if ever "complete." Here, for instance, the student could have done more with the sounds: Whitman's diminuendo in "dismasted . . . disabled, done" or his finality in "haul'd up at last and hawser'd tight," to mention but one possibility. Nor does this explication preclude other readings with a somewhat different emphasis. Another student, having read about Whitman's last years, might unfold these meanings more fully than the writer of the essay has. And, in fact, if a second student were to interpret the poem mainly as a picture of the poet's old age, this reading would supplement, not contradict, the first reading. The two readings would constitute hypotheses about the poem to be compared in relation to the evidence—the words of the text.

Now, having read the poem, the explication, and our comments, try working with the words of another of Whitman's poems. This one is concerned with youth, beginnings, fullness of power and experience. Read it aloud and analyze it first for its own layers of meaning—its playfulness with motion and speed, light and color, water and wind. Then juxtapose it to "The Dismantled Ship": what is the composite picture, and how is it composed by the contrasting images?

The Ship Starting

Lo, the unbounded sea,
On its breast a ship starting, spreading all sails, carrying
    even her moonsails,
The pennant is flying aloft as she speeds she speeds so stately
    —below emulous waves press forward,
They surround the ship with shining curving motions and foam.

This composite picture of youth and age, beginnings and endings, could just as easily be developed in a single work quite unlike Whitman's two poems. We will close with such a poem, one by Emily Dickinson. In working with her words, you might begin by explicating "quiet dust" and the connections between "Gentlemen and Ladies" and "Lads and Girls." Then try to visualize how "Bloom and Bees / Exist an Oriental Circuit," that is, live out a full cycle. After you have finished with Dickinson's poem, compare it with Whitman's two poems: what are the significant contrasts in the imagery and meanings?

This quiet Dust was Gentlemen and Ladies

This quiet Dust was Gentlemen and Ladies
And Lads and Girls—
Was laughter and ability and Sighing
And Frocks and Curls.

This Passive Place a Summer's nimble mansion
Where Bloom and Bees
Exist an Oriental Circuit
Then cease, like these—

To conclude, let us recall the questions posed at the chapter's beginning and make a final suggestion. The questions: How to understand our relationship to the work? How to share our experience of it most effectively with others. How to convince others that ours is a valid way of looking at the work? The suggestion: Begin with the words. In and through them alone you have experienced "the noble accents" and "lucid, inescapable rhythms" you have known.

18c

Exercise 1

This first group is designed to give you a chance to question inhibiting assumptions.

1. Write a paragraph on Whitman's "The Dismantled Ship" in which you reduce it to one meaning, that is, make all the images show only the loneliness of old age, *or* its feebleness, *or* its absence of activity. Then write another paragraph in which you show how much you have had to leave out of the poem in order to achieve a single meaning. Now compare the two paragraphs: How radically did you simplify the poem's imagery? What was the greatest reduction in meaning you made? How was it the greatest?

2. Write a paragraph on Whitman's "The Ship Starting" in which you interpret it as, say, a reader beginning an absorbing novel, a crowd moving across a field, or a rocket accelerating off its pad. Then write a paragraph which questions the plausibility of your interpretation as a hypothesis. Now compare the two paragraphs: What is the most telling evidence you cited to question the interpretation? How is it the most telling?

Exercise 2

18c

This second group is designed to give you practice with interpretive, evaluative, and integrative questions.

1. Pick a work—a poem, play, or piece of fiction—that you like and know well and that has an effective title. Write several paragraphs in which you show *how* the title acts as a governing image to unify elements of the work—its plot and characters, themes and development, images and details, etc. Make as many connections as you can, even if a few of them seem a bit strained or far-fetched. When you have finished, reread the paragraphs critically and revise them by concentrating on the most important connections that should be made. Now compare the two sets of paragraphs: How much of the first version did you discard? What elements of the first version became more unified in the second?

2. Choose a short story or novel and write several paragraphs in which you imagine how the work would be different if told from another point of view— for instance, *The Adventures of Huckleberry Finn* through Jim's eyes, or *Heart of Darkness* through Kurtz's eyes. Then write an analysis of what changes you have had to make, what new aspects of the story you have discovered or highlighted, and what modifications in meaning and theme your version entails.

3. Do the same with a short poem, for instance, Thomas Hardy's "Had You Wept" from the woman's point of view, Frost's "Mending Wall" through the neighbor's eyes, or Robinson Jeffers's "Hurt Hawks" through the "terrible eyes" of the bird or "the wild God."

4. Write a paragraph on Dickinson's "This quiet Dust" in which you visualize as fully as you can *how* dust permeates the poem. For instance, how does cloth ("Frocks") look, feel, and smell as it turns to dust, or how do summer flowers ("Bloom") fade and dry?

5. Choose some type of literature you read purely for pleasure—Harlequin romances, science fiction, sports stories, fantasy, whatever. Then evaluate by

describing as precisely as you can the kind(s) of pleasure you look for and make a case for such reading by specifying the ways it can be successful.

6. Thumb through the editors' headnotes or introductions to the authors in your literature anthology and find some critical judgment that you disagree with. Try to choose one that points to some limitation or failure in the work or writer—for instance, remarks like "Hardy's novels and poems are too often marred by pessimism" or "Sylvia Plath's poetry is too painful for most readers." Then write a thoughtful response in which you perhaps concede part of the criticism but find other grounds for valuing the writer or work.

7. Jot down three or four integrative questions that you might be interested in answering—for example, what connection there is between a writer's work and life, between a historical period or event and a work, between a religious or philosophical idea and a work, etc. Then review your questions critically with the following in mind: (1) Is the question, as worded, answerable? If not, can it be rephrased to become so? (2) What more would you have to know to answer the question? (3) What significant similarities and differences might an educated guess lead you to expect?

8. Using the paper "Why Old Hilse?" as a model, write an essay in which you analyze how a character is used primarily to provide some larger perspective on or understanding of a play, poem, or novel.

Exercise 3

18c

This third group is designed to give you practice in working with useful strategies.

1. Keep a journal faithfully for at least a month, making at least two entries a week of 150 words each. Write on whatever aspects of the literature you wish—how it's related to your experience, what ideas you find most interesting, why you like or dislike a particular work, whatever you find most congenial. At the end of the month, reread your entries with the following questions in mind: (1) Did you have any new insights or make any discoveries while writing? (2) Did writing about the literature increase your pleasure in it?

2. For an assigned work (preferably a longer one) try summarizing its parts, sections, or chapters at the end of each division. Then, after you have finished the work, reread your summaries with the following questions in mind: (1) Did the summarizing help you understand the whole section more clearly? (2) As you review your summaries, do you find you have a firmer grasp on the entire work?

3. Choose two poems that deal with the same theme—love and loss, men and women misunderstanding each other, delight in a natural setting or living creature, suffering and recovery, the passage from adolescence to adulthood, etc. Write an analysis in which you first explicate each work and then compare and contrast the two as treatments of the theme.

4. Choose a short poem (of no more than 25 lines) you like. Then write as complete an explication of it as you can, unfolding every image as fully as possible and looking for the ways the images support and develop the theme. After you have finished, read your analysis with the following questions in mind: (1) Can you find images you want to do still more with? (2) How much has your explication changed your understanding of or feelings about the poem? Why?

5. The same as 4, but use the lyrics to a popular song (rock, country, folk, whatever). Pose yourself one question in addition to those for 4: What happens to the lyric when you consider the words without the music?
6. Choose a page of a short story or novel you like and analyze it carefully with the following in mind: Do you find the kinds of images that you expect in poetry? If so, what are they and how are they used? If not, what evidence of craft or technique do you find? How, as best you can determine, are these effects achieved? How do they affect you as a reader?

The
Research
Paper

Part V

19 *The Research Process*

When we open a newspaper at the end of a busy day, we may not think that we are doing research, but we are. We are doing research as we scan the paper for reports about the mayor's latest conflict with the city council, or about the response of the stock market to the Federal Reserve Board's new monetary policy. We are doing research when we copy a recipe out of the food section, check the standings of our favorite team, read a movie review, or hunt through the classified ads for a good used lawnmower. Research is part of the texture of our lives. It answers one of our deepest needs as thinking human beings—our need for information.

Gathering information is not a mechanical task; on the contrary, it constantly calls forth our powers of judgment and evaluation. After we have seen a baseball game or a new movie, we want friends to discuss it with, newspaper accounts or reviews to read. Why? By considering the opinions of people around us, we come to understand our own judgments better. Which play was really the turning point in the game? Which actor gave the film its emotional force? We engage in heated arguments not only in the noisy cafeteria or the crowded bar, but also in our silent interaction with the printed opinions of others.

Writing papers based on research calls us into such a silent dialogue with other thoughtful men and women, sharing their concerns, agreeing and disagreeing with their opinions, reflecting and expanding upon their conclusions. If we consider the research assignment as an opportunity to gather and evaluate information in order to enter into a kind of informed conversation with researchers who have preceded us, then the experience can be genuinely fulfilling.

Research satisfies not merely our curiosity but our more profound desire to understand. Behind every fact that engages our attention lies our natural wish to comprehend its meaning, our impulse to fit it into a context or pattern. Consider the research of Max Weber, the noted sociologist. He observed that the great period of industrial growth in Western Europe occurred after the Protestant Reformation of the sixteenth century, but he was not content with the mere fact of this observation. The search for its significance led him to phrase a new question for investigation: Did the Reformation *cause* the Industrial Revolution, and if it did, what factors of the Reformation were the most important? The answer to this question was one of the fine books of our century, *The Protestant Ethic and the Spirit of Capitalism.*

Whether or not your research raises an entirely new set of issues for scholarly discussion, as Max Weber's did, it should satisfy your desire to know and to understand. And it will offer you a place of your own in the dialogue among well-informed people.

19a Choosing a topic for research

If doing research is new to you, your first impulse may be to choose a topic that you already know well. Such a choice, however, is almost certain to rob your research of any interest or satisfaction, leaving you only with tedious and meaningless busywork. Research is a process of discovery. You can participate in this process only if you select a subject that is a genuine question for you, a problem, a mystery, an unknown quantity. The purpose of research, after all, is not to document what you already know, but to discover what you do not. As disturbing as it may sound at first, you are doing real research only if you do not know where it will lead.

The fundamental requirement for a topic to research is the same as that which should guide the choice of any subject for writing: your interest in it. In a freshman writing course, your instructor may leave the subject for your research paper entirely up to you, or may allow you to choose from a list of subjects or a general subject area. Even if your instructor limits the range of subjects more narrowly, you should seek out a specific angle or focus that appeals to you for some reason. In other courses, you will most likely be left on your own to identify a workable subject for research. Writing a research paper in your freshman composition class offers you a chance to experiment with the selection of a good topic and to learn what goes into the process of making such a choice.

In earlier chapters, we observed that the process of writing itself alters a writer's topic. Sometimes it becomes narrower, as the writer becomes aware of the need to balance completeness with limitations on length. Sometimes it changes focus, as related subjects and ideas occur to the writer. In a research paper, many of these modifications in your topic occur *before* you begin writing, during the research process itself.

The writer of the paper on pages 303–17 began only with a general interest in the subject of natural disasters, a subject he began to explore by looking up articles in the *Readers' Guide to Periodical Literature* (see **20d**). Gradually he decided to focus on a specific type of natural disaster—floods—and then on one specific flood—the flood that devastated Florence, Italy in 1966.

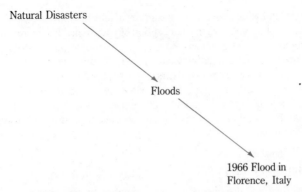

At first this subject seemed sufficiently narrow for a research paper of average length. But as the student found and read additional sources of information about the flood in Florence, he realized that even this subject could be developed in a number of different ways:

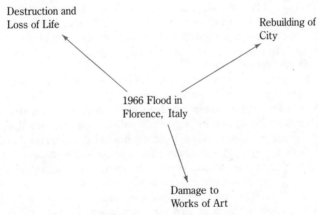

19a

Because he had taken a course in art history, the writer found the damage done by the flood to Florence's vast collections of Renaissance art an especially intriguing subject. But as he read further, he found an even narrower and more effective focus for his paper: the *restoration* of the works of art damaged by the flood. Now he could continue his research more efficiently, picking out sources that dealt with this precise subject and taking notes with a new sense of purpose and direction. The final result was his paper, "Recovery from the Florence Flood: A Masterpiece of Restoration."

As you start to explore a tentative subject, you should be ready to accept similar changes in your original plan. You may expect your research to lead in directions you had not anticipated, to new sources of information and new ideas that will inevitably affect your original conception of your topic. The opinions of others will modify your early ideas, leaving you with new perspectives to consider. On other occasions, unfortunately, you will find that the libraries available to you do not have enough material on your subject from which to construct a serious research report, and you will be forced to modify your original subject radically or to abandon it altogether. Such is the life of the dedicated researcher—a combination of excitement and frustration, of discovery and disillusionment.

19b Planning the long paper

Perhaps the most disconcerting requirement of a research paper is its length—often five or more times longer than most of the other papers you have written in freshman composition. Your shorter papers provided a good introduction to the writing process, but a long paper offers valuable practice in the kinds of writing that you will be called on to do in upper-level courses and later in life. A long paper is a typical assignment in seminars and independent study courses. Business people write formal reports; lawyers write legal briefs; social workers write case histories; journalists write feature articles. People in many professions must be able to compose long pieces of writing that draw on material from several different sources.

The first step in all of these cases, of course, is gathering information. For your purposes, that will mean doing substantial research in a library. You can't understand or focus your topic until you have a firm grasp of what others have written about the subject. In Chapters **20** and **21**, therefore, we will spend a good deal of time discussing some basic approaches to locating material in the library and some strategies for taking effective notes from the sources you find.

You will also need to know some of the conventional methods of documentation, that is, the formal ways of acknowledging to the reader the sources of your material. If you fail to indicate the source of an idea accurately, you may lead the reader to believe that it is your own conclusion, and you will be guilty of **plagiarism.** Presenting other people's words, sentences, or ideas as your own, whether deliberately or accidentally done, is a serious offense. In college it can lead to dismissal; in life after college it can lead to a damage suit. We will deal at length with the important matter of careful documentation in Chapter **22**.

The finest library facilities and the best ideas for a research paper will not be of much use to you if you do not leave yourself enough time for working on your paper. You may have been able to write a first draft of your other essays in freshman composition in just a few sittings—one devoted to exploring the subject, one to outlining and planning, one to composing. That will not be sufficient for a serious research paper, which usually involves at least a few weeks of preliminary work even before you begin writing, and several composing sessions as you assimilate and structure the material you have accumulated. You can never begin researching too early, for you must be prepared for all the setbacks that accompany research, from the topic that grows increasingly complex to the critical book missing from your library. And the task of fusing your final set of notes into a coherent whole may also be more difficult than you expect. The most important rule for research, then, is to plan ahead, leaving yourself plenty of time to gather information and several sessions for writing and typing. The research paper completed in a single coffee-soaked night is not likely to be very successful, no matter how thorough the research that it is based on.

19b

20 *The Library*

A good subject for a research paper, as we have said, is one about which you have unanswered questions, one that remains to be explored and focused. Once you have tentatively decided on such a subject, you won't be able to make much progress sitting at your desk. Your next stop is the library.

20a Using the library

When most people think of libraries, they think of books—and with good reason, for books are the most visible of any library's holdings. When you use a library for serious research, however, you need to be familiar with the many other kinds of materials available—especially with standard reference works, magazines, journals, newspapers, and government publications. Since most American libraries use the same basic system for filing and organizing materials, we can offer some guidelines below that will apply to almost any library that you have access to. But we should perhaps stress that this is only an introduction to library use. To get the most out of your library, you will have to discover its own particular strengths—its large microfilm holdings, for example, or its outstanding record collection. You will need to know where various holdings are kept and what library policies govern their use. You can learn about these and other features of your library through the official tours that many college libraries offer at the beginning of the semester. Or you can give yourself a tour. Ask at the main desk for a map of the building and its features, or simply wander from floor to floor at a leisurely pace, identifying the materials available and noting their locations. Becoming familiar with the arrangement and system of your library is your first task as a serious researcher, one that will help to make your work more efficient and satisfying.

20b The card catalog

The card catalog in a library is the major index to its holdings. Usually, all the books, reference works, indexes, and periodicals received by a library are indexed alphabetically here on 3 x 5 cards. Each book is ordinarily listed in at least three different places: under its author's name (under each author's name if

20b

there are more than one); under its title; and under the subject or subjects it covers. In some university libraries, author and title cards are collected in a single alphabetical catalog, while subject cards are filed separately, also in alphabetical order.

Catalog cards contain a good deal of potentially important information, including the publication date of a book, the number of its pages, and notes about such features as indexes and illustrations in the book. The more you use the card catalog, the more skilled you will become in assessing this information before you actually examine the book itself. When you identify a book that you wish to look at, make a note of its *call number*, also found on the catalog card. The call number, which is based on a nationally used classification system, is your guide to the location of the book in your library. Two principal systems of classification are used by American libraries: the Dewey Decimal System (a numerical system) and the Library of Congress System (an alphabetical classification). At your library's main desk, you can get further information about the system your library follows. If your library has open stacks—that is, if library patrons are allowed to browse through the shelves and select books themselves—you will also find information here about the location of books throughout the library.

When you want to know where a specific book is located in your library, the author or title card will lead you to it fastest. When you don't know authors or titles, look through the cards under the subject you are interested in. Since both the Dewey Decimal System and the Library of Congress System are based on subject matter, you will usually find that the books your library has on a particular subject are shelved together. You can use the subject cards, therefore, not only as a listing of the library's holdings on a subject but also as a guide to the appropriate section of the book stacks. If your library has open stacks, some browsing around in this area will usually lead you to a number of useful books. Feel free to pull down from the shelves any books that look interesting, but respect your library's policies about reshelving books. To avoid the chaos created by accidental misshelving, many libraries ask that you do not put books back yourself, but leave them instead on a table or at some other designated place for library staff members to reshelve.

20b

Increasingly, libraries are developing computer systems that enable patrons to bypass the card catalog and locate books and other materials simply by typing the author or title into a computer terminal, which then displays all of the information normally found on a card in the card catalog. Some such systems also make it possible to search for books by subject. If your library has put its holdings "on line" with such a system, you should definitely learn how to use it, for it will save you valuable time. However, because subject searches on these systems can sometimes be hard to use effectively and because a library may not have all of its holdings on line, you will probably also want to be sure that you know how to locate books through the card catalog if you have to.

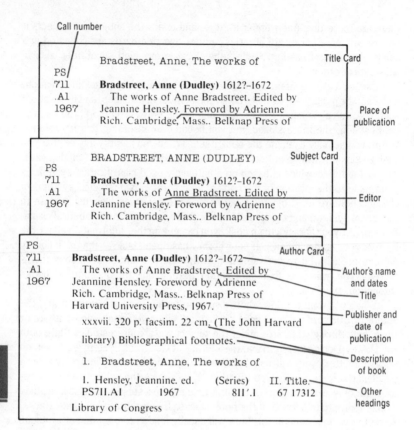

Call number

Bradstreet, Anne, The works of   Title Card

PS
711   **Bradstreet, Anne (Dudley)** 1612?-1672
.A1   The works of Anne Bradstreet. Edited by
1967   Jeannine Hensley. Foreword by Adrienne   Place of
        Rich. Cambridge, Mass.. Belknap Press of   publication

BRADSTREET, ANNE (DUDLEY)   Subject Card
PS
711   **Bradstreet, Anne (Dudley)** 1612?-1672
.A1   The works of Anne Bradstreet. Edited by   Editor
1967   Jeannine Hensley. Foreword by Adrienne
        Rich. Cambridge, Mass.. Belknap Press of

PS
711   **Bradstreet, Anne (Dudley)** 1612?-1672   Author Card
.A1   The works of Anne Bradstreet. Edited by
1967   Jeannine Hensley. Foreword by Adrienne   Author's name
        Rich. Cambridge, Mass.. Belknap Press of   and dates
        Harvard University Press, 1967.   Title

        xxxvii. 320 p. facsim. 22 cm. (The John Harvard   Publisher and
            date of
        library) Bibliographical footnotes.   publication

        1.   Bradstreet, Anne, The works of   Description
            of book
        1. Hensley, Jeannine. ed.   (Series)   II. Title.
        PS711.A1   1967   811'.1   67 17312   Other
        Library of Congress   headings

Catalog cards

20b

This is a good place to mention one other way of finding materials in books. The *Essay and General Literature Index* (1900–), whose location you can find in the card catalog, is an annual subject index of books that are collections of essays on different subjects, often written by different authors. This index is usually the only way to locate such essays, since the title and subject classification of these books in the card catalog will ordinarily not be specific enough to help you.

Suppose, for example, that you are interested in the subject of women and art. If you look under the two headings "Women" and "Art" in the card catalog, you will find dozens of books on each subject, but you might spend days—or even weeks—looking through the books on women for those that also deal with art, and searching in the books on art for material on women artists. A few minutes of browsing in a recent issue of the *Essay and General Literature Index,* however, will lead you to the heading "Women in Art," and under it, entries like the following:

> Withers, J.   Judy Chicago's Dinner party: a personal vision of women's history.
>   *In* Art the ape of nature, ed. by M. Barasch and L. F. Sandler p789–99

What this entry means is that an essay by J. Withers entitled "Judy Chicago's Dinner Party: A Personal Vision of Women's History" is included on pages 789–99 of the book *Art, the Ape of Nature,* edited by M. Barasch and L. F. Sandler. The complete publication information for any book that you find listed is included at the back of the volume of the *Essay and General Literature Index* that you are using. With this information, you can go to the card catalog and determine whether the book is available in your library. The library in which we located this book listed it in the card catalog only under its title, the names of its two editors, and the broad subject heading "Art—Addresses, Essays, and Lectures." Without the *Essay and General Literature Index,* we would have had no easy way of finding Withers's valuable essay.

20c Standard reference works

You can use the card catalog to locate not only individual books by a specific author or on a particular subject, but also the standard reference works owned by your library—encyclopedias, dictionaries, indexes, and bibliographies. Your personal library no doubt includes a number of reference books, such as a dictionary and a desk encyclopedia; a college or public library, however, may own hundreds of specialized and useful reference works. These works fall into two general categories: books that offer facts (usually in the form of compact essays on various subjects), and books that provide bibliographies (lists of other books and articles on a given subject). Books in the first category are often useful when you are beginning a research project; they give you basic information on a subject, so that you can begin research with at least general knowledge of the field in which you are working. Books in the second category will lead you to further sources of information as your research efforts begin in earnest.

Reference works, like other books, are shelved according to call number, but most libraries conveniently place their reference books together in a single section of the library, or even in a separate reference room. (The catalog card will indicate if this is your library's practice.) As you become familiar with the reference works in your library, you may want to keep your own list or card file of the ones that you have found especially useful, so that you can locate them quickly for future research work. Skill in using your library's reference collection, like skill in most other areas of life, will come from frequent practice.

Below is a list of some standard reference works, grouped by type and subject. You will no doubt find many more in your library

Guides to reference books

Guide to Reference Books.
Guide to the Use of Books and Libraries.
The Reader's Adviser.

General information

Chambers' Encyclopedia.
Colliers' Encyclopedia.
Encyclopedia Americana.
Encyclopaedia Britannica.
Encyclopedia International.
New Columbia Encyclopedia.

Gazetteers and atlases

Columbia-Lippincott Gazetteer of the World.
National Geographic Atlas of the World.
Rand McNally Atlas of World History.
The Times Atlas of the World.

Reference books for special subjects

Art and architecture

Bryan's Dictionary of Painters and Engravers.
Encyclopedia of World Art.
Haggar, Reginald C. *Dictionary of Art Terms.*
Hamlin, T. F. *Architecture Through the Ages.*
Myers, Bernard S., ed. *Encyclopedia of Painting.*
Zboinski, A., and L. Tyszynski. *Dictionary of Architecture and Building Trades.*

Biography

American Men and Women of Science. This set includes scholars in the physical, biological, and social sciences.

Current Biography. Monthly since 1940, with an annual cumulative index, and brief bibliographic entries.

Dictionary of American Biography. Has bibliographic entries at the end of each article.

Dictionary of National Biography (British). 22 vols. and supplements. Each article is accompanied by a bibliography.

Directory of American Scholars. This set includes scholars in the humanities.

James, Edward T., and Janet W. James, eds. *Notable American Women 1607–1950.* Has bibliographic entries.

National Cyclopedia of American Biography. Includes supplements.

Webster's Biographical Dictionary.

Who's Who (British), *Who's Who in America, International Who's Who.* Brief accounts of living men and women, frequently revised.

Who's Who of American Women. 1958–.

Classics

Avery, C. B., ed. *New Century Classical Handbook.*

Hammond, N. G. L., and H. H. Scullard, eds. *Oxford Classical Dictionary.*

Harvey, Paul, ed. *Oxford Companion to Classical Literature.*

Current events

20c

Americana Annual. 1923–. An annual supplement to the *Encyclopedia Americana.*

Britannica Book of the Year. 1938–. An annual supplement to the *Encyclopaedia Britannica.* Some entries have a brief bibliography.

Facts on File. 1941–.

Statesman's Year Book. 1864–. A statistical and historical annual giving current information (and brief bibliographies) about countries of the world.

World Almanac. 1968–.

Economics and commerce

Coman, E. T. *Sources of Business Information.* A bibliography.

Greenwald, Douglas, et al. *McGraw-Hill Dictionary of Modern Economics.* Has bibliographic references.

Historical Statistics of the United States: Colonial Times to 1970. Includes indexes and bibliographies.

International Bibliography of Economics. 1952–.

Munn, Glenn G. *Encyclopedia of Banking and Finance.* Has bibliographic entries.

Sloan, Harold S., and Arnold Zurcher. *A Dictionary of Economics.*

Statistical Abstract of the United States. 1897–.

Wyckham, Robert G. *Images and Marketing: A Selected and Annotated Bibliography.*

Education

Burke, Arvid J., and Mary A. Burke. *Documentation in Education.*

Deighton, Lee C., ed. *The Encyclopedia of Education.* Has bibliographic entries.

Ebel, Robert L., et al. *Encyclopedia of Educational Research.* Has bibliographic references.

World Survey of Education. Has bibliographic references.

History

Adams, James T., ed. *Dictionary of American History.* A bibliography accompanies each article.

American Historical Association: Guide to Historical Literature.

Cambridge Ancient History. Bibliographic footnotes.

Cambridge Medieval History. Bibliographic footnotes.

Langer, William L., ed. *Encyclopedia of World History.*

Martin, Michael R., et al. *An Encyclopedia of Latin-American History.*

Morris, Richard B., and Graham W. Irwin, eds. *Harper Encyclopedia of the Modern World.*

New Cambridge Modern History. Bibliographic footnotes.

Literature, drama, and film

A. American

Hart, J. D. *Oxford Companion to American Literature.*

Leary, Lewis. *Articles on American Literature.*

Spiller, Robert E., et al. *Literary History of the United States.* Entries include bibliographic essays.

B. British

Baugh, A. C., et al. *A Literary History of England.* Has bibliographic entries.

Harvey, Paul, ed. *Oxford Companion to English Literature.*

20c

Sampson, George. *Concise Cambridge History of English Literature.*

Watson, George, ed. *The New Cambridge Bibliography of English Literature.*

Wilson, F. P., and Bonamy Dobree, eds. *Oxford History of English Literature.* Excellent bibliographic essays at the end of each volume.

C. Continental and general

Fleischmann, Wolfgang Bernard, ed. *Encyclopedia of World Literature in the Twentieth Century.* Brief bibliographies.

Grigson, Geoffrey. *The Concise Encyclopedia of Modern World Literature.* Brief bibliographic entries.

Leach, Maria, and Jerome Fried, eds. *Funk & Wagnall's Standard Dictionary of Folklore, Mythology, and Legend.*

MacCulloch, John A., et al. *Mythology of All Races.* Bibliography at end of each volume.

Preminger, Alex, F. J. Warnke, and O. B. Hardison, eds. *Encyclopedia of Poetry and Poetics.* A brief bibliography accompanies each article.

D. Drama and film

Gassner, John, and Edward Quin, eds. *Reader's Encyclopedia of World Drama.*

Hartnell, Phyllis, ed. *Oxford Companion to the Theater.* A bibliography accompanies each article.

The International Encyclopedia of Film.

20c

Music and dance

Apel, Willi. *Harvard Dictionary of Music.* Has brief bibliographic entries.

Beaumont, Cyril W. *A Bibliography of Dancing.*

De Mille, Agnes. *The Book of the Dance.*

Ewen, David. *The World of Twentieth Century Music.* Brief bibliographic entries.

Grove, George. *Dictionary of Music and Musicians.* This work and the *Harvard Dictionary of Music* are the authorities in the field. Excellent bibliographies.

Hanna, Judith Lynne. *To Dance Is Human.*

Scholes, P. A. *Oxford Companion to Music.* Includes bibliographies.

Thompson, Oscar. *International Cyclopedia of Music and Musicians.* Brief bibliographies.

Westrup, J. A., ed. *The New Oxford History of Music.* Includes bibliographies.

Philosophy

Copleston, Frederick. *A History of Western Philosophy.* Bibliography at
end of each volume.

Edwards, Paul, ed. *Encyclopedia of Philosophy.* Bibliographies.

Urmson, J. O. *The Concise Encyclopedia of Western Philosophy and
Philosophers.* Brief bibliography at end of volume.

Political science

Morgenthau, Hans. *Politics among Nations.*

Political Handbook of the World. 1927–.

Smith, Edward C., and A. J. Zurcher, eds. *Dictionary of American
Politics.*

White, Carl M., et al. *Sources of Information in the Social Sciences.*

Psychology

Beigel, Hugo. *A Dictionary of Psychology and Related Fields.*

Drever, James. *Dictionary of Psychology.*

The Harvard List of Books in Psychology. Annotated.

Psychological Abstracts. 1927–.

20c

Buttrick, G. A., et al. *Interpreter's Dictionary of the Bible: An Illustrated
Encyclopedia.* Has bibliographic entries.

Cross, F. L., and Elizabeth A. Livingstone. *Oxford Dictionary of the
Christian Church.* Has brief bibliographies.

Ferm, Vergilius. *Encyclopedia of Religion.* Brief bibliographic entries.

Hastings, James, ed. *Encyclopedia of Religion and Ethics.*

Jackson, S. M., et al. *New Schaff-Herzog Encyclopedia of Religious
Knowledge.*

McDonald, William J., et al., eds. *New Catholic Encyclopedia.*
A bibliography follows each article.

Werblowski, R. J. Z., and Geoffrey Wigoder, eds. *The Encyclopedia of
the Jewish Religion.*

Science

A. General

McGraw-Hill Encyclopedia of Science and Technology.

Newman, James R., et al. *Harper Encyclopedia of Science.* Brief
   bibliographic entries.

Van Nostrand's Scientific Encyclopedia.

B. Life sciences

Benthall, Jonathan. *Ecology in Theory and Practice.* Includes
   bibliographic references.

De Bell, Garrett, ed. *The Environmental Handbook.* Bibliography at end
   of volume.

Gray, Peter, ed. *Encyclopedia of the Biological Sciences.* Brief
   bibliographic entries.

Smith, Roger C., and W. Malcolm Reid, eds. *Guide to the Literature of
   the Life Sciences.*

C. Physical sciences

The International Dictionary of Physics and Electronics.

Kemp, D. A. *Astronomy and Astrophysics: A Bibliographical Guide.*

*Larousse Encyclopedia of the Earth: Geology, Paleontology, and
   Prehistory.*

Universal Encyclopedia of Mathematics.

Van Nostrand's International Encyclopedia of Chemical Science.

Sociology and anthropology

Biennial Review of Anthropology.

International Bibliography of Sociology. 1951–. Annual.

International Encyclopedia of the Social Sciences. Each article is followed
   by a bibliography.

Social Work Year Book. 1929–. Includes bibliographies.

20d   Indexes to periodicals

Many students new to research rely heavily—or even exclusively—on
books as their sources of information. Such a strategy has its pitfalls. For one
thing, books are not usually as well focused as a narrowly defined research
topic, and finding the precise information you need in a towering stack of general
books on a subject can become an exercise in frustration. Moreover, the time
involved in producing a book means that current information—the most recent
developments in Middle Eastern politics, for example, or the newest advances

in cancer treatment—may not be available in book form. To find such information, in addition to material on virtually any other kind of topic, you can turn to articles in periodicals.

Just as the card catalog provides an author, title, and subject index to your library's book holdings, periodical indexes offer a fast and easy way of locating articles in magazines, journals, and newspapers. Usually, you will find your library's periodical indexes grouped together in the reference collection. It is important to know the scope of at least the major indexes described below, because they cover different kinds of periodicals. However, since many of these indexes are produced by the same publisher in similar formats, you will discover that after you have become familiar with the layout of one, you can move easily to the others.

Once you have used the indexes below to locate potentially useful articles on the subject you are researching, determine whether or not your library subscribes to the journals you need by looking them up in the card catalog. Most libraries bind back issues of periodicals like books and shelve them together in a periodical room or by call number among books in the stacks. Current issues are usually on display in a periodicals reading room. For assistance in locating the periodicals you need, ask at your library's main desk.

If your library does not have a specific periodical that you need, ask at the Interlibrary Loan department about acquiring a photocopy of the article you're interested in from another library. Most libraries offer this service for a small charge. However, you should try not to depend on articles that you must order in this way, since the process can take several weeks, and the article, when it arrives, may turn out to be of less value to you than its title promised.

20d

General periodical indexes

Readers' Guide to Periodical Literature. 1900–.
> An author and subject index to over 200 magazines of general interest, such as *Consumer Reports, Ms., Newsweek, Sports Illustrated,* and *Popular Electronics.* Bound volumes cover a year or more; paperback supplements keep the index current usually to within a few weeks.

Humanities Index and *Social Sciences Index.* 1974–. Formerly a single
> index, published as the *Social Sciences and Humanities Index* from 1965 to 1974, and as the *International Index* from 1907 to 1965. The major general index to professional journals in the humanities (for example, *American Literature, Harvard Theological Review, Journal of Philosophy, New England Quarterly*) and the social sciences (for example, *Crime and Delinquency, Geographical Review, Journal of Economic Theory, Political Science Quarterly*). Same format as the *Readers' Guide,* though usually somewhat less current.

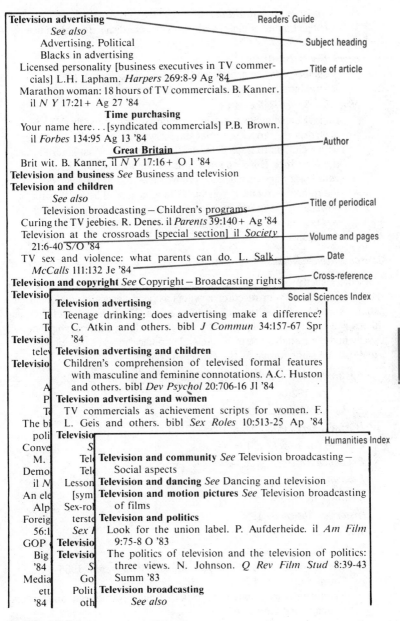

Television advertising — Readers' Guide — Subject heading
    See also
    Advertising. Political
    Blacks in advertising
Licensed personality [business executives in TV commer- — Title of article
    cials] L.H. Lapham. *Harpers* 269:8-9 Ag '84
Marathon woman: 18 hours of TV commercials. B. Kanner.
    il *N Y* 17:21+ Ag 27 '84
            Time purchasing
Your name here...[syndicated commercials] P.B. Brown.
    il *Forbes* 134:95 Ag 13 '84 — Author
            Great Britain
Brit wit. B. Kanner. il *N Y* 17:16+ O 1 '84
Television and business *See* Business and television
Television and children
    See also
    Television broadcasting—Children's programs — Title of periodical
Curing the TV jeebies. R. Denes. il *Parents* 39:140+ Ag '84
Television at the crossroads [special section] il *Society* — Volume and pages
    21:6-40 S/O '84
TV sex and violence: what parents can do. L. Salk. — Date
    McCalls 111:132 Je '84
Television and copyright *See* Copyright—Broadcasting rights — Cross-reference
Television

Social Sciences Index

Television advertising
    Teenage drinking: does advertising make a difference?
    C. Atkin and others. bibl *J Commun* 34:157-67 Spr
    '84
Television advertising and children
    Children's comprehension of televised formal features
    with masculine and feminine connotations. A.C. Huston
    and others. bibl *Dev Psychol* 20:706-16 Jl '84
Television advertising and women
    TV commercials as achievement scripts for women. F.
    L. Geis and others. bibl *Sex Roles* 10:513-25 Ap '84

Humanities Index

Television and community *See* Television broadcasting—
    Social aspects
Television and dancing *See* Dancing and television
Television and motion pictures *See* Television broadcasting
    of films
Television and politics
    Look for the union label. P. Aufderheide. il *Am Film*
    9:75-8 O '83
    The politics of television and the television of politics:
    three views. N. Johnson. *Q Rev Film Stud* 8:39-43
    Summ '83
Television broadcasting
    See also

Periodical indexes

20d

Poole's Index to Periodical Literature. 1802–81, 1882–1906.
> A subject index of nineteenth-century periodicals, harder to use than the *Readers' Guide,* but irreplaceable nonetheless.

Biography Index. 1946–.
> A subject index to articles and sections of books that are biographical in character. Same format as the *Readers' Guide.*

New York Times Index. 1913–.
> An invaluable subject and author index to one of the world's great newspapers. Provides a brief summary of most articles, together with a citation to issue date, section, and page. Most libraries carry the *New York Times* on microfilm; for the location of microfilms in your library and instructions on their use, ask at the main desk or in the reference room. If you live in an area served by another major newspaper, your library may also have an index for it that will help you find information on significant current and past events in your community.

Subject periodical indexes

Many disciplines produce thorough indexes to a variety of specialized journals in the field. Whenever your research is within a specific academic discipline, you should check to see whether such an index exists. The indexes that follow, and others like them, can be located through the library's card catalog; you will usually find them shelved near the general periodical indexes described above. Most use the same format as the *Readers' Guide.*

20d

Applied Science and Technology Index. 1957–.

Art Index. 1929–.

Biological Abstracts. 1926–.

Business Periodicals Index. 1958–.

Current Anthropology. 1960–.

Economic Abstracts. 1953–.

Education Index. 1929–.

Engineering Index. 1884–.

Historical Abstracts. 1955–.

Music Index. 1949–.

Philosopher's Index. 1940–.

Modern Language Association International Bibliography. 1956–.
> Formerly the *MLA American Bibliography,* 1921–55.
> The major bibliography of articles on English, American, and foreign language and literature.

Psychological Abstracts. 1927–.

Public Affairs Information Service. 1915–.

> A valuable index of articles, books, pamphlets, government documents, and other reports on public administration, international relations, and a broad range of economic and social issues.

Sociological Abstracts. 1955–.

Zoological Record. 1864–.

20e Database searches

An increasing number of libraries offer their patrons computerized access to lists of articles, unpublished papers, and other sources of information on a wide variety of subjects. Such computerized files are known as databases. Typically, a library will subscribe to the services of a database "vendor," a company that makes available by computer the contents of many different databases compiled and updated by independent companies and associations. For example, DIALOG, one of the largest such vendors, currently offers access to nearly two hundred separate databases in business, technology, the humanities, the social sciences, and the natural sciences. In all, a DIALOG subscriber may search through over seventy-five million records for titles relevant to a specific subject.

To perform a database search in most libraries, you will be asked by the reference librarian to complete an information form on your subject. The librarian then enters one or more "descriptors," or relevant subject headings, into a computer terminal, and the computer searches through all of the databases on the system and compiles a list of appropriate sources. On some systems, moreover, you can order a printed copy of the full text of an article. Some libraries also subscribe to simplified searching systems that library patrons can use directly, without the intermediary help of a librarian.

Perhaps the most serious drawback to such on-line searching is the cost, which is usually calculated according to the length of time that you are connected to the computer system. Although a ten-minute computer search may cost only a few dollars, a search that takes considerably longer can become an unrealistically expensive proposition for undergraduate research. On the other hand, database searches offer enormous savings of time. In just a few minutes, a computer can scan bibliographies that might take weeks to examine by hand. Databases are also more current than printed reference works can be. The new Wilsonline databases, for example, which offer computerized access to the Wilson family of periodical indexes (*Readers' Guide, Humanities Index, Social Science Index, Biography Index, Education Index,* etc.), are updated twice each week, whereas the corresponding bound indexes usually lag several weeks to several months behind the current date.

20e

20f Government documents

One of the most often overlooked and yet one of the most valuable sources of information on a wide range of subjects is the United States Government. Each year, the agencies of the national government publish thousands of pamphlets, booklets, magazines, and books on hundreds of subjects. Many libraries routinely receive and catalog much of this material, which is usually collected together in a single location.

The Subject Index in the *Monthly Catalog of United States Government Publications* is a good place to begin discovering the range and variety of government documents. The subject headings in one recent issue include everything from *Acid Rain* to *Airplane Inspection,* from *Computer Graphics* to *Chippewa Indians,* from *Lake Trout* to *Literacy,* from *Radioactive Waste Disposal* to *Retirement* to *Rhetoric* to *Rocket Engines.* Once you have located some promising titles in the subject index, the government documents librarian in your library can show you how to use the index to the documents on file and how to find items in your library's collection.

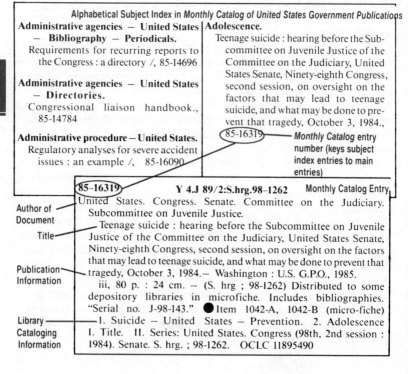

21 Working with Sources

A list of books, articles, and other sources of information on a given topic is called a bibliography. Most research papers end with a bibliography or with a list of works cited in the paper. But the research process also *begins* with the compilation of a "working bibliography," that is, a list of sources that the writer intends to examine. Only after assembling such a preliminary list of sources do most researchers move to the next important stage of research, taking notes.

21a The working bibliography

The working bibliography is valuable for a number of reasons. First, it becomes your master list of sources. Over a period of several weeks of research, you will not be able to remember all of the books and articles that you consulted, some of which were useful and some of which you found irrelevant to your topic. The working bibliography offers a systematic way of keeping track of all of these sources. Because it contains references to sources that you must still check, it provides an outline of the research work that remains for you to do; and since it includes the sources you have looked at, it helps to eliminate accidental backtracking. Second, the working bibliography gives you a place to make potentially useful notes about your sources as you examine them. Later, when you are putting your paper together, you will often find it helpful to be able to recall what an author's main point in an article was, or what your reactions to a book were as you read it.

Use common sense in choosing items for your working bibliography. Don't waste time, for example, in collecting references to obscure publications not available in your library. Interlibrary loans are possible but may be time-consuming, unpredictable, and expensive; you will usually find it more rewarding to explore the resources of your own library. Look for information in the most likely places. If your topic is a recent event or living person, for instance, start with newspapers and periodicals rather than with books.

The most sensible way to compile your working bibliography is to enter each potentially important source that you identify on a separate 3 x 5 card or slip of paper. On the back of each card, make your brief notes about the source. The separate cards can be sorted in any number of handy ways; for example, you might place all the sources remaining to be consulted on the top, all those that you have already examined on the bottom. When you are at last ready to compile your paper's list of works cited, you can simply remove cards for the sources not used in the paper, alphabetize the remaining cards, and type the list of works cited directly from them.

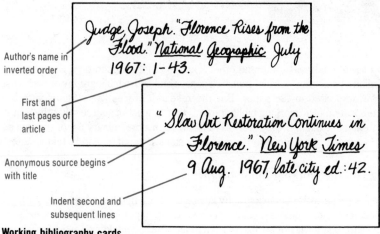

Author's name in inverted order

First and last pages of article

Anonymous source begins with title

Indent second and subsequent lines

Working bibliography cards

21a

In order to be able to use your working bibliography cards as the basis of your paper's final list of works cited, you must be careful to include all the information needed for the bibliography entries when you fill out each card. Otherwise, you will find yourself trekking back to the library at the last minute to look up a missing year of publication or to double check an illegibly written author's name. Even better, when you first fill out each bibliography card, use the precise bibliographic *form* described below, in order to expedite typing the list of works cited from your original cards.

Bibliography forms vary from discipline to discipline, but most systems of citing and listing sources aim for clarity and simplicity, and none is inherently superior to another. In this book we will follow the popular system of documentation prescribed by the Modern Language Association of America. Your instructor may give you another model to use. The most important thing about using any system is that you must follow it precisely and consistently. Though its rules may be arbitrary, they cannot arbitrarily be broken.

Below are model bibliographic entries, in MLA format, for most of the kinds of sources you will encounter. You might want to remember to have these samples handy when you are doing your library research so that you can refer to them as you fill out your bibliography cards. Note that the author's name is always given last name first for easy indexing. For the same reason, the second and subsequent lines of each entry are always indented.

Book by one author

White, Elizabeth Wade. Anne Bradstreet: "The Tenth Muse."
New York: Oxford UP, 1971.

[The abbreviation *UP* means *University Press*. For non-academic publishers, use a shortened form of the company's name (e.g., *Heath* for D. C. Heath and Company; *Knopf* for Alfred A. Knopf, Inc.).]

Book by one author, revised or later edition

Morison, Samuel Eliot. The Intellectual Life of Colonial
New England. 2nd ed. New York: New York UP, 1956.

Book by one author, reprint of an older edition

Bailey, Elmer Jones. Religious Thought in the Greater
American Poets. 1922. Freeport: Books for Libraries, 1968.

[As the copyright page indicates, this book was originally issued in 1922 by a different publisher.]

Book by one author, edited by another

Bradford, William. Of Plymouth Plantation: 1620–1647.
Ed. Samuel Eliot Morison. New York: Knopf, 1952.

Hutchinson, Robert, ed. Poems of Anne Bradstreet. New
York: Dover, 1969.

[In the first case, the work of primary interest is Bradford's original text; in the citation, therefore, the author's name precedes the editor's. In the second case, the editor's work is being cited.]

21a

Translated book

Brumm, Ursula. American Thought and Religious Typology.
Trans. John Hoaglund. New Brunswick: Rutgers UP,
1970.

Book by one author, part of a series

Piercy, Josephine K. Anne Bradstreet. Twayne's United
States Authors Series 72. 1965. New Haven: College
and UP, 1965.

Waller, George M., ed. <u>Puritanism in Early America</u>. 2nd
ed. Problems in American Civilization. Lexington:
Heath, 1973.

[The name of the series and, if given, the number of the volume in the series follow the title and edition, and are not underlined.]

Multivolume book

Sturzo, Luigi. <u>Church and State</u>. 2 vols. Notre Dame: U of
Notre Dame P, 1962.

Book by two or more authors

Miller, Perry, and T. H. Johnson. <u>The Puritans</u>. 2 vols. New
York: Harper, 1963.

[Note that the second author's name is given in normal rather than reversed order. When the source is a work by more than three authors, you need give the name only of the first, following it with the Latin abbreviation *et al.* (*and others*): Walker, Stephen A., et al.]

Essay in book of essays by different authors

Martin, Wendy. "Anne Bradstreet's Poetry: A Study of
Subversive Piety." <u>Shakespeare's Sisters: Feminist
Essays on Women Poets</u>. Ed. Sandra M. Gilbert and
Susan Gubar. Bloomington: Indiana UP, 1979. 19–31.

[The title of the essay is followed by the title of the book in which it is contained and the book's editor or editors. At the end of the citation come the pages on which the essay is found.]

Unpublished dissertation

Requa, Kenneth Alan. "Public and Private Voices in the
Poetry of Anne Bradstreet, Michael Wigglesworth, and
Edward Taylor." Diss. Indiana U, 1971.

Article in a weekly or monthly magazine

Cotter, J. F. "Women Poets: Malign Neglect?" <u>America</u>
17 Feb. 1973: 140–42.

[Underline the name of the magazine, abbreviate the month, and give the first and last pages of the article at the end of the citation. The citation for an anonymous article begins with the title.]

21a

Article in a professional journal

Laughlin, Rosemary M. "Anne Bradstreet: Poet in Search of
Form." American Literature 42 (1970): 1–17.

[Most periodicals issued less frequently than monthly, like this one, use continuous
pagination for all the issues published in a single year; that is, if the first issue ends on
page 125, the second issue begins with page 126. In the citation of a periodical with
continuous pagination, it is not necessary to include more than the volume number, the
year, and the page numbers of the article. If the journal above did not number pages in
each volume continuously, it would be necessary to add the issue number after the
volume number: 42.1 (1970): 1–17.]

Article in a newspaper

Donoghue, Denis. "Does America Have a Major Poet?" New York
Times 3 Dec. 1978, late city ed., sec. 7: 9+.

[The page citation 9+ indicates that the article begins on page nine and continues on
nonconsecutive pages later in the newspaper. Specify the edition of the paper when it is
given on the masthead. If the newspaper is divided into sections with separate
pagination, specify the section as well; if the sections of a newspaper are lettered, the
section can be incorporated into the page citation: 11 Nov. 1982, early ed.: C23. The
citation for an anonymous newspaper article begins with the title.]

Article in an encyclopedia

21a

"Bradstreet, Anne Dudley." Encyclopaedia Britannica:
Micropaedia. 1974 ed.

[Unless the article is signed, begin with the subject heading as it appears in the
encyclopedia, enclosed in quotation marks. For standard reference works like encyclopedias, full publication information is not required in the citation.]

Interview

Toulouse, Teresa A. Personal interview. 31 Mar. 1985.

Book review

Pettit, Norman. Rev. of American Puritanism: Faith and
Practice, by Darrett B. Rutman. New England Quarterly
43 (1970): 504–06.

Government document

United States. Superintendent of Documents. <u>Poetry and Literature</u>. Washington: GPO, 1978.

[Unless the name of the author of a government publication is known, begin as above with the name of the government and the name of the agency issuing the publication. The abbreviation *GPO* stands for *Government Printing Office.*]

<u>21b</u> Taking notes

After you have identified several likely sources of information on your topic, your next impulse may be to arm yourself with packages of looseleaf paper or piles of legal tablets to be filled up with notes. But remember that you will be writing your paper directly from your notes, not from the books you've consulted, which are hard to refer to, or from the periodicals you've read, which usually cannot leave your library. The basic consideration for note taking, then, is this: how can you take notes that will be most useful and most accessible later, as you compose the paper?

For most people, the answer to this question is to take notes on separate cards or slips of paper, 4 x 6 or larger (regular typing paper cut in half works very well). The rationale for such a system is simple. Note taking is an exploratory act, not a definitive one; as you are taking notes, you can never be certain which notes you will later use and which you will not need. If your notes are on separate cards, you will later be able to sort them out, clip them together, arrange some and discard others. You will gain a flexibility that will enormously simplify the task of organizing and writing your paper.

For such a system of note taking to work, though, it should be clear that each note card must be *self-contained.* To insure that you will later be able to cite sources accurately in your paper, you must include on each note card a reference to the source from which that note was taken. You can accomplish this simply by numbering your bibliography cards in sequence, and then copying the correct source number onto each of the note cards that you complete while you are working with that source. In addition, you must be sure that the page number or numbers from which the note was taken also appear on the card, for you will need to be able to cite those page numbers in your final paper. Finally, you must be certain that the single note you place on each card is complete and clear, so that it will make sense to you later, when you no longer have in front of you the entire article or book from which it was taken.

Before we discuss the content of your notes, let's consider the types of notes that you might take. There are four basic types of notes, and a single note card may contain just one or a combination of all four:

21b

Text of Source

essentially a struggle for survival. The amenities of gracious behavior
could hardly be expected to flourish in the midst of the damp and
dirt of the hastily built, overcrowded shelters, the crippling illnesses,
and the spiritual disabilities of homesickness, sorrow, and discourage-
ment. But the Puritan's code of good manners was an integral part
of his standard of Christian conduct, and for these devout colonists,
especially those among them who had been privileged to live gently
in England, it must have been disheartening to see the formality of
every-day communication, the respect for individual privacy, the quick
concern for a troubled neighbor, and the dignity of innate self-
possession, too often falter and fail under the weight of outrageous
circumstance.

Tho
failed
was be

Bibliography Card

White, Elizabeth Wade. *Anne Bradstreet*:
"*The Tenth Muse.*" New
York: Oxford U P, 1971.

Source

Page

Paraphrase

Quotation

Researcher's
Note
to Self

Note Card

21b

White, p. 116
 Crude living conditions particularly
hard for Puritan colonists to endure,
since "the Puritan's code of good manners
was an integral part of his standard
of Christian conduct...."
 (another example of moral tone of
life in Massachusetts Bay Colony)

Source, bibliography card, note card

1. Direct quotation

Copying direct quotations onto note cards may at first seem to be the easiest way to take notes, but often it actually creates more work for you later on. Mounds of undigested quotations lacking their original contexts are usually harder to work with as you are writing your paper than incisive and thoughtful notes in your own words (see *Paraphrase,* below). Sometimes, however, you will find a writer who states his or her point so forcefully or cleverly or succinctly that you believe you might want to quote the author's own phrasing in your paper. In such cases, when you copy an author's exact words onto your note card, be certain to enclose them in quotation marks so that later, as you compose your paper, you will be able to distinguish between your own words on your note cards and the words that belong to others. Be certain, too, that everything within the quotation marks is exactly as it appears in the original quotation; you are not free to omit or add words randomly, or to change punctuation or spelling. If you have to add a word or phrase for clarity, you must enclose the added material in square brackets ([ ]—not parentheses). If you wish to delete part of an overly long quotation, you must show the deletion with three spaced periods (. . .) called ellipses. Quotations, in short, must be handled with precision. If you fail to set them off with quotation marks, you leave yourself open to the serious charge of plagiarism, to be discussed further below. If you alter them without indicating the change, you may be penalized by your instructor for the sloppiness of your research procedures.

21b

2. Paraphrase

A paraphrase is a restatement of another writer's ideas in words which are entirely your own. Paraphrasing takes thought and care, for it must reflect the meaning of the given text but must be wholly original in phrasing. You may not simply replace some of the words in another writer's sentence with your own; instead, the very structure of your sentence should be different from your source's. Good paraphrasing takes time when you are doing it, but it can save time later: if you have paraphrased well, you may be able to write your paper directly from material on your note cards, though you will still need to acknowledge the source of the ideas contained in your prose (for more information on acceptable paraphrase, see **22b**).

3. Summary

As you get further and further along in your research, you will be better able to decide when you need to note all of the details given in a passage in one of your sources, and when you can simply summarize the passage in a sentence or two. Look for opportunities to reduce your work without sacrificing important information by using summary effectively.

4. Notes to yourself

Have you found a quotation that might make an attention-getting introduction to your paper? Are you reading a source whose ideas contradict other articles that you've examined? Is the book in front of you the best survey of your subject that you have located so far? You can't expect to remember all the peripheral ideas that occur to you as you do your research, so write them down on your note cards as they come to mind. Later, when you review your cards in preparation for outlining the paper, you'll be glad for the clarifying or explanatory or suggestive notes that you made to yourself while you were deep in the research process.

• • •

As this description of notes suggests, note taking is far from being a mechanical task. It is a thoughtful, even creative, act that demands your alertness and care.

If research is new to you, you may be wondering how you will recognize a "note" when you encounter one in your reading. When you are just beginning to research a topic, after all, almost everything you read about it may be new. Is everything, therefore—every page, every paragraph, every sentence—a note waiting to be jotted down? If that is so, you may be thinking, note taking will mean paraphrasing or summarizing the complete contents of every article or book you pick up.

Although there are no secret tricks that will unfailingly enable you to spot potential notes hidden among the closely packed lines of an article in the *New York Times,* note taking is fortunately a more selective process than that description of it suggests. You might keep the following general guidelines in mind as you decide what information to commit to your note cards. *First,* a good note will make a clear point. If you can't understand what the author you're reading is saying, copying down a quotation from the article or a paraphrase of the text will not help you later. The notes you take should each be clear enough for anyone looking over your note cards—even a person who had not read the original sources—to understand. *Second,* good notes often reflect the particular attitudes or opinions of the author whom you are reading. Try to write notes that capture the essence of an author's argument, concisely restate the main point, or indicate his or her biases. *Finally,* good notes will present specific information—facts, places, descriptions, examples, statistics, case histories. Like all good essays, successful research papers are grounded in specific information, information that must exist on your note cards when you begin to compose your paper.

In the early stages of your work, you should expect to take many notes that you will later discard. This is an inevitable part of research work since, as we said earlier, it is only through the research process that you will be able to define and focus your subject clearly. Taking notes and rethinking your original topic are two processes that go hand in hand. To put it more brutally: you'll have to take many notes that you will ultimately throw away before you'll know which ones to keep.

21b

Exercise 1

Write a bibliographic entry in correct MLA format for each of the following sources.

1. An article entitled Of Time and Mathematics, published by Philip J. Davis in the Southern Humanities Review, volume 18, 1984. It appears on pages 193 to 202.
2. Frances Gray's article The Nature of Radio Drama, in a book entitled Radio Drama and edited by Peter Lewis. The book was published in London by Longman. The year of publication is 1981. The article appears on pages 48 to 77.
3. Sheila A. Egoff's book Thursday's Child: Trends and Patterns in Contemporary Children's Literature, published in Chicago by the American Library Association. The year of publication is 1981.
4. Cost Estimate Jumps for Music Center Expansion, an article in the September 12, 1984 issue of the Los Angeles Times. It appears on page 1 of section VI.
5. An article in the Journal of Broadcasting by Joanne Cantor, Dean Ziemke, and Glenn G. Sparks. The title is Effect of Forewarning on Emotional Responses to a Horror Film. It appears on pages 21 to 31 of volume 28, 1984.
6. A two-volume book by Joseph N. Ireland entitled Records of the New York Stage from 1750 to 1860. It was originally published in 1866 and was reissued in 1966 by Benjamin Blom, Inc. of New York.
7. An anonymous article on page 23 of the August 6, 1984 issue of Business Week. The title is Job Safety Becomes a Murder Issue.
8. An article written by James A. Winders entitled Reggae, Rastafarians and Revolution: Rock Music in the Third World. It appears on pages 61 to 73 of the Journal of Popular Culture, volume 17, 1983.
9. A book by Charles J. Maland entitled Frank Capra. It is a volume in Twayne's Theatrical Arts Series and was published in 1980 in Boston by Twayne.
10. The article Sleep in the 1980 Encyclopedia Americana. Ian Oswald wrote the article, which appears on pages 31 to 33 of volume 25.

21b

22 Writing the Research Paper

The more you learn about your subject from note taking, the more you may feel that you will never be able to stop examining sources without the risk of missing some potentially important new piece of information. Strictly speaking, of course, that's true. But the realities of research—whether in college or in business life—dictate that you must at some point call a halt to your research and consciously consider ways of shaping the material that you have collected into a coherent whole. At this point in the research process, your attention naturally turns to questions of organization and documentation.

22a Organization and structure

How can you know when you've collected enough information and can safely end your note taking? Although it may be difficult to be certain that you have reached this stage in your work, you might expect your research to progress along lines something like the following. First, you will examine all of your "major" sources, that is, all of those that you initially expected to be important sources of information on your topic. Once you move beyond that list and start looking at other sources, you will probably discover a number of the same specific topics surfacing in many of your sources, and you will begin to see connections among your note cards for the first time. Source Y has an opinion different from source X's; source B's recent research confirms the earlier hypothesis of source A. As the same major issues surface repeatedly in your work, you may gradually begin to develop a vague mental outline of some of the key points you think your paper should cover. Eventually, the sources you examine may begin simply to duplicate those that you have already looked at, and the time you spend locating an obscure book or article is no longer repaid by the information you glean from it.

At about this point, you will no doubt realize that you have developed ideas of your own about your subject based on the reading and note taking that you have done. This, too, may be an indication that your note taking is nearing an end. The best researchers, after all, are less interested in mere piles of accumulated data than in ways of using the data they have collected to support their own observations and ideas. Once you are able to see beyond your separate notes to the ways in which these notes can be used to support a larger argument of your own, a sense of the completeness of your work may begin to grow upon you. When the material you've accumulated begins to seem rich and full enough to be the basis of a sophisticated and original paper, it may be time to retire from the library—for a while, at least—and have a try at writing the paper.

The first stage in writing your paper is reviewing and sorting out all of the notes you have taken, bringing together notes from different sources that explain, comment on, or give evidence for the same specific points. If you have put your notes on separate cards or slips of paper, you will find this easy to do. As you read each one, decide which aspect of your subject it pertains to, and group it with others that deal with the same issue. Don't be surprised if you have a large "miscellaneous" category made up of notes whose value may seem questionable; many of your early note cards may indeed not be important anymore, now that your subject has become more clearly limited. Of course, while sorting out your note cards will help you define the main issues to focus on, it may also help you to see which points need further research. Some additional trips to the library in search of specific pieces of information may still be necessary before your paper is finished.

As they sort out their note cards, some writers compose a "comment card" to go with each note card, reminding them of their reasons for taking the note or briefly indicating the way they expect to use the note in the paper. Later, when they have begun writing, they can easily expand the comment card into a sentence or two that establishes a clear context for the material on the note cards. This practice helps to guarantee that the finished paper will not be a mere splicing together of facts or quotations; instead, the notes will function as part of a larger argument created by the researcher.

22a

Few writers can progress beyond this point in composing a long paper without making at least an informal outline. The piles of note cards before you will help. Each of the large piles may be one of the main points in your paper, a main heading in your outline. Within each pile you will find notes that will make up the subpoints to be covered. With your usable notes organized in groups before you, sketch out an outline of your paper on a separate sheet of paper, including all the subpoints that you have notes to support. Some writers like to mark each of their note cards to correspond with the points in their written outline, so that they will know just which cards to pick up as they compose the paper.

Armed with an outline and groups of note cards that support it, you are ready to begin writing. Often, students mistakenly approach the writing of a research paper as if it were entirely different from the other writing that they have been doing in freshman composition. Instead of composing a thesis with a clearly stated subject and focus, they open their paper with a formula like, "This paper will deal with. . . ." Instead of writing well-organized paragraphs structured around topic sentences and specific evidence and detail, they will let some paragraphs run on for a page or more, while they cut others off after only a few lines. Perhaps the most important advice to keep in mind as you begin writing is that the research paper, though it may be longer than other papers you have written, is more like a typical expository essay than it is unlike one, and its success will depend largely on the same principles of effective writing that you have already encountered. If you have learned how to formulate a thesis and introduction, how to write clearly structured paragraphs, how to use specific diction and development effectively, how to ensure coherence and maintain consistency of tone, then you should be able to write a good research paper.

Below we will discuss some guidelines for using and citing in your paper the material you take from your note cards. Apart from those hints and the information on composing presented elsewhere in this book, most of the advice we can offer at this point on writing your research paper is based on common sense. Write your first draft in any way that will help you move along quickly, whether that means using a soft pencil, a ballpoint pen, a typewriter, or a word processor. Your main goal at this stage should be to get your ideas down on paper while they are hot. Skip lines if you write by hand, so that you will have room for additions and changes to be made later. In your first draft, don't take the time to copy down quotations that you want to use in your text; instead, simply clip the note card with the quotation on it to the appropriate page of your draft. Try to divide your planned paper up into segments; if you get stuck in one section, leave it temporarily and work on a different one. The time to worry about tight organization will come later, as you revise your early drafts.

22a

When you do begin revising, you should probably be prepared to make more changes than you might have made in other papers you have written. The length of a research paper and the number of different materials on which it is based open up a variety of possibilities for its organization, and you need to be ready to reassemble your material in several ways before you find it completely satisfactory. Transitional words, phrases, and sentences will be more important than ever as you attempt to link together smoothly the information gathered from your various sources and your own observations and conclusions.

The best advice we can offer is, for many students, the hardest to follow: leave enough time to write your earliest draft in several sittings, to put it away for a day or two (or at least overnight), and then to return to it fresh for thorough revision. A research paper is a complex project, and you should not expect to be able to dash off a draft one evening, patch it up the next, and hand it in on the following morning. Apart from matters of composition—formidable enough in a paper of this length—you will need time to double-check your use of sources, make sure your citations are accurate, type up the paper in the correct format, and proofread carefully. Leave yourself time enough to assemble a paper worthy of the weeks of research you have completed.

22b Avoiding plagiarism

Although it is similar in many respects to the other writing you have done, the research paper presents you with at least one major new task: accurately citing the sources of your research. If you fail to distinguish between your own words and thoughts, and those of your sources, you mislead your reader into assuming that everything in the paper is your own work. To pass off the language or ideas of someone else as your own is plagiarism, and it can have serious consequences. In the section below we will discuss the proper format for citing sources in your paper. Before we do that, however, we need to look more closely at the concept of plagiarism itself.

There are two basic situations in which you must cite your sources in order to avoid plagiarizing, and we will examine them separately.

1. Every direct quotation must be enclosed in quotation marks, and its source must be cited.

This rule is easy enough to understand. If you did not enclose the direct quotations that you take from your sources in quotation marks, your reader would have no way of knowing which words were yours and which were those of your sources. And once you do use quotation marks to set off these phrases or sentences, your reader's natural question will be, "Who wrote this?" Your citation of the source answers that question.

The logic behind acknowledging direct quotations is clear, but the precise difference between quotation and acceptable paraphrase is harder for many writers to grasp. *In general, several words in succession taken from another source may be said to constitute direct quotation.* Thus you cannot turn a quotation into an acceptable sentence of your own simply by changing a few words in the original. Consider the following examples.

Source

"In a given area the plague accomplished its kill within four to six months and then faded, except in the larger cities, where, rooting into the close-quartered population, it abated during the winter, only to reappear in spring and rage for another six months."

— Tuchman, Barbara W. *A Distant Mirror: The Calamitous 14th Century.* New York: Knopf, 1978. [p. 93]

Unacceptable paraphrase

In a specific area the plague killed its victims in four to six months and then receded, except in big cities, where it declined in the winter, only to reappear in spring and

flourish for another six months.

[This writer has merely substituted a few words of his own for words in the source. The structure of the sentence, however, is Tuchman's. The result is plagiarism.]

Unacceptable paraphrase

The plague accomplished its kill within four to six months

in most places, but in the cities it abated during the winter

and would rage again in the spring.

[The structure of this writer's sentence is original, but she has used several phrases taken directly from Tuchman: *accomplished its kill within four to six months, abated during the winter.* Borrowing such phrases without enclosing them in quotation marks makes the writer guilty of plagiarism. Just the word *rage* as used here would constitute plagiarism in most readers' eyes, even though it is not part of a longer phrase taken from Tuchman, because it is such a distinctive verb in Tuchman's original sentence.]

Acceptable paraphrase

In the crowded cities, the plague never completely disap-

peared; though relatively dormant in the winter, it returned

in full force when the weather turned warm again.

[This writer has captured the exact meaning of Tuchman's passage, but in a sentence that is original in structure and diction. The only major words taken from Tuchman are *cities, plague,* and *winter;* such duplication is acceptable, since it would be impossible to find synonyms for these basic terms.]

22b

But even a quotation converted into acceptable paraphrase will need to have its source cited in your paper if it falls under the second rule for citing sources, which deals not with the *language* of the original source, but with the *ideas* in the texts you read:

2. Even if they are acceptably paraphrased, all ideas taken from a source must be documented unless they are considered common knowledge.

The critical term in this rule is, of course, "common knowledge." In practice, we often find it simply impossible to give sources for everything we write. Where, for example, did we get these rules for avoiding plagiarism? We really don't know. For years we have heard plagiarism talked about, have read about it, and have recognized examples of it in student papers. In short, our knowledge of what the term means is common knowledge, part of our understanding for which we have no single source.

If you are unsure whether an idea you encounter in your research qualifies as common knowledge, you might keep in mind the following two-step test. An idea is common knowledge and need *not* be cited only if

a. you found it repeated in many sources, rather than stated in only one, *or*
b. you believe it would be familiar to the average educated person, even one who had not researched the subject (a person, for example, like one of your classmates).

Thus the fact that the Olympic Games originated in Greece would not need citation, since it is information that would be found in many books and articles on the Olympics, and it is a fact known by most people. Nor would the fact that the modern Olympic Games were begun in 1896 require citation; although most people you asked would probably not be able to give you this date, anyone doing research on the Olympics would encounter it over and over again in a variety of sources. But a single writer's opinion about the propaganda value of the 1936 Olympics in Berlin *would* probably need a citation, even if it were acceptably paraphrased. Such a statement would not meet either of the conditions above. As a specific writer's opinion, it would appear only in a single source (though if you found a great many writers who shared this opinion, it would then qualify as common knowledge after all). And as the statement of a presumed authority on the Olympics, it would not be information that we could expect others who had not studied the subject to know.

22c

22c Citing sources

Above we described the situations in which you must indicate the sources of the material—whether quoted or paraphrased—that you have used in writing your research paper. In this section, we turn to the method of making such citations in the text of your paper.

The Modern Language Association of America has adopted a system of documentation that eliminates the elaborate footnotes used for years by both students and scholars. The simplicity of this new system and the academic prestige of its proponent, the MLA, suggest that it will come into increasingly widespread use, and it is therefore the method of documentation that we describe below. Keep in mind, however, that systems of documentation vary arbitrarily from discipline to discipline. The best advice we can offer you is to follow closely whatever model your instructor suggests.

The new MLA system reduces documentation to two components. First, at the end of each passage whose source must be noted, the last name of the author and the page or pages on which the material is found are inserted in parentheses:

(Alexander 197—98)

At the end of the paper, on a separate sheet with the heading **Works Cited,** a complete bibliographic entry is provided for each of the sources cited in the text (see the sample lists of works cited on pages 317 and 333). These entries, which follow the forms for the bibliography cards described on pages 277–80, are arranged alphabetically according to the last names of the authors:

Alexander, Edwin P. On the Main Line: The Pennsylvania Rail-
road in the 19th Century. New York: Potter, 1971.

If you properly filled out a bibliography card for each of your sources as you took notes, you will be able to alphabetize the cards for the sources you used and copy your works cited entries directly from them.

The examples below illustrate some variations on this method of citing sources.

Quotations

Typically, the parenthetical citation in a text comes *after* the quotation marks that close a quotation but *before* the sentence's end punctuation:

22c

Citation in text

The definitive biography of Mahatma Gandhi remains to be
written. As one Gandhi scholar has explained, "Multivolume
works written by Gandhi's former colleagues and published
in India are comprehensive in scope, but their objectivity
suffers from the authors' reverent regard for their subject" (Juergensmeyer 294).

Citation in works cited

Juergensmeyer, Mark. "The Gandhi Revival—A Review Article." Journal of Asian Studies 43 (1984): 293—98.

A quotation of more than four lines is commonly set off from the text and indented ten spaces from the left margin. Such a quotation is usually introduced with a colon, and the parenthetical citation is placed *after* the end punctuation:

Citation in text

One editor suggests that photographers trying to publish their work should aim to surpass—not just equal—the photographs they see in print:

> Editors know where they can get pictures like the ones they've already published. If you want to get noticed, you have to take pictures better than those. This is especially true if you are looking for assignments rather than to sell existing pictures. Why take a chance on a new photographer who will come up with no better than what you already have, an editor might reason? (Scully 33)

Citation in works cited

Scully, Judith. "Seeing Pictures." <u>Modern Photography</u> May 1984: 28–33.

22c

You can often fit quotations into your text smoothly by introducing the author's name before the quotation or by placing it at some point in the middle of the quotation. In such cases, only the page number of the source needs to appear in the parenthetical citation. The following examples illustrate both of these techniques:

Citation in text

The English, notes Richard Altick, are obsessed by love for their dogs. "Walking dogs is a ritual that proceeds independently of weather, cataclysms, and the movements of the planets; they are led or carried everywhere, into department stores, fishmongers', greengrocers', buses, trains" (286).

Citation in works cited

Altick, Richard D. <u>To Be in England</u>. New York: Norton, 1969.

Citation in text

> "After watching a lot of music videos," Holly Brubach
> observes, "it's hard to escape the conclusions that no one
> has the nerve to say no to a rock–and–roll star and that most
> videos would be better if someone did" (102).

Citation in works cited

> Brubach, Holly. "Rock–and–Roll Vaudeville." <u>Atlantic</u>
> July 1984: 99–102.

If the author of the material you are quoting is not given, use the title, or a shortened form of the title, in your text citation. Place the titles of articles in quotation marks; underline the titles of books. Remember, whenever you quote, that you may use part of an author's sentence rather than the whole, as long as the section you have chosen fits into the syntax of your own sentence and does not misrepresent the author's original meaning:

Citation in text

> Environmentalists protested that a recent study of the plan
> to spray herbicides on marijuana "systematically under–
> estimated the possibility of damage from such spraying and
> exaggerated the benefits to be achieved by a spraying
> program" ("Marijuana Spraying" 14).

22c

Citation in works cited

> "Marijuana Spraying Opposed." <u>New York Times</u> 22 Aug.
> 1984: 14.

In the case of a one-page article like that above, the page number may be omitted in the text citation.

The text citation to a work in more than one volume includes the volume number and a colon before the page citation:

Citation in text

> The medieval manor–house dominated nearby cottages "not
> only because it was better built, but above all because it
> was almost invariably designed for defence" (Bloch 2: 300).

Citation in works cited

> Bloch, Marc. <u>Feudal Society</u>. Trans. L. A. Manyon. 2 vols.
>
>   Chicago: U of Chicago P, 1961.

When two or three persons wrote the material that you wish to quote, include the names of all. Follow the same order in which the names are printed in the original source:

Citation in text

> Selvin and Wilson argue that "a concern for effective
>
> writing is not a trivial elevation of form over content.
>
> Good writing is a condition, slowly achieved, of . . . being
>
> what one means to be" (207).

Citation in works cited

> Selvin, Hanan C., and Everett K. Wilson. "On Sharpening
>
>   Sociologists' Prose." <u>Sociological Quarterly</u> 25
>
>   (1984): 205–22.

When your source is a work by more than three authors, give the name only of the first in your text citation, followed by the abbreviation "et al." ("and others"), for example: (Leventhal et al. 54).

If your list of works cited includes more than one work by the same author, your text citations to this author must indicate which work you are referring to. In such cases, add a shortened version of the relevant title. In the list of works cited, substitute three hyphens and a period for the author's name in the second citation.

22c

Citation in text

> "Of America's eastern rivers," writes one historian, "none
>
> was longer or potentially more important than the one the
>
> Indians accurately described as the 'Long–reach River'––
>
> Susquehanna" (Hanlon, <u>Wyoming Valley</u> 17).

Citations in works cited

> Hanlon, Edward F. <u>The Wyoming Valley: An American Portrait</u>.
>
>   Woodland Hills, CA: Windsor, 1983.

———. "Urban—Rural Cooperation and Conflict in the Congress:

      The Breakdown of the New Deal Coalition, 1933—1938."

      Diss. Georgetown U, 1967.

Paraphrasing

A successful research paper, as we suggested earlier, is more than a string of quotations. Although a strategically placed quotation can help to focus a paragraph or emphasize a point, an extended series of quotations in a research paper often creates the impression of disjointedness and confusion. Look instead for opportunities to express in your own words the ideas that you have discovered during your research.

As the following examples illustrate, the rules described above for acknowledging the sources of quotations also apply to paraphrased material.

Citation in text (author's name in parenthetical citation)

The steadily growing role of television in politics has

helped to shift attention away from the politicians' stands

on issues to the way they appear before the camera

(Meyrowitz 51).

Citation in works cited

Meyrowitz, Joshua. "Politics in the Video Eye: Where Have

      All the Heroes Gone?" Psychology Today July 1984:

      46—51.

22c

Citation in text (author's name in text)

One effect of the microscope's development in the late

1600's, Paul Fussell points out, was to change attitudes

toward insects. Whereas people in the seventeenth century

had considered insects innocuous creatures, eighteenth—

century men and women, exposed for the first time to

drawings of magnified insect bodies, regarded them as

hideous and contemptible (235—36).

Citation in works cited

> Fussell, Paul. <u>The Rhetorical World of Augustan Humanism:</u>
> <u>Ethics and Imagery from Swift to Burke</u>. London:
> Oxford UP, 1965.

Citation in text (anonymous article)

> Some airport delays, it appears, can be blamed on govern-
> ment deregulation of the airlines. On at least one weekday
> at Kennedy International Airport, for example, airlines
> have now scheduled over sixty arrivals between four and
> five o'clock, even though the airport can accommodate only
> forty-nine landings each hour ("Not Quite Ready" 25).

Citation in works cited

> "Not Quite Ready When You Are." <u>Time</u> 9 July 1984: 25.

Citation in text (source with two authors)

> Computers may be dominating the modern office, but archi-
> tects are beginning to counter this technological takeover
> by designing comfortable and inviting office interiors
> (Davies and Malone 73).

Citation in works cited

> Davies, Douglas, and Maggie Malone. "Offices of the
> Future." <u>Newsweek</u> 14 May 1984: 72+.

The page citation "72+" above indicates that this article begins on page 72 and continues on nonconsecutive pages in the rest of the magazine.

Although footnotes have been eliminated from the citing of sources in the new MLA system of documentation, they may still be used to add supplementary information to the text of a research paper. Such notes, often referred to as "content notes," are indicated in the text with consecutive superscript numerals and are placed either at the bottom of the appropriate page or together on a separate sheet, with the heading **Notes,** inserted after the text of the paper and before the Works Cited page. If you collect your notes together on a separate sheet, as most instructors prefer, double-space between and within the notes. Indent the first line of each note five spaces.

Content notes offer a convenient means of including explanatory material or referring the reader to additional sources of information:

Text with superscript

> The art of biographical writing in nineteenth–century
> England has generally been undervalued,[1] with the result
> that modern readers tend to regard Victorian biographies
> with a certain condescension and smugness.

Note

> [1] A few recent authors, however, have recognized the
> artistic merit of at least some nineteenth–century bio–
> graphical writing. For useful readings of several major
> biographies of the period, see Gwiasda and Reed.

The full publication information for sources mentioned in notes is supplied in the list of works cited:

Citations in works cited

> Gwiasda, Karl E. "The Boswell Biographers: A Study of 'Life
>   and Letters' Writing in the Victorian Period." Diss.
>   Northwestern U, 1969.
> Reed, Joseph W., Jr. English Biography in the Early
>   Nineteenth Century, 1801–1838. New Haven: Yale UP,
>   1966.

22d

<u>22d</u> Format

The physical appearance of a research paper makes its own contribution to the paper's effectiveness. A meticulously prepared paper naturally inclines the reader to expect content of equal quality. Haphazard typing, on the other hand, can undercut the authority of even the best research and writing by giving a reader the impression of hasty and careless work. Proper format, therefore, is more than a superficial concern.

The format guidelines below are based on those suggested by the Modern Language Association. Your instructor may give you supplementary or alternative instructions to follow.

1. Paper

Using a typewriter with a fresh ribbon, type your research paper on standard 8½ x 11 white bond. Do not use onion-skin paper, which is hard to read, or eraseable typing paper, which easily smears. For convenient reading, most instructors prefer that the pages of a research paper be held together with a paper clip rather than stapled or fastened in a folder.

2. Spacing and margins

Double-space everything in your paper—text, long quotations, notes, and list of works cited. Double-space as well between page headings such as Works Cited and the first line of text on the page. Only notes placed at the bottoms of pages, rather than on a separate sheet at the end of the paper, are single-spaced; separate such notes from the text on the page by quadruple-spacing, and double-space between them.

Leave a one-inch margin on the top, bottom, and sides of each page. Page headings such as Notes and Works Cited are centered just within this margin, one inch from the top of the page. Page numbers are placed outside the top margin, one-half inch from the top of the page and one inch from the right side of the page. Number all pages, including the first. You should not use punctuation or abbreviations such as "p." with page numbers; however, to guard against pages becoming separated and misplaced, you may precede the number on the top of each page with your last name: Smith 2.

22d

3. Title page

Do not include a separate title page unless your instructor specifically requests it. Instead, on four separate double-spaced lines in the upper left corner of the first page, type your name, the name of your instructor, the course number, and the date. Double-space, center the title of your paper, and quadruple-space before you begin the text of the paper. Double-space between lines of your title if it runs onto a second line. (See sample title pages on pages 303 and 319.)

Exercise 1

Treat each of the passages below as if it were to become part of a research paper that you are writing. In each case, compose (1) an acceptable paraphrase of one or more of the ideas in the passage; (2) a few sentences that incorporate a quotation taken from the passage; (3) a citation of the source in proper form for a list of works cited. Remember to include appropriate text citations in (1) and (2).

1. "In the second half of the seventeenth century, Holland, a term used to describe the seven United Provinces of the Northern Netherlands, was at the peak of its world power and prestige. With its dense, teeming population of two million hard-working Dutchmen crowded into a tiny area, Holland was by far the richest, most urbanized, most cosmopolitan state in Europe. Not surprisingly, the prosperity

of this small state was a source of wonder and envy to its neighbors, and often this envy turned to greed. On such occasions, the Dutch drew on certain national characteristics to defend themselves. They were valiant, obstinate and resourceful, and when they fought—first against the Spaniards, then against the English and finally against the French—they fought in a way which was practical and, at the same time, desperately and sublimely heroic." [Passage is on page 178 of Peter the Great: His Life and World, by Robert K. Massie, published in 1981 in New York by Ballantine Books. The book was first published by Alfred A. Knopf in 1980.]

2. "The music of every generation has been profoundly shaped by changing technology. Although we think of crooning as 'natural' pop music, in fact singing intimately with a large orchestra works only with a microphone. It was not until the rock era, however, that large numbers of people took an interest in the relationship between music and machines. Whereas the younger generation recognized that high-volume rock could be cathartic, older people found it threateningly loud. Once in full bloom the sixties rock culture ignored a basic contradiction in its chosen art form—that it depended on technology just as much as warfare did." [Passage is on page 102 of an article entitled Machines as Collaborators and published in the June, 1984 issue of Atlantic. The article runs from page 102 to page 103 and was written by Stephen Holden.]

3. "Pity the Pilgrims, who stepped ashore to confront a wall of forest and a cruel joke beneath the trees. New England stands on granite. Except for the silted beaver meadows and alluvial valleys like the Connecticut, the glaciers left the colonists only a thin mantle of hilly, stony soil. The Southeast also was of mineral-poor rock, and it had weathered too long in the rain. Save for the river deltas and the limestone valleys, its old soils were largely pooped out before the first ax rang in the forest." [Passage is on page 376 of an article by Boyd Gibbons on pages 350 to 388 of National Geographic, September, 1984. The title of the article is Do We Treat Our Soil Like Dirt?]

22d

23 *Sample Research Papers*

The sample research papers that follow are somewhat shorter than a typical research assignment, but they illustrate techniques of writing and documentation that are characteristic of all sound research. The first paper, on the flood that damaged Florence's priceless art treasures in 1966, draws heavily on accounts of the restoration work found in contemporary newspaper and magazine articles. The second, a paper on the early American poet Anne Bradstreet, blends critical appraisals of Bradstreet's work with the writer's own reading of her poetry.

In both cases, notice how the writers have used their research to support a clearly focused argument. Neither writer moves mindlessly from one note or quotation to another; instead, the research cited throughout each of these papers serves a purpose that the writer has consciously defined. In their ability to use the ideas of others as the foundation for an original essay, these writers exemplify the goal of all serious researchers.

Note the effective movement of Geary's introductory paragraph. It begins with a brief but specific survey of the flood's devastating impact on Florence, then moves to the damage done to the city's art, then (with the Batini quotation) shifts to the narrower subject of art restoration, the focus of Geary's paper.

Compare the version of the Batini quotation given in the paper with the original, on Geary's note card:

23

> Batini, p. 90
>
> "Despite the various complex restoration methods briefly explained above, the havoc played by the flood among works of art in Florence presented many new problems. For example, never before had so many and diverse works of art been damaged at the same time, all of which needed to be restored at once by an army of specialists, unfortunately a rarity today."

In Geary's paper, the bracketed capital N at the start of the quotation and the ellipses at the end indicate that only part of the original sentence is quoted here.

1″

½″

1

1″

Emmet Geary

Professor J. V. Catano

History 244

October 18, 1985

Recovery from the Florence Flood:

A Masterpiece of Restoration

quadruple-
space

On November 4, 1966 the swollen Arno River inundated
Florence, Italy. Nineteen inches of rain had fallen in two
days, causing flood waters to reach depths of twenty feet in
some parts of the city. The damage was devastating: six
thousand of the city's ten thousand shops were destroyed,
five thousand families were left homeless, and over a
hundred people drowned. But the primary reason why most
outsiders grieved for Florence was the damage to its unique
collection of Renaissance art treasures and rare books. As
Giorgio Batini noted, "[N]ever before had so many and
diverse works of art been damaged at the same time, all of
which needed to be restored at once . . ." (90). The story of
this restoration is a story of commitment and ingenuity.
Though the Florence flood destroyed some priceless master-
pieces and heavily damaged others, it inspired valiant
efforts among professional restorers and untrained volunteers alike, and even occasioned some discoveries in the
field of art that would otherwise never have been made.

23

If we compare Geary's paraphrase of Horton with the original text, we can see that he has effectively and accurately summarized the source in his own words:

> A few days after the disastrous floods that occurred in Italy on November 4, 1966, a group of art lovers in the United States organized the Committee to Rescue Italian Art (CRIA). One of their first acts was to send, on November 8, two art historians to Florence and Venice, the areas where the art losses were reported to be the greatest, to assess the damage and to find out what could be done to help. Word was received from them by transatlantic telephone that restoration experts and materials were urgently needed. By November 14, there were 16 conservators on their way to Florence. Within the next week, they were joined by four more conservators. This group of 20, headed by Lawrence Majewski, acting director of the Conservation Center, Institute of Fine Arts, New York University, included: a chemist; 13 conservators of paintings, frescoes, mosaics, and furniture; two conservators of prints and drawings; one librarian; and three bookbinders, specializing in the restoration and conservation of books, manuscripts, and other library materials.

23

2

As the floodwaters rose, the first exhibition of
dedication to art was shown by fourteen members of the staff
of the Uffizi Gallery, who risked their lives to rescue
twenty-four paintings stored in the museum's basement
(Rhode 20). When the floodwaters had subsided, generous
contributions from all over the world arrived in Florence,
and hundreds of volunteers—mainly students from throughout Europe and North America—came to undertake the messy
cleanup that would return Florence to normal and salvage
the city's damaged treasures. They were led by an international team of art historians and conservators. Within
only a few days of the flood, for example, one group of
American art lovers had organized the Committee to Rescue
Italian Art and two weeks later had dispatched to Florence a
team of twenty experts, including specialists in paintings, mosaics, furniture, prints, book bindings, and
manuscripts (Horton 1035).

23

Two distinct types of damage to art had resulted from
the flood: that due to submersion, and that due to water
pressure, turbulence, and friction. Submersion caused the
flood's most significant artistic loss—the great Cru-
cifix by Giovanni Cimabue, painted at the end of the
thirteenth century—as well as most of the other damage to
paintings and books. Compounding the problem of submersion
was the oil spilled from ruptured fuel tanks around the
city, which rode the top of the floodwater and coated

By inserting the citation to Ricci in the middle of his sentence, Geary makes it clear that only the information in the first half of the sentence—the specific data about the size and speed of the floodwaters—comes from this source.

Geary found his information about the damage to Ghiberti's baptistry doors in many sources; consequently, it could be considered common knowledge and did not require specific documentation.

In his paragraph describing the flood's damage to Florence's libraries, note Geary's effective integration of related material from different sources.

23

everything it touched. Having never before worked on paintings stained by fuel oil, restorers were forced to
experiment with a number of solvents, including benzene
and carbon tetrachloride (Judge 39). Water pressure and
turbulence created a different kind of devastation. Sweep-
ing through the city at forty to fifty miles an hour, the
twelve-foot wave of water (Ricci 25) knocked sculptures
from their pedestals and damaged the altarpieces of
churches. The famous baptistry doors of the city's cathedral, cast by Lorenzo Ghiberti in the fifteenth century,
were violently battered by the water, which dislodged five
of the doors' bronze panels.

 The first task that restoration workers faced was
collecting the objects to be restored. Since the last
serious threat to Florence's art had come from German
artillery bombardment during World War II, many of the most
valuable books and manuscripts had been stored below
ground for safety (Horton 1036). Now these books had to be
pulled from library basements full of water and mud. In the
Biblioteca Nazionale alone, over 300,000 volumes had been
damaged; in the library of the Gabinetto Vieusseux, another 250,000 had been under water and needed immediate
attention ("Florentine Flood Disaster" 194). All told,
nearly two million books had been damaged by the flood
(Horton 1036).

A quotation of more than four typed lines is usually set off by indenting ten spaces. Double-space between the last line of the text and the first line of the quotation, and double-space the quotation itself. No quotation marks are used when a quotation is set off in this way.

Again, the information given here about methods of restoring and drying books was available in several sources and therefore did not require documentation in Geary's paper.

23

4

Not only the floodwaters but the subsequent growth of destructive mold spores threatened Florence's priceless books. As Carolyn Horton explains, mold endangered even books that had escaped direct damage from the flood:

> Books are hygroscopic, i.e. have the capacity
> for absorbing water from the air around them.
> Therefore any books stored in conditions of high
> humidity are in danger of being damaged by mold.
> We had received reports that the flooded area of
> Florence had become, in effect, a huge humidity
> chamber. The wet books in rooms that were only
> partially flooded were humidifying the dry
> books on the upper shelves. (1035)

Salvaged books, covered with mud and oil and soaked with water, were first washed with mild soap and then treated with fungicides and antibiotics that would inhibit the growth of mold and bacteria. Then came the drying, by any means available: heating in tobacco ovens and brick kilns, interleaving pages with absorbent paper, spraying with powder.

23

Like books, paintings on wooden panels were particularly susceptible to damage from submersion in water. As one observer described the problem:

> [W]hen the water has soaked into the wood, the
> priming layer of glue and gesso [plaster] dis-
> solves, and the colours dissolve with it. . . .

Compare Geary's version of the quotation from the anonymous article "The Florentine Flood Disaster" with the original text:

> The situation regarding panel paintings has not changed much since the preliminary reports. The return to health will be slow and laborious. As is well known, when the water has soaked into the wood, the priming layer of glue and gesso dissolves, and the colours dissolve with it. This is not only the case with panels that were entirely submerged, as at Santa Croce (Fig. I). Even in cases where a few inches along the bottom were submerged, those parts buckle, and crack the part that seemed safe. More unexpected still, some panels which seemed quite undamaged when the flood subsided, developed blisters two or three days later, and the paint began to fall.

Note the editorial changes that Geary has made: (1) he has enclosed the initial W of his quotation in brackets to indicate that the first words of the original quotation have been omitted; (2) he has inserted the word "plaster" in brackets to define the unfamiliar term "gesso" for the reader; (3) he has inserted ellipses to indicate an omission after his third sentence (note that a fourth period—the period of the sentence—follows the usual three periods); (4) he has inserted the word "only" in brackets to make the sense of the original quotation clearer. Geary has retained the unorthodox punctuation and the British spelling ("colours") of the original text.

23

5

> Even in cases where [only] a few inches along the
> bottom were submerged, those parts buckle, and
> crack the part that seemed safe. More unexpected
> still, some panels which seemed quite undamaged
> when the flood subsided, developed blisters two
> or three days later, and the paint began to fall.
> ("Florentine Flood Disaster" 193)

To prevent wooden panels from drying too fast and shrink-
ing, thus causing the pigment to flake off, restoration
workers had to reduce the humidity around the panels
gradually. Within twelve days of the flood, the Limonaia, a
large greenhouse in one of Florence's public parks, was
converted to a sophisticated drying facility complete with
an elaborate humidity control system. Initially set at
ninety percent, the humidity level inside was gradually
lowered, and the panels were constantly checked to insure
sufficiently slow drying (Batini 90–91). Only after complete drying, a process that sometimes took many months,
could the painted panels be moved to laboratories for
further restoration, which usually involved planing down
the back of the panels until only the pigment and priming
layers remained, and then attaching a laminated, shrink-
proof panel to the back of the painting ("Road Back" 80).

Even more difficult to restore were Florence's
frescoes, paintings originally executed directly on damp
plaster, so that the pigment fused with the surface of the

When parts of a sentence derive from different sources, insert the appropriate parenthetical citations in mid-sentence, as Geary has done here, for accurate documentation. Consider his note cards below.

"Florentine Flood Disaster," p. 193

Damage to frescoes more serious than people thought at first: dampness penetrated plaster even above the level of the flood water, causing "a breaking down of the adhesion between the plaster layers and the wall."

"Slow Art Restoration," p. 42

Salt dissolved in the flood waters "had become lodged inside and under wood panels and frescoes, causing tiny explosions to tear the paint."

23

wall. Besides damage from submersion and floating fuel
oil, frescoes were affected by dampness, which caused the
plaster layers to separate from the wall ("Florentine Flood
Disaster" 193), and by salt contained in the floodwaters,
which penetrated the plaster and caused "tiny explosions"
in the painted surface as the wall dried ("Slow Art Restoration" 42). To save frescoes, restorers used a technique
called "strapo," which involves applying a coating of glue
and a canvas sheet to the wall. After the glue has dried, the
painting can be pulled from the wall intact on the canvas.
Difficult as this process is, it yielded an unexpected
reward: when the painted surfaces were removed, over three
hundred sinopias, or preliminary drawings for the frescoes, were uncovered on the walls ("Church Found" 35).

Surprisingly, sculpture seems to have received more
benefit than harm from the flood. Some statues were actually cleaned by the swirling water, whose mud acted as a
gentle abrasive, removing the grime of hundreds of years.
The restorers themselves used mud to clean sections of
statues that were untouched by the floodwaters (Batini
103–05). Fuel oil, on the other hand, did pose a serious
threat to sculpture. Since marble is a porous stone, the
oil penetrated beneath the surface and had to be drawn out
and absorbed by talc applied to the statues. But such
thorough cleaning of these statues actually left them
cleaner than they had been before the flood and led to a few

The Ricci quotation provides the foundation for an effective concluding paragraph. It not only echoes ideas from the paper's introduction but also gives Geary the opportunity to reiterate his main idea—the importance of the volunteer efforts to save Florence's art.

23

7

surprises. For example, the restoration revealed for the
first time that Donatello's statue The Magdalen had originally had gilded hair ("Florentine Flood Disaster" 194).

Only a few months after the floodwaters had devastated
Florence, as the frantic restoration work continued,
Leonardo Ricci aptly described the world's reaction to the
disaster. "Many floods indeed and natural tragedies have
happened everywhere in the world," he wrote. "But never have
we heard such a cry as for Florence. As if, instead of a city
it were a person, a loved one who in a way belongs to everybody and without whom it is impossible to live" (25–32). In
a real sense, the rescued art of Florence does belong to
everyone: without generous contributions of money from
around the world and the tireless efforts of an international corps of volunteers, Florence's treasures could not
have survived.

23

Anonymous works are included in the list of works cited alphabetically according to the first important word in the title.

Ricci's article begins on page 25 but continues on nonconsecutive pages later in the magazine.

The March 12, 1967 issue of the *New York Times* is a Sunday edition divided into sections; the section number must therefore be included in the citation. The August 9, 1967 issue, a weekday issue, is paged continuously without section divisions; no section number is necessary, since there is only one page 42 in the issue.

½″

8

1″

double-space

Works Cited

Batini, Giorgio. 4 November 1966: The River Arno in the
    Museums of Florence. Trans. Timothy Paterson. Flor-
    ence: Bonechi Editore, 1967.

"Church Found Under Basilica in Florence." New York Times
    4 Nov. 1967, late city ed.: 35.

"The Florentine Flood Disaster." Burlington Magazine 109
    (1967): 193–94.

Horton, Carolyn. "Saving the Libraries of Florence."
    Wilson Library Bulletin 41 (1967): 1034–43.

Judge, Joseph. "Florence Rises from the Flood."
    NationalGeographic July 1967: 1–43.

Rhode, Eric. "Good News from Florence." New Statesman
    6 Jan. 1967: 20.

Ricci, Leonard. "Exploratory Research in Urban Form and
    the Future of Florence." Arts and Architecture Feb.
    1967: 25+.

"Road Back is Long for Florentines." New York Times 12 Mar.
    1967, late city ed., sec. 1: 80.

"Slow Art Restoration Continues in Florence." New York
    Times 9 Aug. 1967, late city ed.: 42.

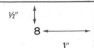

23

For the origin of Conlon's title, see her analysis of Bradstreet's poem "The Author to Her Book" in the fifth paragraph of the paper.

Conlon has quoted rather than paraphrased Rich's words because they offer an especially vivid impression of the Massachusetts Bay Colony. The themes of desolation and hardship that the quotation introduces will be important to Conlon's analysis of Bradstreet's poetry.

Compare Conlon's excerpt from Bradstreet's letter to her children with the original text:

> After a short time I changed my condition and was married, and came into this country, where I found a new world and new manners, at which my heart rose. But after I was convinced it was the way of God, I submitted to it and joined to the church at Boston.

23

Conlon has selected only the passage in these sentences that directly relates to Bradstreet's reactions to the New World and has inserted in brackets the words "in revolt" to clarify the intended meaning in Bradstreet's somewhat ambiguously worded sentence. The ellipses at the end of the quotation indicate the omission of the final words of the original text. The superscript 1, raised half a line, refers the reader to the content note after the last page of the paper.

Conlon's second paragraph introduces her thesis, the competing themes of revulsion and submission in Bradstreet's work.

1"

½"

1"

1"

1" ←

Suzanne E. Conlon

Professor Leslie Perelman

English 344

April 28, 1986

Anne Bradstreet's Homespun Cloth:

The First American Poems

quadruple-
space

In 1630 a young Englishwoman sailed for the New World
with her husband and parents aboard the Arbella, the
flagship of the Winthrop fleet carrying Puritan settlers
from Southampton to the Massachusetts Bay Colony (White
103). The voyage was rough and uncomfortable, and the
landing was not quite the relief that the eighteen-year-old
bride had expected; she had been brought, in Adrienne
Rich's words, to "the wild coast of Massachusetts bay, the
blazing heat of an American June, the half-dying, famine-
ridden frontier village of Salem, clinging to the edge of
an incalculable wilderness" (ix). Forty years later
Bradstreet was to write in a letter to her children that she
"found a new world and new manners, at which my heart rose
[in revolt]. But after I was convinced it was the way of God,
I submitted to it . . ." ("To My Dear Children").[1]

In its combination of revulsion and submission, Anne
Bradstreet's poetry represents an American variation of
the "Puritan dilemma" (Miller and Johnson 2: 287) as it was
experienced by a sensitive, cultivated, and pious woman of

23

The long Richardson quotation has been cut down by the two omissions indicated with ellipses. The omitted words are irrelevant to Conlon's point here. Note that a quotation with ellipses must make grammatical and logical sense without the omitted words.

23

The factual information about the publication of Bradstreet's book is available in many sources and may therefore be considered common knowledge. It does not need specific documentation.

early New England. As one scholar explains, "The Puritan was always trying to achieve a balance between this world and the next. . . . One could not safely turn one's back on this world, for the simple reason that God has made it and found it good; yet one could not rely upon . . . an earthly life which was, at last, insubstantial" (Richardson 317–18). Anne Bradstreet's dilemma involved a similar conflict between opposite impulses. Instead of loving the New World, she at first hated the harsh life it imposed on colonists, but this feeling went against her conviction that God's will demanded her to stay there and submit. Eventually she managed to strike her own balance: despite periods of doubt and depression, she bore and raised eight children in the wilderness near Andover and in intervals stolen from her scanty leisure time, she wrote five long didactic poems. The poems had been collected in manuscript as a present for her father, Thomas Dudley, and they were not meant to be published. But her brother-in-law took the manuscript with him on a journey to England and had it printed, as a surprise, under the title The Tenth Muse, Lately Sprung Up in America. With its publication in 1650, Bradstreet became America's first poet.

Anne Bradstreet's poetic accomplishment is par-ticularly surprising when one considers the handicaps that a woman on the frontier had to overcome. Early in their new life, the Dudleys and the Bradstreets, though among the

23

The citation "qtd. in Hutchinson 4" indicates that the words of Bradstreet's father are directly *quoted* by Hutchinson on page 4 of his book. Compare with "Hutchinson 4," which would indicate that the words were Hutchinson's own.

Conlon has skillfully fitted the lines of verse that she quotes into the grammatical structure of her sentence. Compare her excerpt with the complete stanza in Bradstreet's poem:

> I am obnoxious to each carping tongue
> Who says my hand a needle better fits,
> A poet's pen all scorn I should thus wrong,
> For such despite they cast on female wits:
> If what I do prove well, it won't advance,
> They'll say it's stol'n, or else it was by chance.

In Conlon's text, a slash (/) indicates the line division, and her citation provides the title of the poem and the lines she has quoted. (See Conlon's content note after the last page of the paper.)

23

richer founders of the Bay Colony, probably lived in
wigwams or caves dug into the hillside. Anne Bradstreet's
father reported that they had "no table, nor other room to
write in than by the fireside upon my knee" (qtd. in
Hutchinson 4). Even when living conditions improved, the
unending labor of caring for eight children must have left
little time for poetry.

In addition, a good Puritan woman was supposed to base
her life on submission to God and husband. It was her duty
to love God and to subordinate her own interests to the
welfare of her father, husband, and family. Anne Bradstreet
was fully aware of "each carping tongue / Who says my hand a
needle better fits" ("The Prologue" 27–28). Such critics
held that it was an aberration for a woman to write at all.
It was even more unseemly, if not actually sinful, for a
Puritan woman to write poetry. To the Puritan mind, poetry
represented attachment to the things of this world: to
words rather than to the dogma that words were meant to
communicate, to the natural world rather than to the
Heavenly Kingdom, to loved ones rather than to God. Cotton
Mather, the great Puritan preacher, announced magiste-
rially that poets were "the most numerous as well as the
most venomous authors" in the Devil's Library on earth
(qtd. in Hoffman 253). Any woman who attempted to join this
company was apt to come to a bad end, like the wife of the
governor of Hartford, Connecticut, who had suffered

Anne Bradstreet's poem, "The Author to her Book," is reprinted below. Note that Conlon has selected from it just those phrases she needs and has fitted them smoothly into her own sentence structure to create a concise and effective summary.

The Author to Her Book

Thou ill-formed offspring of my feeble brain,
Who after birth didst by my side remain,
Till snatched from thence by friends, less wise than true,
Who thee abroad, exposed to public view,
Made thee in rags, halting to th' press to trudge,
Where errors were not lessened (all may judge).
At thy return my blushing was not small,
My rambling brat (in print) should mother call,
I cast thee by as one unfit for light,
Thy visage was so irksome in my sight;
Yet being mine own, at length affection would
Thy blemishes amend, if so I could:
I washed thy face, but more defects I saw,
And rubbing off a spot still made a flaw.
I stretched thy joints to make thee even feet,
Yet still thou run'st more hobbling than is meet;
In better dress to trim thee was my mind,
But nought save homespun cloth i' th' house I find.
In this array 'mongst vulgars may'st thou roam.
In critic's hands beware thou dost not come,
And take thy way where yet thou art not known;
If for thy father asked, say thou hadst none;
And for thy mother, she alas is poor,
Which caused her thus to send thee out of door.

Here Conlon is moving from the first main section of her paper, which dealt with Anne Bradstreet's earlier poems and the background against which she wrote them, to the second main section, which will be concerned with a closer look at Bradstreet's later poetry. She makes her transition effectively, using a quotation from Bradstreet's early work to introduce the point that there is "another voice" in the first volume of poems, "forceful, ironic, intelligent."

4

insanity because, it was alleged, of her devotion to
reading and writing. There was also the example of the
sister of Bradstreet's husband, disgraced in her family for
"Irregular Prophecying" and preaching in England, as well
as Bradstreet's friend Anne Hutchinson, expelled by the
Massachusetts Bay Colony for listening to the inner voice
of God rather than to the elders of the Church (White
173–76).

 Such consequences of speaking out may have prompted
Bradstreet's humility in her early verse, which she describes meekly as the "ill-formed offspring of my feeble
brain." She had hoped, she continues, to trim her "rambling brat" in better dress, though "nought save homespun
cloth i' th' house I find" ("The Author to Her Book" 1, 9,
19). It is an apt phrase to describe the mixture of pedantic
learning, dull moralizing, and poetic cliché that made the
book popular in its own time. But another voice also speaks
out in this first volume, a forceful, ironic, intelligent
voice, as in these lines from "In Honour of Queen Elizabeth":

 Now say, have women worth? or have they none?
 Or had they some, but with our Queen is't gone?
 Nay masculines, you have thus taxed us long,
 But she, though dead, will vindicate our wrong.
 Let such as say our sex is void of reason,
 Know 'tis a slander now but once was treason.
  (100–04)

23

Since the title of the poem being quoted is given at the start of this paragraph, it does not need to be repeated in the citations later in the paragraph, which indicate only the appropriate line numbers.

23

5

As she set about revising her poems and adding to them in
the second edition, Anne Bradstreet drew upon this voice.
Instead of writing what she thought was expected of a
Puritan poet, she now wrote what she felt, drawing for
material on the timeless events of a woman's personal life.
The tension generated by the persistent conflict between
the duty owed to God and the loyalty and love given to her
family gives strength and vitality to these later poems.

A typical example is "Before the Birth of One of Her
Children" which expresses her fears, well founded in the
seventeenth century, of dying in childbirth. Her sadness
arises not from terror of the afterlife, for she had the
Puritan's confidence in salvation, but from imagined grief
at leaving her husband. The tears that dropped on her
manuscript, she writes, fell also for her children, and she
begged her husband to "protect [them] from step-dame's
injury" (26).

"Contemplations," by common agreement the most successful of her poems, has as its underlying theme the truth
that earth as well as heaven declares the glory of the Lord.
Looking at the autumnal splendor of the New England land-
scape, Bradstreet asks:

> If so much excellence abide below,
> How excellent is He that dwells on high,
> Whose power and beauty by his works we know?
>   (10-12)

23

Again, ellipses and brackets indicate Conlon's changes in the original text of Bradstreet's poem:

> But plants new set to be eradicate,
> And buds new blown to have so short a date,
> Is by His hand alone that guides nature and fate.

23

6

Though the poem unflinchingly faces the passing of fragile
beauty and human life into the everlastingness of God, the
poet nevertheless lingers for a long, loving look by the
river's bank with her senses full and a "thousand fancies
buzzing in my brain" (178). "Contemplations" has been
called the first American nature poem (Waggoner 8).

Another theme that evokes the best in Bradstreet is
the terrible mystery of the early death of children. Three
of her grandchildren died within five years, and
Bradstreet's protest at this eradication of "plants new set
. . . [a]nd buds new blown" ("In Memory of My Dear Grand-
child Elizabeth Bradstreet" 17–18) is at first bitter,
revealing a dark root of anger and grief. In the end, as
always, she submits:

> Such was His will, but why, let's not dispute,
> With humble hearts and mouths put in the dust,
> Let's say He's merciful as well as just.
>> ("On My Dear Grandchild Simon Bradstreet"
>> 10–12)

Along with the submissiveness, one hears in such poems as
this the persistent protest of her heart against the
desolate life in this new world.

One of the senseless accidents of life that the
Puritan was bound to accept as part of God's merciful
Providence was the loss of wordly goods. When the
Bradstreet house burned down through the carelessness of a
servant, she lost not only her shelter from the New England

No colon is needed to introduce the quotation after the word "places," because the quoted lines are grammatically part of the sentence that introduces them.

If a verse quotation begins in the middle of a line, indent the first line several additional spaces. Again, no introductory colon is needed here, because the quoted lines complete Conlon's own sentence.

23

Conlon's deft conclusion neatly pulls together the main ideas of her paper—the contrast between Bradstreet's early and later poems, the typical themes of her later work, and her importance as the first American poet.

7

weather but all the little personal possessions that had
helped to make her new life tolerable. Compared to the
modest wealth she had known in England, her American
treasures must have been paltry, but losing them was still
painful, and her grief was real as she looked at the places

> Where oft I sat and long did lie:
> Here stood that trunk, and there that chest,
> There lay that store I counted best.
>> ("Some Verses Upon the Burning of Our
>> House" 28–30)

But Bradstreet well knew the Puritan's answer to such trib-
ulation. She might feel sorrow at the sight of her treasures
now in ashes, but

> when I could no longer look,
> I blest His name that gave and took,
> That laid my goods now in the dust. (17–19)

Bradstreet's later poems, in which the Old World and
its old history are forgotten and the New World and its
trees and small graves are remembered, assure her a prominent place in the American tradition. The recognition that
came with the publication of her first poems seems to have
freed her to write poetry about what she saw and touched and
lost. These later poems still stand, three hundred years
after she wrote them, as honest testaments of the human
condition as one woman saw it.

23

1″   ½″

8

Note

[1] Quotations from Bradstreet's works are taken from the Hensley edition. Line numbers are given for verse quotations.

23

1"   ½"

9

Works Cited

Bradstreet, Anne. The Works of Anne Bradstreet. Ed.
 Jeannine Hensley. Cambridge: Harvard UP, 1967.

Hoffman, Daniel G., ed. American Poetry and Poetics.
 Garden City: Anchor, 1962.

Hutchinson, Robert, ed. Poems of Anne Bradstreet. New
 York: Dover, 1969.

Miller, Perry, and T. H. Johnson. The Puritans. 2 vols. New
 York: Harper, 1963.

Rich, Adrienne. Foreword. The Works of Anne Bradstreet.
 Ed. Jeannine Hensley. Cambridge: Harvard UP, 1967.
 ix–xx.

Richardson, Robert D., Jr. "The Puritan Poetry of Anne
 Bradstreet." Texas Studies in Literature and Language 9 (1967): 317–31.

Waggoner, Hyatt H. American Poets from the Puritans to the
 Present. New York: Dell, 1968.

White, Elizabeth Wade. Anne Bradstreet: "The Tenth Muse."
 New York: Oxford UP, 1971.

23

Letters, Résumés, Essay Examinations

24 *Business Letters*

The process of composing a business letter naturally involves many of the same issues that are important in other writing tasks. What is your main point, and what do you wish to accomplish? How much do you know about your readers and their probable response? What tone should you adopt? How much specific detail must you include? But beyond these matters of content, the appearance of a business letter is also critical. An effective business letter *looks* like a business letter; it wins its reader's attention partly by following the conventions that characterize business correspondence. This chapter, therefore, deals not only with questions of content but also with important matters of form.

24a The rhetoric of business correspondence

We write business letters for many reasons—to request information, to place orders, to voice complaints, to offer thanks. Each business letter takes shape in a unique rhetorical situation, a specific relationship to be developed between writer and reader. The best letters build on that relationship to accomplish their writers' purposes.

Whenever possible, address your letter by name to a specific person rather than to a mere job title such as "Personnel Director" or "Customer Relations Manager." Particularly for application letters or letters of complaint, it may well be worth the small cost to telephone a company and ask the name of the person to whom you should write. Letters addressed impersonally to a mere title will eventually land on the correct desk, but they lack the impressive sense of direct contact conveyed by letters written to a specific individual.

Think carefully about your reader, and try to strike an appropriate tone. A snarling letter of complaint may offer a temporary outlet for your frustrations, but it is less likely to resolve your problem than a letter that suggests your patience and reasonableness. As you organize the contents of your letter, keep in mind the suggestions for effective writing discussed elsewhere in this book. Provide your reader with specific information, and arrange it in paragraphs that are coherent and complete; no reader making his way through a stack of incoming correspondence will be willing to puzzle over your intended meaning.

Give your letter the attention to style that suggests a sophisticated writer, and proofread the final copy with professional accuracy.

Business letters, even short ones, are usually typed, single-spaced, on one side of 8½ x 11 paper. Neat centering on the page is more important than adherence to standard margins. In what is called **block style,** all the parts of a letter are typed flush against the left margin, and the first lines of paragraphs are not indented (see sample on page 344). In the less formal **indented style,** by contrast, the inside address and the close are typed on the right side of the page and the first line of each paragraph is indented five spaces (see sample on page 341). The **modified block style** follows the general arrangement of the indented style, but without indentation of the first lines of paragraphs (see sample on page 340).

<u>24b</u> Parts of a business letter

A typical business letter has five parts.

1. The heading

The heading consists of your address and the date, usually typed on three lines, and placed either flush against the upper left margin (block style) or in the upper right corner (indented style). It is included so that the person who receives your letter will be able to respond to you even if your envelope is lost or discarded.

The first line of the heading contains your street address; the second, your city, state, and zip code; the third, today's date. If you abbreviate your state, use the standard two-letter abbreviation (without periods) prescribed by the U.S. Postal Service. Double-space or quadruple-space after the last line of the heading.

2. The inside address

The inside address is identical to the address that you type on the envelope. Including it inside the letter insures that your letter will reach its addressee even if it is opened by someone else in an office and becomes separated from its envelope.

On the first line of the inside address, use the appropriate abbreviated title with the full name of the person you are writing to: Mr. David Hunt, Dr. Elizabeth Aikers, Ms. Harriet Sweeney, Rev. Stephen Jules. If the person has an official position within a company, the title of the position and the name of the company are given on the second line, separated by a comma, or on the second and third lines.

```
Mr. Robert O'Malley
Editor-in-Chief, The Indianapolis Courier
```

```
Ms. Margaret Wilson
Vice President
Blindex Corporation
```

The next line of the inside address contains the street address, followed on the concluding line with the city, state, and zip code. Again, if you abbreviate the state, use the U.S. Postal Service abbreviation. Double-space after the inside address.

3. The salutation

The salutation repeats the name given on the first line of your inside address, omitting the person's first name. In business letters the salutation is followed by a colon:

```
Dear Mr. O'Malley:
```

```
Dear Ms. Wilson:
```

If you are unable to obtain the name of the person to whom your letter should be addressed, use one of the following salutations:

```
Dear Sir or Madam:
```
[used when you are writing to a specific person whose name you do not know—for example, the editor of a newspaper or the chief of surgery in a hospital]

```
Ladies and Gentlemen:
```
[used when you must address your letter to a company or organization rather than to a specific person]

If you know the sex but not the name of the person to whom you are writing, you may use the salutation "Dear Sir" or "Dear Madam."

Avoid the older salutations "Dear Sirs" and "Gentlemen," both of which illogically exclude women. And never open a standard business letter with the phrase "To Whom It May Concern"; this salutation is used only in letters such as personal recommendations that are intended for distribution to various people unknown to the writer.

Double-space after your salutation.

24b

4. The body

Clearly state your purpose for writing—to apply for a job, or to order a replacement part, or to express a complaint—as early as possible in your letter. Major corporations and large government offices receive hundreds—if not thousands—of letters every day, and your correspondence will get the fastest possible treatment if the person who opens your letter can immediately determine what you want. For the same reason, be concise, specific, and clear.

5. The close

Double-space or quadruple-space after the last line of the body of your letter and type an appropriate close, either very formal ("Very truly yours,") or formal ("Yours truly," "Sincerely yours," "Sincerely,") or relatively informal ("Best wishes,"). The close is positioned under the inside address, either flush left (block style) or at the right side of the page (indented style). Capitalize only the first word, and follow the close with a comma. Leave room for your signature by quadruple-spacing, and type your name exactly as you will sign it:

```
Sincerely yours,
```

William A. Quinn

```
William A. Quinn
```

Business letters are usually mailed in long (9½″) envelopes. Type your name and address in the upper left corner, and center the name and address of your correspondent, just as they appear in your letter's inside address:

```
Maureen Brown
218 East 10th Street
Columbus, OH 43202



           Mr. Stephen Lunsford
           Circulation Manager, Book Collectors' Digest
           2772 Kankakee Boulevard
           Chicago, IL 60607
```

24b

Sample business letter / modified block style

```
                                   218 East 10th Street
                                   Columbus, OH 43202
                                   February 8, 1986

Mr. Stephen Lunsford
Circulation Manager, Book Collectors' Digest
2772 Kankakee Boulevard
Chicago, IL 60607

Dear Mr. Lunsford:

For the second consecutive month, I have not received my
issue of Book Collectors' Digest. Since my address has not
```

changed, I am inclined to think that a mailing problem exists somewhere in your office, and I would appreciate your looking into the matter. My subscription number is B2184–886.

Because I have missed two issues of my subscription through this delivery problem, may I ask that you extend my subscription by two months, until October of this year? I enjoy your magazine and look forward to remaining one of your subscribers.

Sincerely,

Maureen Brown

Maureen Brown

Sample business letter / indented style

90 North Thomas Avenue
Kingston, New York 12401
May 16, 1986

Catalog Department
Gillespie Furniture Creations
3101 Fontaine Road
Denver, CO 80203

Ladies and Gentlemen:

On April 26 I ordered a chrome and glass coffee table (model C261/LY) from your Spring 1986 catalog. When it arrived yesterday, I discovered that several pieces of hardware needed for assembly were missing. Would you please send me the following missing parts:

6–#17 metal screws
1–connecting rod "B"
2–chrome finishing caps

For your information, I have enclosed a copy of the shipping invoice. I appreciate your assistance and look forward to hearing from you.

Yours truly,

Mark Wallace

Mark Wallace

24b

25 Résumés and Job Applications

Job applications are among the most important letters that anyone writes. When you compose a résumé and write an accompanying letter of application, you must rely on your writing to persuade a potential employer that your qualifications, personality, and interests make you the best candidate for the job.

25a Designing a résumé

A **résumé,** sometimes called a *vita* (the Latin word for "life"), lists chronologically the activities of your life that qualify you for a job. It is an essential part of every job application.

There is no fixed format for a résumé, but you should keep in mind a few general guidelines. Above all, make the content of your résumé clear and easy to follow, and arrange it attractively. Résumés should generally not exceed a single page in length, but when you have a good deal of important information to include, continuing on a second page may be a better alternative than crowding everything together on a single sheet.

Every résumé should begin with your full name (avoid nicknames), your current address, and your telephone number (include both a home and office number if you are willing to receive calls from potential employers at your present place of work). Typically, the major categories under which the remaining material on a résumé is placed are "Education" and "Experience." List items in reverse chronological order, and provide accurate dates, so that a reader can see what you have done in each recent year of your life. A résumé usually ends with a brief list of references, persons whom the reader can contact for more information about you. Some employers also like to find something about a candidate's outside interests on a résumé; some consider such information irrelevant padding. Use your best judgment, based on what you can learn and surmise about your reader. In any case, you should not include such personal information as height, weight, or marital status unless it has direct bearing on the job you are applying for. (See the sample résumé on page 345.)

25b Letters of application

A résumé is usually accompanied by a cover letter personally addressed to a potential employer. Such a cover letter should be complete but should normally not exceed one page. We can summarize the essential contents of a **letter of application** by considering its main parts:

1. Introduction

Use your introductory paragraph (which may be no longer than a sentence or two) to accomplish three things. First, make it clear that you are writing a letter of application. Businesses receive many kinds of letters every day, and you want to be sure that yours is immediately grouped with those of other job applications. Second, state the specific job that you are applying for. Often a company will advertise several positions at once; it is to your advantage, obviously, to be sure that your letter correctly places you in competition for the job you want. Finally, indicate how you learned of the opening you are applying for—whether you read a newspaper advertisement, for example, or were referred by a friend who knew of the company's hiring plans.

2. Body

The body of your letter should summarize your qualifications clearly and specifically. Don't simply repeat all the facts on your résumé; instead, use your letter to *comment* on the résumé, emphasizing your most important qualifications and providing additional information about your background where appropriate.

At the same time, let the style of your writing reveal something about your personality. Ideally, the tone of an application letter should be businesslike but not stuffy, natural but not chatty. Be positive, but without being pushy or insistent; most employers, like most general readers, are impressed by confidence but not by raw aggressiveness. Don't make insupportable assertions about your suitabililty for the job in question ("I am unquestionably the candidate you are looking for"). Similarly, don't offer glowing evaluations of your accomplishments ("My course work in economics has given me outstanding mastery of the field"). Take a more objective stance instead, and let the facts in your background speak for themselves ("At my graduation I was named 'Outstanding Student in Economics' on the basis of the 4.00 grade point average that I earned in my economics course work"). Finally, avoid a highly idiosyncratic style or an unorthodox approach in your letter unless you are certain that it is appropriate for your potential employer.

25b

3. Conclusion

Use the brief conclusion of your letter to direct the reader's attention to the résumé that you have enclosed, to state your willingness to be interviewed for the position, and to provide information about when and where you would be available for a possible interview. Some employment counselors recommend that a letter of application end with the applicant's offer to call the reader in the near future in order to arrange an interview; others argue that such calls are presumptuous and will only alienate a potential employer. You must decide which approach is suitable for the employers you address. (See the sample application letter below.)

Sample cover letter / block style

2094 Neil Avenue, Apt. 45
Des Moines, IA 50312
June 17, 1985

Mr. William Prewett
Personnel Director, A&G Associates
1212 Milliken Drive
Cedar Rapids, IA 52401

Dear Mr. Prewett:

I wish to apply for the position of Public Relations Assistant that you advertised in the Des Moines Register last week.

I received my B.A. in May from the University of Iowa with a major in history and a minor in communications. My major field has given me not only the broad intellectual background of a liberal arts curriculum, but also substantial experience in research and report writing. Through my minor in communications, moreover, I have gained experience in the areas of interpersonal communication, group dynamics, and organizational and small group communication.

From my extra-curricular work, I have gained practical experience in publications and editing. As managing editor of the University of Iowa student literary magazine for the last two years, I shared responsibility for all editorial decisions with the magazine's editor-in-chief. In addition, I had primary responsibility for overseeing the actual production of each semester's issue. During my junior year, I was one of two student assistants employed by the Office of the Dean of Students to type, duplicate, and distribute office memoranda throughout the campus.

My résumé is enclosed. Although I am currently living in Des Moines, I would be happy to come to Cedar Rapids at any time for an interview. I appreciate your consideration and look forward to hearing from you.

Sincerely,

Phyllis Wainwright

Phyllis Wainwright

25b

Sample résumé

RÉSUMÉ

Phyllis Wainwright
2094 Neil Avenue, Apt. 45
Des Moines, IA 50312
(515) 555–6682

Education B.A., cum laude, University of Iowa, 1985.
Major: History
Minor: Communications

Experience Managing Editor, Iowa Literary Journal,
1983–85.
Solicited student submissions of fiction and poetry; shared responsibility
for all editorial decisions; supervised
proofreading, design, and layout of
magazine.

Student Assistant, Dean of Students' Office,
University of Iowa, 1983–84.
Responsible for typing and distributing
office memoranda, distributing incoming
mail, and helping to maintain office
files.

Hostess, Macmillan's Restaurant, Des Moines,
Iowa, Summer, 1983.

Peer Tutor, Department of History, University
of Iowa, 1982–83.
Tutored freshman students in History
121, 122 (European History I, II).

References Dr. Rosemary Eddins
Faculty Adviser, Iowa Literary Journal
Department of English
University of Iowa
Iowa City, IA 52240

Mr. Nathaniel Robinson
Dean of Students
University of Iowa
Iowa City, IA 52240

Dr. Alice Voros
Chair, Department of History
University of Iowa
Iowa City, IA 52240

25b

26

Answering Essay Questions

Sometimes, we don't have the time to plan, write, and revise with the leisure we would prefer. Pop quizzes, short-answer essays, the hour-long test with two questions to be covered, the three-hour final with four questions to be covered—these examples should remind us of the limits often imposed. Here, we will stress the techniques for effective economizing, that is, working intelligently to one's best advantage within such restrictions. And because the paragraph, *not* scattered sentences, is the usual form expected of the writer for essay examinations, it helps to know certain relevant principles and techniques for working under pressure—for the efficient use of limited time and space.

A few preliminary words about these principles and techniques follow. First, none of them are substitutes for having mastered the material; they will not conceal the fact that a writer has little to say, given ten minutes or two hours, one page or five. Second, although some of these aids may seem obvious or general, *that* is their value. Because they are obvious, they are often ignored or forgotten; because they are general, they can be applied to a number of writing situations. Third, although several of them may seem like formulas, that also is a value: while being learned, they may help give confidence; once mastered, they can be modified by experience.

26a Preparations for the essay examination

Last-minute cramming may work for some students, but it won't for most. Plan your time so that you can review systematically and fully. Begin by going over your class notes and your underlinings in your text or texts. In doing so, pay special attention to the concepts and ideas that have been stressed and the information or key examples that flesh out these primary ideas. For instance, in an introductory film course you would need to know the concept of "shooting angle" and to be able to illustrate it by a concretely detailed reference to Hitchcock or some other master. Take the time to work through any methods of analysis you are uncertain about. For instance, in a course on educational tests and measurements, you would want to be able to explain *how* to determine the validity and reliability of a test. Start, then, by reviewing the major course topics, techniques of analysis, and key illustrations.

You can also prepare by trying to anticipate the kind of question you are likely to be asked. One way of doing this is to pose such questions for yourself and to think through how you would answer them. For example, if you had just finished a long unit on the Civil War in an American history course, you could easily frame questions on the Civil War's early roots, its more immediate causes, and its major phases. Posing such questions is excellent preparation in two ways: it facilitates your reviewing, and it enables you to synthesize the materials into your own understanding of them. Many students have found that it helps to work together in framing and answering possible essay examination questions.

26b Reading the examination

Once the examination has been handed out, *plan on reading it through carefully.* As you read, keep in mind the number of questions you are expected to answer and the suggested time limits, if any, for each question. If the teacher has not indicated the weight of each question by suggesting time limits, you will have to make these choices yourself. Usually, you will have a pretty good idea of which questions are harder and therefore require more time, and which are easier and require less.

After having read the examination and tentatively allocated your time, *go back* and *reread* the *questions* you *plan* to *answer* with *special attention to the directions* for each. If you don't understand what is called for, ask the instructor. Your doubts or bewilderments may be shared by other students. Further, in reading the *topic, attend* to the *verb* that *tells* you *what you are required* to *do:*

Explain = **Spell out** the reasons, causes, connections.

> ("Explain why Britain adopted the V.A.T." = spell out the reasons Britain adopted the value-added tax.)

Analyze = **Break up,** separate, segment into parts, steps, phases, sections, causes.

> ("Analyze the effects of the Cold War on French foreign policy" = separate into phases the effects of the Cold War on French foreign policy.)

Compare = **Place side by side** and **point out** significant similarities, differences, or both.

> ("Compare the role of the government in Keynesian and monetary economic theory" = place the roles of government in Keynesian and monetary economic theory side by side.)

26b

Summarize = Reduce, abbreviate to the major aspects, features, events, arguments, without distortion

("Summarize Hume's views on causation" = abbreviate Hume's major arguments on causation.)

Evaluate = Judge, take a position on the merits of, adequacy of, reasons for or against, consequences of.

("Evaluate Piaget's views on how children learn" = judge the merits or adequacy of Piaget's views on how children learn.)

But what about *discuss,* that open-ended verb so often used for exam questions? Broadly, *discuss* means to open up, reflect on, show that you know about and have thought about the subject. Sometimes, the context makes clear what is called for. "Discuss the pros and cons of federal intervention in abortion," for instance, means "Summarize, compare, and evaluate the case for and against federal intervention in abortion." If you are in doubt, try turning the command into a question in order to discover which analytic skills are called for. To take a few examples:

1. Discuss the plausibility of Jung's doctrine of the collective unconscious = How convincing is Jung's doctrine? = **Evaluate.**
2. Discuss the major therapies in the treatment of autistic children = **What are** the major therapies? = **Summarize** and **Compare.**
3. Discuss the significant changes in Hester Prynne's attitude towards her sin in *The Scarlet Letter* = What **are** the major changes? = **Analyze.**

Once you are clear on what is called for, *plan your answer.* This is the most important step you can take before you begin writing. Except for brief quizzes, you always have at least a few minutes to think before answering; take them. Strategies for planning answers vary: some students jot down an informal outline, with major headings and subheadings; others simply list key terms, phrases, names, or details, and then look for a pattern or case; still others reflect, work out a thesis, a case to argue, and then dive in. Any of these techniques is valuable. The point is to get *inside* the topic *before* writing, so that you don't use up half your time in desperate false starts or chewing on your pen and vaguely wondering what to say. By planning you not only gain focus; you also make yourself a searcher in pursuit of an answer instead of remaining a spectator waiting for something to happen.

26c Writing the essay

In writing your answer, you should strive for the same qualities of effective exposition that are expected in papers written out of class. Obviously, though, time won't always allow you to polish and review your answer as fully as you and your teacher would like. Sometimes, you will be pushed just to finish and to have a few minutes for proofreading. Nevertheless, while writing you should try to keep the following principles in mind, a minimal list of the characteristics of an effective answer.

Don't begin with long, prefatory remarks, but *get directly to the question.* Answers which begin with sentences like "This is a very controversial issue on which people hold many different viewpoints" or "This is a very complicated subject and solutions are hard to find" and which run on this way for a whole paragraph are mere throat-clearing. If the issue is controversial, your analysis should make this clear in its treatment of the viewpoints; if the issue is complex, your analysis should reflect this complexity. Similarly, don't begin with a long digression on something you haven't been asked about. If, for instance, you were asked to discuss the effects on the Vietnam War on America in the 1960s, you would simply be avoiding the question if you started with a long paragraph on French colonial policy or the history of the Monroe Doctrine. Such false starts are rather like the complaint of one of Saul Bellow's characters in *Seize the Day:* "If you wanted to talk about a glass of water, you had to start back with God creating the heavens and earth."

Your beginning is a promise to yourself and the instructor about your intended direction. Often, your opening will be framed by the terms of the topic: "Discuss three causes of," "Compare Tweedledum's and Tweedledee's theories of," "Summarize the symptoms of," and the like. Go directly *to* the causes, theories, or symptoms, in an orderly enumeration and discussion. In cases where the wording of the topic is more open-ended, try turning the directions into a question. Thus, for example, if you were directed to "Write an essay on some significant aspect of Cézanne's achievement as a painter," you could easily ask yourself "What *is* a significant aspect of his achievement as a painter?" If, as sometimes happens, you do find yourself off to a false start, stop immediately. Return to the question and redirect your thinking to it.

The body of your essay is the heart of your answer. Your instructor will, naturally, look for coherent connections and transitions and for adequate development and relevant detail. One of the more common but easily avoidable failures in essay answers is the substitution of summary for analysis. If, for instance, you are asked to compare two major historical figures, a mere description, which only outlines each, will not do: you are asked to bring prominent similarities and differences together—to highlight these features. So, also, if you are asked to analyze or evaluate a case, a plot, or an event, don't give a summary. A sure sign that thought is absent is the writer's stating what happened without shaping an argument, making connections, or offering an interpretation—the summary that all too often runs: "This was said and that happened and this was the result, so thus and such also was said and led to another result, and. . . ."

The crucial choices you face in the body of the answer concern examples: what kind? how many? how thoroughly discussed? First, unless asked to give all

26c

examples, be selective, not exhaustive. Pick the most telling or typical ones. For instance, if you were discussing Huck Finn's essential decency, his humaneness, you couldn't list all cases—the novel is full of them—but you could focus on his growing awareness of how much he cares for Jim and his resolve to help Jim escape, and you could point to the risks Huck takes to help the Wilks girls. Perhaps other examples interest you more—Huck's shock at the feud or pity for the tarred-and-feathered Duke and King, despite their treachery. Whatever the case, *limit* your choices to a few pointed ones.

Second, *do* something with your evidence. Merely mentioning an example or two in a sentence is not enough. Until you show by concrete development how the example applies, how it makes your point, *how it fits the terms of the question,* you have no depth. For instance, if you were discussing why German and more recently Japanese car manufacturers have taken over a significant part of the American market, you couldn't merely drop the names Volkswagen and Toyota. What about them—better engineering and design? quicker anticipation of the demand for small cars and flexibility in planning and retooling? lower cost to the consumer because of gas economy and cheaper production costs? better marketing and servicing? Any or several of these may be relevant. However, until you specifically discuss, say, what is better in the engineering of a major foreign model, you haven't done anything with your evidence or answered the question "Why?"

As you come to the end of your essay, look over what you have written to determine whether you need a conclusion or not. Usually, a short summary paragraph that restates your argument or recapitulates your main points will serve well enough. Finally, when finished take a few minutes to proofread, not just skimming for obvious errors but considering changes in wording, insertions, even the renumbering of paragraphs. You haven't really finished until you turn the bluebook in.

26d · A miniature overview

We will conclude by illustrating the differences between an ineffective answer and an effective answer. Here are two examples in miniature as answers to the following question:

> What did William James mean by "the moral equivalent of war" and how does his idea illustrate pragmatism as a philosophy?

First, an ineffective answer:

> William James was the brother of the novelist Henry James and was Gertrude Stein's teacher. James taught at Harvard for many years along with such other notables as Santayana and Royce. James was one of the founders of pragmatism, a philosophy which judges ideas by their practicality. By "the moral equivalent of war," James meant something to replace war with. James speaks of war as "a

school of strenuous life and heroism." He believed war was destructive and hardened soldiers. He also believed war promoted discipline and was a universal model of heroism. He wanted to discover a peaceful equivalent of war. That was what he meant by "the moral equivalent of war."

You can easily see why this answer is ineffective. The opening two sentences are a false start; they have nothing to do with the question. The third sentence—on pragmatism—is brief, unclear, and left dangling, unrelated to the question or the answer. The rest of the paragraph consists of choppy, disconnected sentences that lack focus. And except for the quotation from James, there isn't much concreteness. Now, by contrast, an effective answer:

By "the moral equivalent of war," James means a spiritual or social equivalent that would appeal as universally to our capacity for discipline and bravery as war does, but without its terrible destructiveness. Defining war as "a school of strenuous life and heroism," James recognizes how it hardens soldiers but also how it is the only model of selflessness available to the mass of men. He observes that voluntary poverty might be one example of a disciplined life that does not rely on hurting others. Pragmatism, a philosophy which tests concepts by looking at their actual consequences in life, is clearly expressed in James's suggestion. In effect, he looks at the facts—the consequences—and says that if something as vicious as the idea of war can still draw out heroic qualities, then we ought to be able to find a noble idea—"a moral equivalent of war"—that brings out the best in us.

This effective answer begins by defining James's idea and develops it clearly and coherently. The answer is much more tightly organized and precisely worded than the first. And it *connects* James's idea to pragmatism, as directed by the question, while also defining pragmatism more adequately than the first answer defines it. Finally, the answer closes strongly with a firm restatement of James's idea. The second paragraph isn't much longer than the first, but it contains far more and is much easier to follow. It answers the question.

26d

Grammatical
Usage

Part VII

27

Agreement

As in many other languages, most of the nouns, pronouns, and verbs in English have different forms that indicate their relation to one another in a sentence. Most nouns and all verbs, for example, have different singular and plural forms; for a sentence to make grammatical sense, singular verbs must be used with singular subjects, and plural verbs with plural subjects. Pronouns, too, have separate forms to indicate number (singular or plural) and person (first person: *I, we;* second person: *you;* third person: *he, she, it, they*). The matching of subjects and verbs, pronouns and nouns, according to person and number in a sentence is called **agreement.**

The rules of agreement sound simple enough in theory, but in practice they can sometimes be a bit confusing. One reason for this is that most speakers of English are not very sensitive to questions of agreement, because English has relatively few inflections, or different forms, to begin with. The verb *walked,* for example, remains the same whether its subject is singular or plural, or first, second, or third person:

I walked   you walked   they walked

A more unusual grammatical construction may therefore momentarily puzzle even the most meticulous user of English:

Either Susan or Alan is?/are? going to be nominated.

Athletics is?/are? in danger of being cut from the school budget.

To complicate matters further, dialectical variations among speakers of English often affect the rules of agreement, since various dialects may form singulars and plurals in different ways. Speakers of such dialects have two sets of rules to keep in mind: those that apply in their dialect and those that operate in what is called Edited English, the English commonly used in business, journalism, academics, and professional life.

<u>27a</u> Agreement of subject and verb

The subject and verb of a sentence must agree in person and number. For example, if the subject is in the first-person singular (*I*), the verb must be also (*am*). The only highly inflected verb in English, that is, the only verb with several different forms, is *to be:*

I *am*	we *are*
you *are*	you *are*
he/she/it *is*	they *are*

In most other English verbs, the only inflection is the *s* or *es* added to the third-person singular in the present tense:

I know	we know
you know	you know
he/she/it knows	they know

What is sometimes confusing here is that plural nouns and singular verbs in the third-person singular present usually end in *s,* whereas singular nouns and plural verbs usually do not:

Singular (verb ends in s)	Plural (noun ends in s)
The clock ticks loudly.	The clocks tick loudly.
The star shines faintly.	The stars shine faintly.
That contestant has talent.	Those contestants have talent.

This rule holds most of the time, but English includes some nouns whose singular *and* plural forms end in *s,* as well as a few irregular nouns whose plural forms do *not* end in *s* (for example, *man, woman, child, tooth, sheep, goose, criterion*). These unusual noun forms do not affect the correct form of the verb.

Singular (some nouns end in s)

That bus looks unreliable.

Gas sells for less now than it did last month.

Plural (some irregular nouns do not end in s)

Her feet feel tired.

Those phenomena seem to be inexplicable.

These, then, are the basic rules for subject-verb agreement in English. But we must also consider several grammatical situations that are sometimes confusing. Note that these are not exceptions to the rules above; they are simply cases where it may be difficult at first to see how to apply those rules.

27a

1. Modifying phrases after the subject

Uncertainty about which word is the subject of the sentence can result in an agreement error. A modifying phrase placed between the subject and verb may seem to change the number of the subject, but it does not.

Incorrect A program of two Bergman films were shown last night.

Correct A *program* of two Bergman films *was shown* last night.

> [Because *films* is the noun closest to the verb, it may appear at first that the verb in this sentence should be plural. But *films* is simply the object of the preposition *of.* The subject of the sentence is *program,* and the verb must always agree with its subject no matter what words or phrases come between them.]

Phrases such as *accompanied by, as well as,* and *together with* suggest a plural idea, but they do not change the number of the subject. When you are determining whether your verb should be singular or plural, disregard these phrases and remember what your subject is.

Incorrect The prisoner, accompanied by guards and her lawyer, were in the courtroom.

Correct The *prisoner,* accompanied by guards and her lawyer, *was* in the courtroom.

Incorrect The mansion, along with the guest house and garages, were up for rent.

Correct The *mansion,* along with the guest house and garages, *was* up for rent.

2. Compound subject

When two subjects are joined by *and,* they are usually considered to be plural.

> *Science* and *math are* my best subjects.

> The *screening, hiring,* and *training* of each applicant *are* left to the Personnel Department.

Sometimes, though, two nouns are used together to indicate a single idea; in those cases the verb is singular.

> Bacon and eggs *is* a typical American breakfast.

27a

Similarly, when the two nouns of a compound subject both refer to the same person or thing, the verb is also singular.

> This young bachelor and man-about-town *was* finally discovered to be an imposter.

Finally, when *each* or *every* is used to modify a compound subject, a singular form of the verb is also used.

> Each soldier and sailor *was* given a complete examination.
>
> Every camera and light meter *has* been reduced in price.

3. Collective nouns

Collective nouns, such as *class, committee, team, family,* and *number* are treated as singular when they refer to the group as a unit. But if you want to emphasize the individual members of the group, you may use the plural form of the verb.

> The committee *was* unanimous in its recommendation.
>
> The number of correct answers *was* small.
>
> The team *were* unable to agree on a date for the party.
>
> [Many writers would find this last sentence awkward, even though it is correct, and would rephrase it: *The members of the team were unable to agree. . . .*]

There is a strong tendency in English to treat Latin plurals like *data* and *strata* as collective nouns that may be either singular or plural.

> We must classify all the data that *have* been collected.
>
> This data *was* collected in last week's survey.
>
> These strata *go* back to an even earlier period.

4. Nouns ending in *s*

Some abstract nouns that are plural in form are grammatically singular—for example, *aesthetics, economics, linguistics, mathematics, news, physics, semantics.*

> Physics *was* the hardest course I had in high school.
>
> The news *is* better than we had expected.

Note that certain other nouns ending in *s* have no singular form and are always plural—for example, *trousers, scissors, measles, forceps.* Finally, some nouns ending in *-ics*—such as *athletics, politics,* and *statistics*—may be either singular or plural, often with a distinction in meaning.

27a

> Athletics [the collective activity] *builds* the physique.
>
> Athletics [particular activities] *are* her favorite pastime.
>
> Statistics *is* my most difficult course.
>
> Statistics *suggest* that his argument is weak.

5. Linking verbs

When two nouns in a sentence are connected by some form of the verb *to be,* remember that the first noun is the subject and that the verb always agrees with it.

Correct   The first *thing* visible on the horizon *was* the tuna boats.

Correct   The tuna *boats were* the first thing visible on the horizon.

6. Inverted sentence order

Sometimes the subject of a sentence may follow the verb. In these cases of inverted word order, the subject and verb still agree.

Incorrect   Beyond the old mud fort was the endless sands of the desert.

Correct   Beyond the old mud fort *were* the endless *sands* of the desert.
[*Fort* is the object of the preposition *beyond* in this sentence. The subject is *sands,* and the verb must therefore be plural, *were.*]

In sentences beginning with *there is* or *there are, there* is an element called an **expletive** and is not the subject. The real subject of the sentence always follows the verb in these cases.

There *is* only one correct *solution* to this problem.

There *are* a million *laughs* in that movie.

There *is* a long *list* of jobs to be done before we leave.

There *are* many *jobs* to be done before we leave.

In informal or spoken English, a singular verb is occasionally used in these constructions even when a compound subject follows the verb.

Formal   In the office there *are* a desk, a chair, and a filing cabinet.

Informal   In the office there *is* a desk, a chair, and a filing cabinet.

7. *Or/nor*

When two subjects are joined by *or* or *nor,* the verb is singular if both subjects are singular and plural if both are plural.

Neither the *manufacturer* nor the *consumer was* treated fairly.

Poor testing *procedures* or inadequate safety *standards were* responsible for the accident.

When one subject is singular and one is plural, the verb agrees with the subject nearer it.

Neither Sam nor his *sisters have* ever been abroad.

Either good grades or an outstanding *recommendation is* needed for admission to the honors program.

27a

8. Indefinite pronouns

Indefinite pronouns, such as *each, every, either, neither, any, some,* and their compounds with *-one* or *-body* are always singular in number and are correctly followed by singular verb forms.

Each of the boys *was* tested.

Either of these candidates *is* qualified for the job.

Anyone not admitted *is* guaranteed a refund.

None, some, more, most, and *all* may be singular or plural, depending on the context and the intended meaning.

None of the money *was* wasted.

None of the dresses *were* paid for.

Most of the food *has* been eaten.

Most of the students *have* read that play.

9. Relative pronouns as subjects

The relative pronouns *who, which,* and *that,* when used as subjects of subordinate clauses, take a singular verb when their antecedent in the sentence is singular and a plural verb when it is plural.

Betsy is a *woman* who *loves* life in the country.

This is one of those *motors* that *were* imported from Japan.

Exercise 1

Give reasons for using the singular or the plural verb form in the following sentences.

1. Every one of the nine men on the team (is, are) important.
2. The close relationship with professors and fellow students (makes, make) the small college the choice of many entering freshmen.
3. Doug sprawled in the chair and knocked over one of the lamps which (was, were) on display.
4. There (has, have) never been hard feelings between the families on this street.
5. The symptoms of lead poisoning (varies, vary) with each individual case.
6. Next in the waiting line (was, were) an elderly lady and her grandson.
7. He believes that athletics (improves, improve) school morale.
8. Up goes the starter's gun, and each of the runners (becomes, become) tense.
9. The doctor said that there is always a possibility that the infection will return but that so far there (has, have) been no signs of its recurrence.
10. The family (takes, take) its annual vacation during August.
11. Each of the hospital's patients (has, have) some kind of medical insurance.
12. Either the *Times* or the *Tribune* (is, are) a reliable source of news.
13. The catcher, as well as the pitcher and the coach, (was, were) arguing furiously with the umpire.
14. Her chief interest in life (was, were) politics.
15. Slater is one of those legislators who (has, have) always opposed spending.

27a

Exercise 2

In the following sentences, determine the cause of the faulty agreement and supply the correct form of the verb.

1. In addition, there is the students who cheat because they have never been taught differently.
2. The author's portrayal of the guests and the games add up to an extremely vivid picture of that particular society, with its petty concerns and rituals.
3. Another of the unpopular activities that take place during freshman week are the roll calls.
4. The theme of suffering, its causes and its consequences, are treated by Shakespeare, Tolstoy, and Conrad.
5. The first thing that catches your eye are the headlines.
6. The fact that the children are so beautiful and so intelligent add to their goodness and make the ghosts appear even more evil.
7. Everyone else in the story have readjusted to their roles, and Pam is the only one who is injured by the experience.
8. Even more important than Laura's skill was her interest in the job and her concern for other workers.
9. These products of automation may have made life more pleasant but has reduced the population from hardworking pioneers to button-pushing time-servers.
10. She is one of the women who has made this country what it is.

27b Agreement of pronoun and antecedent

Pronouns agree in number with their antecedents, the words in a sentence that they refer to.

Many *people* pay a genealogist to look up *their* ancestry.
[*People*, the antecedent, is plural, so the pronoun *their* must also be plural.]

My *uncle* paid a genealogist to look up *his* ancestry.
[*His* agrees with *uncle.*]

Like subject-verb agreement, the basic principle of agreement between pronouns and antecedents is easy enough to understand. But again, a few unusual constructions may at first seem puzzling.

27b

1. Compound antecedents

Compound antecedents, like compound subjects, are usually considered plural when joined by *and* and singular when joined by *or* or *nor.*

My father encouraged *Henry* and *David* to postpone *their* trip.

Neither the *dog* nor the *cat* had touched *its* food.

2. Collective nouns as antecedents

When the antecedent is a collective noun, the singular pronoun is used to emphasize the cohesiveness of the group, the plural to emphasize the separate individuals.

The *audience* showed *its* approval by applause.

The *audience* were on *their* feet, booing and whistling.
[Note that in the second sentence the verb *were* is also in the plural form. Be consistent. If the verb form indicates that the antecedent is singular, the pronoun must also be singular. If the verb is plural, the pronoun must be plural too.]

> **Incorrect** The panel *is* ready to give *their* opinions.
>
> **Correct** The panel *is* ready to give *its* opinions.
>
> **Correct** The panel *are* ready to give *their* opinions.
> [The second sentence here suggests that the panel members all hold the same opinions; the last sentence suggests that various members of the panel have different opinions to offer.]

3. Indefinite antecedents

In informal usage, indefinite pronouns like *each, either, neither, everyone, everybody, someone, somebody, anyone, anybody, no one,* and *nobody* are often treated as if they were plural.

> **Informal** Almost *everyone* eats some fruit as part of *their* baisc diet.

Strictly speaking, though, all of these pronouns are singular, and pronouns that follow them in Edited American English must also be singular. The problem is that English lacks singular personal pronouns that can refer to both males and females. Consequently, sentences such as the following, while grammatically correct, illogically exclude half of the human population.

> **Illogical** *Anyone* returning merchandise must present *his* sales receipt.
>
> **Illogical** *No one* in line for the cancelled tennis match got *her* money back.

Women, as well as men, may need to return merchandise, and men, as well as women, attend tennis matches. One solution to this problem is to use two pronouns, one masculine and one feminine, when the antecedent can be either male or female.

27b

> **Correct** *Anyone* returning merchandise must present *his or her* sales receipt.
>
> **Correct** *No one* in line for the cancelled tennis match got *his or her* money back.

However, some writers might consider this construction awkward, and most writers would probably reject the following similar sentence as unacceptably clumsy:

> **Correct but awkward** For once, *everyone* in the class saw *himself or herself* as *he or she* really was.

For all of these cases, a second correct—and less awkward—alternative is simply to rewrite the sentence with plural, rather than singular, nouns and pronouns.

> *Customers* returning merchandise must present *their* sales receipts.
>
> *None* of the people in line for the cancelled tennis match got *their* money back.
>
> For once, the class *members* saw *themselves* as *they* really were.

4. Demonstrative pronouns

When demonstrative pronouns (*this, these; that, those*) are used as adjectives, they must agree in number with the words they modify.

Incorrect	*These kind* of vegetables are grown in the valley.
Correct	*This kind* of vegetable is grown in the valley.
Correct	*These kinds* of vegetables are grown in the valley.

Exercise 3

In the following sentences, determine the cause of faulty agreement and supply the correct form of the pronoun.

1. Either Jim or Les are responsible for the final report.
2. The family was quite frank in stating their opinions.
3. These kind of scrimmages can be very bruising.
4. Each camper was supposed to bring their own bedding.
5. Now that everything was perfect, he was going to make sure they stayed that way.
6. Dorm meetings are always a spectacle because someone always loses their temper.
7. A prisoner's attitude toward society is largely determined by the treatment they receive in prison.
8. Every new proposal was dismissed by the company president because she thought they were impractical.
9. Not a single resident of the town was aware of the threat that the rising river posed for them.
10. The florists all said that they rarely had these type of roses so late in the season.
11. Without a word, my friend turned toward me and opened their hand.
12. The witness insisted that neither the woman nor her daughter had left their place in line.
13. Doesn't anybody recognize their responsibility to other human beings anymore?
14. A child who has grown up with television may not be aware of the impact that TV commericals have on them.
15. If a thorough investigation is conducted, both Eric and Tom should get the reward he has earned.

27b

28 *Case of Pronouns and Nouns*

Case refers to the changes in form of a noun or pronoun that show how it is used in a sentence. English nouns used to have many case forms, but today the only case endings remaining are those that indicate possession (*child's, woman's, year's*). Most pronouns, however, have three case forms: the **nominative** (or **subjective**) case when the pronoun is the subject of a verb; the **possessive** (or **genitive**) case to show possession; and the **objective** case when the pronoun functions as the object of a verb or preposition.

Nominative	I	we	he	she	it	they	who
Possessive	my	our	his	her	its	their	whose
Objective	me	us	him	her	it	them	whom

As with agreement, we usually get the case right without consciously thinking about it. But a few constructions can occasionally cause writers trouble.

28a Compound constructions

A noun and a pronoun used together in a compound construction should be in the same case; the same principle applies to constructions like *we citizens* and to appositives. In most of these situations, you can easily check to determine that you have the pronoun in the right case by reading the sentence without the noun. It should still sound correct.

My *mother* and *I* have a good relationship.

The doctor asked my *mother* and *me* to come in together.
[Because a construction like *my mother and I* is so common, it is easy to slip into it even in the second sentence, where the objective pronoun is needed. The correct case of the pronoun is clear when we delete the noun from the compound construction: *The doctor asked . . . me. . . .*]

Between *you* and *me*, Porter doesn't have a chance to win.
[Both the noun and the pronoun are objects of the preposition *between*, and both must therefore be in the objective case.]

Our parents always rewarded *us children* for getting good grades.

We children always tried to please our parents by getting good grades.
[In both of these appositive constructions, the correct case of the pronoun is clear when we read the sentence without the noun *children*.]

Most of the float was designed by two members of the class, *Howard* and *me*.
[Again, deleting the nouns *Howard* and *members* makes the objective case of the pronoun clear: *Most of the float was designed by . . . me. . . .*]

28b *Who* in dependent clauses and interrogatives

When in doubt about the case of the relative pronouns *who* and *whoever,* try a personal pronoun (*he/him, she/her, they/them*) in its place in the sentence. If *he, she,* or *they* sounds right, use the nominative, *who;* if *him, her,* or *them* fits the grammatical context, *whom* is correct.

Here is a woman *who?/whom?* can explain eclipses.
[We could say *she can explain eclipses,* but not *her can explain eclipses.* Thus, *who* is correct in this case; as the subject of the clause, it is in the nominative case.]

Marshall is the man *who?/whom?* I told you about.
[In this sentence, the pronoun is not the subject of the clause; instead, the clause means *I told you about. . . . Him,* rather than *he,* fits this context; the correct pronoun is thus *whom.*]

Here are the extra bluebooks for *whoever?/whomever?* needs them.
[You could say *he needs them* or *she needs them,* but not *him needs them.* The correct pronoun is in the nominative case, *whoever.*]

Note that inserting an expression such as "I think" or "he says" after the pronoun *who* or *whom* does not change its case.

The man *who?/whom?* I thought would accept the nomination changed his mind.
[The sense of the clause is, *I thought he/him would accept the nomination.* Only *he* fits into this sentence, so *who* is the correct pronoun.]

In formal writing the interrogative pronouns *who* and *whom* are used exactly like the relative pronouns.

Who is coming to the party? [They are.]

Whom are you expecting at the party? [I am expecting *them.*]

In speech and in much informal writing, the tendency is to use *who* as the interrogative form whenever it begins a sentence, no matter what its grammatical place in the sentence. In Edited English it is safer to be formal.

28b

Formal	*Whom* are you expecting for dessert?
Informal	*Who* are you expecting for dessert?
Formal	With *whom* are you leaving?
Informal	*Who* are you leaving with?

28c Complement of *to be*

In formal writing, the complement of the linking verb *to be* is in the nominative case.

> The members of the delegation are *you,* your *sister,* and *I.*
>
> We hoped the speaker would be President Markson, but it was not *he.*
>
> A voice on the telephone asked for Dr. Poynter, and I said, "This is *she.*"

However, in speech and informal writing, the form *It is me* and analogous forms like *I thought it was her* and *It wasn't us* are commonly used.

Note that these cases are all different from one in which a complement follows the infinitive form *to be.* In that situation, the complement is always correctly in the objective case.

> I wouldn't want *to be him.*

28d Pronoun after *than, as,* or *but*

After *than* or *as,* the case of a pronoun is determined by its use in the shortened clause of which it is a part.

> My cousin is taller than *I* [am].
>
> They take more photographs than *we* [do].
>
> I can type as well as *he* [can].
>
> He chooses you more often than [he chooses] *me.*
>
> I thought her [to be] as guilty as [I thought] *him* [to be guilty].

But is sometimes used as a preposition meaning *except.* In such constructions, the object of *but* should be in the objective case.

> By morning everyone had left but *them.*
>
> All the guests at the party had a good time but Judy and *me.*

28e Possessives with gerunds

In grammatical terms, gerunds function in a sentence as nouns. Therefore, a noun or pronoun modifying a gerund, like a noun or pronoun modifying any noun, should be in the possessive case.

> Alan's parents approved of *his* decision.
> [*His* modifies the noun *decision.*]
>
> Alan's parents approved of *his* climbing the mountain.
> [*His* modifies the gerund *climbing.*]
>
> *Julie's* acting amazed everyone in the audience.

28e

Exercise 1

In each sentence, choose the proper case form and be prepared to explain your choice.

1. My sister is a better skier than (I, me).
2. If Harvey hadn't finished college, my parents would never have permitted Betty and (he, him) to get married.
3. There was no comment from the two members (who, whom) I thought were sure to protest.
4. All the students (who, whom) I talked to seemed to like the new coach.
5. My father used to nag us—my sister and (I, me)—about using his pipe cleaners to make bracelets.
6. All the family went to the funeral but (I, me).
7. The new dictator won't be sure of (who, whom) he can trust.
8. His father objects to (him, his) watching sports every spare minute he can.
9. The reward was divided between my older brother and (I, me).
10. The Holes have not lived here as long as (we, us).
11. That year we finally had a teacher (who, whom) won the respect of all of (we, us) students (who, whom) she had in class.
12. Only two members of the family are double-jointed in the thumb, my mother and (I, me).
13. Another good reason for (him, his) joining the Coast Guard is the chance for special training.
14. The ten remaining tickets will be given to (whoever, whomever) applies first.
15. I would hate to be (he, him).

28e

29 *Adjectives and Adverbs*

Adjectives and adverbs are similar types of modifiers with slightly different functions. **Adjectives** modify nouns or pronouns; they provide such information as the color, size, type, or manner of the words they describe.

> The car came to a *sudden* stop.
>
> The performers began an *elegant* dance.
> [In these sentences, *sudden* describes the kind of stop that the car made, and *elegant* describes the dance done by the performers.]

Adverbs, on the other hand, modify verbs, adjectives, or other adverbs. They answer questions like *when? where? why? in what way? to what degree?*

> The car *suddenly* stopped.
>
> The performers began an *unusually* elegant dance.
> [In the first sentence here, the adverb *suddenly* modifies the verb *stopped.* In the second, the adverb *unusually* modifies the adjective *elegant* (not the dance, but its elegance, was unusual).]

Most adverbs are formed by adding -*ly* to the adjective: *clear, clearly; immediate, immediately.* But like other rules of English, this one has its exceptions. Some adjectives and adverbs have the same form: the *far* corner, *much* pleased, I *little* thought, do it *right,* run *fast.* And a few adjectives and adverbs have completely different forms: a *good* job, a job done *well.* Finally, some adjectives already end in -*ly:* a *friendly* gesture, a *manly* appearance, a *leisurely* vacation. In some of these cases, the adverb form is the same; in others, there is no corresponding adverb in English. A dictionary is your best guide.

29a Comparative and superlative forms

Most adjectives and adverbs have three different forms: the **positive** (or dictionary) form, the **comparative** form, and the **superlative** form. Adjectives usually form the comparative by adding -*er* and the superlative by adding -*est.*

tall	taller	tallest
lively	livelier	liveliest

Many adjectives of two syllables and all longer adjectives form the comparative and superlative by adding *more* and *most*.

alert   more alert   most alert

ambitious   more ambitious   most ambitious

Adverbs nearly always form the comparative and superlative with *more* and *most*.

slowly   more slowly   most slowly

In formal writing, the comparative is used for comparisons involving two persons or things, and the superlative when three or more are being compared.

Of my two brothers, Jack was the *taller.*

She was the *quickest* person on the team.

In speech and informal writing, this distinction is not always observed, and the superlative is often used even when only two things are being compared: "Of the two styles offered, the first was the *most* popular."

Some adjectives and adverbs, like *unique/uniquely, perfect/perfectly,* cannot logically take comparative or superlative forms. Since unique means "one of a kind," no object can be more unique than another. Similarly, a thing is either perfect or imperfect; strictly speaking, no degree is possible. Formal writing, therefore, tends to avoid expressions like *more perfect* or *most unique,* although you may use modifiers that indicate an approach to the absolute (a *nearly perfect* performance, an *almost unique* diamond). Informal writing often permits the superlative form *most perfect,* but *rather unique* and *the most unique* were considered unacceptable by 94 percent of the Usage Panel of the *American Heritage Dictionary.*

Formal   Holmes is the *most nearly perfect* actor we have seen this season.

Informal This is the *most perfect* pumpkin in the field.

29b Adjectives with linking verbs

Verbs such as *be, become, seem, appear,* as well as verbs indicating the use of five senses (*look, feel, taste, sound, smell*), are often used to link an adjective to the subject of a sentence. Do not use the adverbial form as the complement of a linking verb.

29b

The swimmer { looked / seemed / felt / sounded / became / was } *cold*

I felt *terrible* about my mistake.

I knew I had played *terribly.*

The melon tasted *sweet,* and my aunt smiled *happily.*

Although the surgeon looked *tired,* he felt my ankle *carefully.*

I smelled the fish *cautiously,* but it smelled *fresh.*

Watching him, Betty felt *uneasy.* [tells something about Betty]

Betty watched him *uneasily.* [tells how she watched him]

I felt *bad* about her illness. [adjective complement of *felt*]

I felt *badly* bruised. [adverb modifying *bruised*]

In speech, the following adjectives are often used to modify a verb or an adjective. Such expressions are considered colloquial.

He looks *real* good in blue.

I slept *good* last night.

I feel *some* better today.

We were *sure* glad to see them again.

In edited writing, however, the corresponding adverbs are expected.

He looks *really* good in blue.

I slept *well* last night.

I feel *somewhat* better today.

We were *surely* (or *certainly*) glad to see them again.

29c Compound adjectives

When a compound adjective is formed from two nouns, from an adjective and a noun, or from two adjectives, the compound is hyphenated when it precedes the noun that it modifies.

The *locker-room* brawl left six players injured.

This book is also available in a *large-print* edition.

Kim looked out over the *blue-green* waters of the gulf.

All the elements of a phrase used as an adjective are also hyphenated.

I wish I had her *never-say-die* attitude.

Peter knew the invitation was a *once-in-a-lifetime* opportunity.

Remember, though, that *-ly* adverbs used with adjectives are a different grammatical situation. Such adverbs are modifiers, not parts of a compound, and they are not hyphenated.

Their first apartment was in an *exceptionally decrepit* building.

However, similar constructions with "well" usually *are* hyphenated when they precede the modified noun: *a well-managed business, a well-done steak* (but *a steak well done*).

Exercise 1

Correct the use of adjectives and adverbs as necessary to bring the following sentences up to the level of formal written English.

1. If you listen close, you should be able to hear it quite distinct.
2. The colors in the living room contrasted harshly and looked shockingly.
3. People today live more secure because of new drugs and antibiotics.
4. I am sure I didn't do too good on the objective part of the final.
5. The sky was clear and the air smelled freshly.
6. In the laboratory we were shown a seemingly impossibility.
7. An exciting documentary affects me quite different from a dramatized story about the same thing.
8. We were real pleased that so many people were willing to help.
9. That disastrous Thursday started out quite normal.
10. The sunset was beautiful that evening, but the sky looked threateningly the next morning.
11. During the whole time that Jane Blaisdel was chairman, business went along very smooth.
12. The trick worked as perfect as we had hoped.
13. By looking real close at the ballot, I could see that somebody had changed it.
14. A small minority of students have given this university a real bad image.
15. At the end of the play, he finds that defeat tastes bitterly.

29c

30 *Verbs*

At the center of every sentence stands a verb, a word describing an action or a state of being. In Chapter **9** we examined the syntactic relationship between the verb and other elements in a sentence. Here we turn our attention to verb forms—in particular, the forms that indicate tense and mood.

30a Tense

By **tense** we mean variations in the form of a verb that indicate time differences. English verbs have six principal tenses.

Present   (describes a current or regularly repeated act)

> I *think* this *is* the right thing to do.
>
> Marcelle *leaves* for class at eight o'clock on Tuesdays.

Past   (describes an act completed in the past)

> I *mowed* the lawn, and my sister *pruned* the bushes.

Future   (describes an act that will happen)

> Next month I *will fly* to Denver.

Present Perfect   (describes an act begun in the past but continuing into the present)

> I *have tried* to discourage him, but he *has insisted* on trying to speak with her.

Past Perfect   (describes an act begun and completed before a specific time in the past)

> She *had finished* the letter by the time I arrived.

Future Perfect   (describes an act that will be completed by a specific time in the future)

> He *will have arrived* before we get to the station.

When two or more verbs are used in the same sentence, the verb tenses follow prescribed patterns:

> When I *press* this button, the motor *begins* to run.
>
> The instant he *pressed* the button, the motor *began* to run.
>
> If you *press* (or *will press*) the button, the motor *will start.*
>
> Now that he *has pressed* the button, *he expects* the motor to start.
>
> Since he *had pressed* the button, he *expected* the motor to start.

If these patterns are not followed, a sentence like the following can result:

> **Incorrect**   When he died, his fellow citizens realized how much he contributed to the community, and since then they collected funds for a memorial.

The tense relationships are more complicated than the sentence indicates. Here is the proper sequence of tenses:

> **Correct**   When he *died* [a particular time in the past], his fellow citizens *realized* [from that time on] how much he *had contributed* [up to the time of his death] to the community, and since then they *have been collecting* [from that time to the present] funds for a memorial.

An infinitive should be in the present tense unless it represents an action earlier than that of the main verb.

> July 14, 1789, must have been a great day *to be* alive [not *to have been* alive].
>
> I realized later that it was a mistake *to have chosen* [not *to choose*] the life of an artist two years earlier.

Statements that are permanently true should be put in the present tense (sometimes called the "timeless present") even though the main verb is in the past.

> Copernicus *found* that the Sun *is* the center of our planetary system. [Not *was;* it still *is.*]
>
> I *insisted* that the Amazon River *is* longer than the Nile.

The present tense is often used in book reviews and criticism for describing a novel, play, or movie. But statements about the facts of a dead author's life are normally in the past tense.

30a

> Oliver La Farge's novel *is* the story of a young Navajo whose wife *seeks* revenge for her mistreatment by a white man.
>
> The setting of Hawthorne's short stories *is* the New England village that Hawthorne *knew* so well. [The setting of the stories is still the same; Hawthorne knew them in the past.]

30b Irregular verbs

Irregular verbs are a small group which, instead of forming their past tenses by adding *-ed* (*start, started*), indicate the past tense and the past participle in varied ways (*begin, began, begun*). The principal parts are (1) the present infinitive (*begin*), (2) the past tense (*began*), and (3) the past participle (*begun*). All tense forms can be derived from the three principal parts. The first principal part is the basis for all present and future tenses, including the present participle; the second principal part is used for the simple past tense—"I began the job yesterday." The third principal part is used in all the compound tenses: "I have begun," "he had begun," "the job was begun."

In the speech of children, errors in the use of principal parts of the irregular verbs are common: "I throwed the ball," "We brung it home," "He has went home." The following list gives the principal parts of some irregular verbs that are sometimes confused.

Infinitive	Past tense	Past participle
arise	arose	arisen
be	was, were	been
become	became	become
begin	began	begun
bid (offer)	bid	bid
bid (command)	bade	bidden
bite	bit	bitten
blow	blew	blown
break	broke	broken
bring	brought	brought
burst	burst	burst
buy	bought	bought
catch	caught	caught
choose	chose	chosen
cling	clung	clung
come	came	come
deal	dealt	dealt
dive	dived, dove	dived
do	did	done
draw	drew	drawn
drink	drank	drunk
drive	drove	driven

30b

Infinitive	Past tense	Past participle
eat	ate	eaten
fall	fell	fallen
fly	flew	flown
forget	forgot	forgotten, forgot
freeze	froze	frozen
get	got	got, gotten
give	gave	given
go	went	gone
grow	grew	grown
know	knew	known
lay (put)	laid	laid
lead	led	led
lie (recline)	lay	lain
ride	rode	ridden
ring	rang	rung
rise	rose	risen
run	ran	run
see	saw	seen
shake	shook	shaken
shrink	shrank, shrunk	shrunk
sing	sang	sung
sink	sank	sunk
speak	spoke	spoken
spin	spun	spun
spring	sprang, sprung	sprung
steal	stole	stolen
swear	swore	sworn
swim	swam	swum
swing	swung	swung
take	took	taken
teach	taught	taught
tear	tore	torn
throw	threw	thrown
wear	wore	worn
write	wrote	written

30b

30c Mood

The **mood** of a verb refers to a verb form that reflects the writer's or speaker's attitude. When you state a fact or ask a question, the verb in your sentence is in the **indicative** mood:

I *am* seated next to Nancy.

Am I seated next to Nancy?

When you give a command, the verb is in the **imperative** mood:

Be seated next to Nancy.

And when you express a wish, your verb is in the **subjunctive** mood:

I wish I *were* seated next to Nancy.

The subjunctive mood is also used in the following other situations:

Condition contrary to fact

If this *were* Saturday, we would be at the lake.

Although the dog has just had his supper, he acts as if he *were* still hungry.

Indirect imperative

The terms of the will require that the funds *be spent* on education.

Her lawyer insists that she *open* a savings account.

Motions and resolutions

I move that the minutes *be approved*.

Resolved, that this question *be submitted* to arbitration.

Subjunctive verb forms are used much less than formerly. In speech, the subjunctive is retained only in formulas like "If I were you. . . ."

Exercise 1

Correct any errors in the use of verbs in the following sentences.

1. She wore a faded blue dress, and her dusty gray shoes were once white.
2. The astronomer said that the moon was approximately 239,000 miles from the earth.
3. For a reader who had never run across advertising of this kind, a further explanation may be necessary.
4. Zephyr, our cat, would lay on the floor for hours and played with a ball of string.
5. He would have liked to have told her what he thought of her.
6. If I had chose physics as my major, I wouldn't have to write all these papers.

7. It was a serious mistake to have been so candid.
8. The book had laid right where I had put it.
9. The water level began to raise, and by noon it had rose 10 feet.
10. She recognized the boy who had spoke to her in her calculus class.

Exercise 2

For each of the following sentences choose the proper verb form and be prepared to justify your choice.

1. I wouldn't tolerate such noise if I (*were, was*) you.
2. He moved that the motion (*is, be*) approved.
3. His mother insists that he (*come, comes*) in right now.
4. If Alaska (*was, were*) a warmer state, its population would be larger.
5. He acts as if he (*was, were*) drunk, and he probably is.

30c

31 Sentence Fragments, Comma Splices, Fused Sentences

Sentences broken into fragments or incorrectly joined together are to be avoided not simply because they violate rules of grammatical usage, but because they distract and confuse any reader. An eye trained to spot subjects and finite verbs and an ear tuned to the intonations of speech are usually sufficient to catch fragmented and run-together sentences. To strengthen your feel for complete sentences, read your writing aloud. Listen to the accents, pitch, and rhythms of the words on the page. Notice the different breath pauses for different marks of punctuation, the rising and falling pitch at different points in the sentence. Read aloud the sentences of other writers for cadence and intonation. Remember that grammar and the human voice often coincide in remarkable ways.

31a Types of sentence fragments

A series of words that does not contain an independent clause, that is, a clause with a subject and a finite verb, is a **sentence fragment.**

Fragment   The purpose of reciting five minutes in French was to encourage imitation of the recording. Thus putting emphasis on intonation, rhythm, and pronunciation.

Correct   The purpose of reciting five minutes in French was to encourage imitation of the recording, thus putting emphasis on intonation, rhythm, and pronunciation.

This statement, which expresses one idea, should be contained in one sentence. The second series of words in the faulty version is a fragment, a participial phrase without a subject or a verb. It should be joined, as it is in the corrected example, to the previous sentence.

Listed below are common types of sentence fragments.

1. Appositive phrase

Fragment The crowd that attended the local track meet was the usual one. Parents, friends of the athletes, and people looking for a good tan.

Correct The crowd that attended the local track meet was the usual one— parents, friends of the athletes, and people looking for a good tan.
[The three nouns *parents, friends,* and *people* are in apposition to *one,* and the appositive phrase should be attached to the rest of the sentence with a dash or a colon.]

2. Prepositional phrase

Fragment The council meeting was to have been conducted in an orderly and democratic fashion, but it was impossible. With demonstrators seizing the microphone and the chair banging her gavel for order.

Correct The council meeting was to have been conducted in an orderly and democratic fashion, but it was impossible with demonstrators seizing the microphone and the chair banging her gavel for order.
[The prepositional phrase that begins *with demonstrators* modifies the adjective *impossible* and must be attached to the preceding sentence.]

Another alternative would be to make the prepositional phrase into an independent clause and write it as a separate sentence.

Correct The council meeting was to have been conducted in an orderly and democratic fashion, but it was impossible. The demonstrators seized the microphone, and the chair banged her gavel for order.

3. Participial phrase

Fragment I was surprised at the commotion in the magazine's office. Reporters and secretaries were rushing all over the place. Running up and down the aisles, conferring with the editors, and talking in little groups.

Correct I was surprised at the commotion in the magazine's office. Reporters and secretaries were rushing all over the place, running up and down the aisles, conferring with the editors, and talking in little groups.
[*Running, conferring,* and *talking* are participles that modify *reporters* and *secretaries.* In other words, they are part of the second sentence and should be attached to it.]

Fragment She had good reason for coming to college, unlike some of her classmates. Having planned for several years to become a doctor.

Correct Unlike some of her classmates, she had good reason for coming to college, having planned for several years to become a doctor.
[The participial phrase modifies *she,* and it is best placed close to the pronoun. To avoid confusion, the *unlike some of her classmates* should begin the sentence.]

31a

4. Infinitive phrase

Fragment   After a long discussion, I finally received permission from my parents. To spend the summer and fall with El Centro de Paz, a work project in Mexico.

Correct   After a long discussion, I finally received permission from my parents to spend the summer and fall with El Centro de Paz, a work project in Mexico.

[*To spend* . . . is an infinitive phrase modifying *permission* and should not be separated from the main clause.]

5. Dependent clause

A dependent clause must either be joined to the sentence of which it is logically a part or be rewritten as an independent clause.

Fragment   Often I stay up late in my room, studying, writing, or thinking about the future. While all the other people in the dorm are asleep.

Correct   Often I stay up late in my room, studying, writing, or thinking about the future while all the other people in the dorm are asleep.

Fragment   I was grateful to learn of the college's loan funds. Because I didn't know where I could turn for help or see how I could take a part-time job.

Correct   I was grateful to learn of the college's loan funds, because I didn't know where I could turn for help or see how I could take a part-time job.

The fragments above might have been eliminated by omitting the conjunctions *while* and *because* to change the dependent clauses into independent clauses. Note, however, that without the conjunction the precise connection between the two clauses in each case is lost.

Correct but weak   Often I stay up late in my room, studying, writing, or thinking about the future. All the other people in the dorm are asleep.

Correct but weak   I was grateful to learn of the college's loan funds. I didn't know where I could turn for help or see how I could take a part-time job.

31b Acceptable incomplete sentences

31b

Certain elliptical expressions are equivalent to sentences because the missing words are clearly understood. Such permissible incomplete sentences include the following:

1. Questions and answers in conversation

Why not? Because it's late.

How much? Two dollars.

2. Exclamations and requests

At last!

This way, please.

3. Informal transitions

So much for the first point.

Now to consider the next question.

In addition, fragments are sometimes deliberately used for particular effects, especially in narrative or descriptive writing. In most expository writing, however, there is seldom a good reason for writing sentence fragments.

Exercise 1

For each of the following sentences, correct the fragment in whatever way seems most effective.

1. When you really get down to it, homework is more likely to be assigned in the academic subjects. Whether they are English, math, science, or some language.

2. One thing that I dislike very much is a person with a mean streak. A person who will go out of his way to do harm to others.

3. During the day the eel lies buried in the mud or concealed under rocks or in seaweed. But at night begins prowling for food.

4. Mary Cassatt was one of the finest American painters of her time. Her work now coming into its own.

5. For some people, life is only boring or painful. Especially if the person has no purpose, no goal in life.

6. The number of the very rich and the very poor having been reduced, leaving most Americans in one large middle class.

7. I now think that my high school was too progressive in some ways. Meaning that it didn't teach how to read and write correctly.

8. The head librarian threatened to close the stacks to all students. Because the cost of replacing stolen books was mounting each year.

9. Tyrone Guthrie's movie production of *Oedipus Rex* was very impressive. Although it took me a while to get used to the masked actors.

10. The City Council's decision to limit speed on a road in the campus but not on a street near an elementary school seemed ridiculous. Since small children are less able to cross streets responsibly.

11. Long hours of practice after classes, the weekends usually taken up with games, and most evenings spent in study. Athletes have little time for working their way through college.

12. Historians are interested only in the more civilized societies that have existed in the past. The ones that have produced great works of art, science, or technology.

13. Every month, the entire research staff spends a full day together in informal conference. To discuss at length current problems and propose and criticize new ideas.

31b

14. A description of being lost in the Grand Canyon when Schuyler's life was saved by a discarded semirotten orange.

15. The distance between the stars is immense. So immense that it is difficult to find a unit of measurement that will help one grasp it imaginatively.

31c Comma splices

A **comma splice**—sometimes called a **comma fault**—occurs when two independent clauses are joined only with a comma. Comma splices are distracting to a reader, and they can often lead to misreading.

> **Comma splice**   My nephew stood in the doorway, soaked from the rain, the stray dog lay at his feet.

Is it the nephew who is soaked from the rain, or the stray dog? The confusion results because the comma by itself is not a strong enough punctuation mark to indicate the end of an independent clause. Two stronger punctuation marks are the period and the semicolon.

> **Correct**   My nephew stood in the doorway, soaked from the rain. The stray dog lay at his feet.
>
> **Correct**   My nephew stood in the doorway; soaked from the rain, the stray dog lay at his feet.

You can sometimes catch comma splices in revision by reading your paper aloud. If you naturally drop your voice or pause substantially at a comma, check to see whether you have mistakenly used the comma to connect independent clauses.

Comma splices can be corrected in several ways:

1. Separation of clauses into sentences

Correct the comma splice by making each main clause into a sentence. Use this method if you want to emphasize the separation between the two statements.

> **Comma splice**   There was an extremely heavy rain on Monday night, after the storm had passed, the streams were overflowing.
>
> **Correct**   There was an extremely heavy rain on Monday night. After the storm had passed, the streams were overflowing.

2. Coordination of clauses by semicolon

Correct the comma splice by using a semicolon to join the two main clauses. This method is appropriate when the relationship between the two statements is to be implied rather than stated explicitly.

31c

Comma splice	Gambling is like a drug, after a while the gambler finds it impossible to stop.
Correct	Gambling is like a drug; after a while the gambler finds it impossible to stop.

3. Coordination of clauses by coordinating conjunction

Correct the comma splice by using a coordinating conjunction to join the two main clauses if you want to give them equal emphasis.

Comma splice	We will add another room to the house this summer, painting will have to wait until next year.
Correct	We will add another room to the house this summer, *but* painting will have to wait until next year.
Comma splice	Reading is partly a matter of personal taste, every reviewer ought to keep this fact in mind.
Correct	Reading is partly a matter of personal taste, *and* every reviewer ought to keep this fact in mind.

The most usual pattern is the coordinating conjunction (*and, yet, but, for, nor, or*) preceded by a comma. When long, complex clauses punctuated internally by commas are joined, a semicolon along with a coordinating conjunction may be needed to show the main division of the sentence.

Comma splice	As the development of the atomic bomb, of computer systems, and of guided missiles shows, technology, indeed basic scientific research itself, is often determined by political and military considerations, many people do not recognize this interdependence and instead regard changes in technology as changes that simply "happen."
Correct	As the development of the atomic bomb, of computer systems, and of guided missiles shows, technology, indeed basic scientific research itself, is often determined by political and military considerations; *but* many people do not recognize this interdependence and instead regard changes in technology as changes that simply "happen."

4. Subordination of one clause

Correct the comma splice by subordinating one of the clauses with a subordinating conjunction like *since, because, although, which, when.*

Comma splice	The banks were closed, John couldn't get the necessary money.
Correct	*Since* the banks were closed, John couldn't get the necessary money.

31c

Comma splice	There are many good reasons for working in the summer, only a few of them can be discussed.
Correct	There are many good reasons for working in the summer, only a few *of which* can be discussed.

5. Semicolon with conjunctive adverbs

Two main clauses linked by a conjunctive adverb require a semicolon or a period between them. One of the most common forms of the comma splice is the use of the comma between two main clauses linked by a conjunctive adverb. Such conjunctive adverbs as *also, besides, hence, however, instead, moreover, then,* and *therefore* should be preceded by a semicolon or period when they introduce a second independent clause.

Comma splice	I hadn't read the test very carefully, therefore I was surprised that I had done so well on it.
Correct	I hadn't read the test very carefully; therefore, I was surprised that I had done so well on it.
Comma splice	To a majority of the economists a gloomy forecast seemed inevitable, however three of the experts were unfashionably cheerful.
Correct	To a majority of the economists a gloomy forecast seemed inevitable. However, three of the experts were unfashionably cheerful.

One way to tell a conjunctive adverb from a pure conjunction is to try to change its position in the sentence. A conjunctive adverb need not stand first in its clause:

We had been told to stay at home; *moreover,* we knew that we were not allowed to play outside after dark.

We had been told to stay at home; we knew, *moreover,* that we were not allowed to play outside after dark.

A pure conjunction will fit into the sentence only at the beginning of its clause:

We had been told to stay at home, *and* we knew that we were not allowed to play outside after dark.

We knew we were not allowed to play outside after dark, *because* we had been told to stay home.

A final exception to what we have said about comma splices should perhaps be mentioned. Short, closely related independent clauses may be joined only by commas. Such punctuation, however, is more common in narratives than in expository writing.

Acceptable	The sky darkened, the wind blew, the cold rain began to fall.

31c

31d Fused sentences

A **fused sentence** is one in which two main clauses are joined with no punctuation between them.

Fused   He took the job he was offered otherwise he would have had to borrow more money.

The fused sentence is a more blatant error than the comma splice because it makes the reader's task extremely difficult. To correct a fused sentence, use any of the means for correcting the comma splice.

Correct   He took the job he was offered. Otherwise, he would have had to borrow more money.

Correct   He took the job he was offered; otherwise, he would have had to borrow more money.

Fused   Congress passed the bill only after long hours of debate there was strong feeling on both sides.

Correct   Congress passed the bill only after long hours of debate. There was strong feeling on both sides.

Correct   Because there was strong feeling on both sides, Congress passed the bill only after long hours of debate.

Exercise 2

In the following sentences, revise the comma splices or fused sentences by whatever means seem most effective. Be prepared to explain the reasons for the means you choose.

1. But why shouldn't carols be played in shops and stores it's all in the spirit of Christmas.
2. Once in her room she did a few dance steps, looked at her unmade bed and shrugged unconcernedly, then she glanced out the window in hopes of catching sight of her little brother.
3. But with the first of September the warm days were over, cold winds began to blow, stirring up freshly turned dirt in the graveyard and causing old Charles to cast apprehensive glances at the sky.
4. Ironically, the population migration has been especially great to places like Arizona, New Mexico, and southern California, these are places with a limited water supply.
5. We found the sea too choppy for sailing or swimming, we stayed on shore.
6. Permission was not granted for the interview, however the reporters never gave up hope.
7. The new dictionary was more than a revision of the old one, the compilers had redefined each entry and included many more examples of usage.
8. The critic wrote that as the commercials became longer and more offensive, the shows became shorter and more innocuous, she also felt advertisers ought to be forced to watch the commercials.

31d

9. In speech class he announced he would give a demonstration-lecture on how not to pack a suitcase, after he was finished, the other students clapped reluctantly.

10. The counselor gathered the paddles, came down to the pier, and untied the canoe then he waited while the campers climbed in.

11. The medical insurance was cheap and comprehensive, according to its advertisers, the people who bought it soon claimed otherwise.

12. Most almanacs have a section on sports and games, this is where track and field records can be found.

13. She usually obeyed her elders, but she always weighed the facts and formed her own opinions, apparently, this independence of hers made some adults angry.

14. Duke Ellington never really retired, instead he kept composing and conducting right up to the end.

15. The day was much too beautiful for staying at home I spent the entire afternoon at the beach.

31d

Punctuation, Spelling, Mechanics

Part VIII

32 *Punctuation*

Punctuation is to writing what notation is to music: it allows the eye to re-create from the page the sounds the author of the composition had in mind. Both are necessary and exacting systems. Just as musicians know the crucial difference between a quarter-note and a half-note, so writers know the crucial difference between a comma and a semicolon, between brackets and parentheses. The brief and moderate and extended pauses noted by punctuation give cadence and rhythm to prose, but, more important, they signal meaning. Only a person who understands punctuation knows how the drop in the voice signaled by the commas makes one of these sentences mean something quite different from the other.

> The students who have worked diligently and completed all the assignments on time will not have to take the final.

> The students, who have worked diligently and completed all the assignments on time, will not have to take the final.

Contrary to popular mythology, there is nothing mysterious or arbitrary about punctuation. There are choices and options and the freedom, within certain unexceptional rules, to write with frequent or infrequent marks, in a liberally or conservatively punctuated fashion, depending upon the writer's taste and style. Only an indifferent writer will sprinkle commas and dashes randomly during a last-minute reading, much as our ancestors sprinkled sand over the paper to dry the ink.

The rules in the following sections specify where punctuation marks are needed and, occasionally, where they are acceptable. Beyond this, you must use your judgment. If you are in doubt and no positive rule covers the point, the habit of less rather than more applies: omit the punctuation mark.

32a End punctuation

1. The period

Use a period to mark the end of a declarative or imperative sentence.

This is an example of a declarative sentence.

Use a period at the end of a sentence like this.

A period is also used after abbreviations, like *Dr*., *Mr*, *Ph*.*D*., *etc*., *A*.*D*., *Calif*., *Inc*. For the proper use of abbreviations, see Chapter **34**.

Three spaced periods (. . .), called ellipsis marks, are used to indicate the omission of a word or words from a quoted passage. If the omitted words come at the end of a sentence, a fourth period is needed.

> We hold these truths to be self-evident: that all men . . . are endowed by their Creator with certain unalienable rights . . . .

Similarly, three (or four) periods are sometimes used in dialogue and interrupted narrative to indicate hesitation and pauses. Beginning writers should use these with caution.

> He inspired uneasiness. That was it! Uneasiness. Not a definite mistrust—just uneasiness—nothing more. You can have no idea how effective such a . . . a . . . faculty can be.

> —Joseph Conrad

2. The question mark

Use a question mark after a direct question.

> Where did you find such information ?
>
> How much of the White Sands is gypsum ?
>
> Looking at me, the officer said, "Where do you live ?

An indirect question should be followed by a period, not a question mark.

> He asked what had caused the delay .
>
> I wonder how many Americans walk to work these days .

A request that is phrased as a question for the sake of politeness is followed by a period.

> Will you please send me your latest catalog .

3. The exclamation mark

Exclamation marks are appropriate only after statements that would be given unusual emphasis if spoken.

> Four hours of taking lecture notes without a break ! Will my fingers ever unbend?

The exclamation mark is seldom suitable to expository writing. Nor is it advisable to use the exclamation mark to underscore flat statements or ironic remarks.

32a

> **Ineffective**   The professor suggested that we take out our notebooks since he was going to give us a little (!) test.

32b The comma

The comma is perhaps the most used and, consequently, the most abused punctuation mark. It separates coordinate elements within a sentence and sets off certain subordinate constructions from the rest of the sentence. Since it represents the shortest breath pause and the least emphatic break, it cannot separate two complete sentences.

A primary function of the comma is to make a sentence clear. Always use commas to prevent misreading: to separate words that might be erroneously grouped together by the reader.

1. To separate independent clauses

Two independent clauses joined by a coordinating conjunction (*and, so, or, nor, but, yet, for*) should be separated by a comma. Note that the comma is always placed *before* the conjunction.

> I failed German in my senior year of high school , *and* it took me a long time to regain any interest in foreign languages.

> She went through the motions of studying , *but* her mind was elsewhere.

Very short independent clauses need not be separated by a comma if they are closely connected in meaning.

> The bell rang and everyone left.

Coordinating conjunctions are often used to join the parts of a compound predicate, that is, two or more verbs with the same subject. In such a sentence a comma is not required to separate the predicates. However, if the two parts are long or imply a strong contrast, a comma may be used to separate them.

> We *measured* the potassium and *weighed* it on the scale.

> Mr. Cowan *demonstrated* the difference between preserving wood with oil and with shellac , *and advised* the use of oil for durable table-tops.

> To our dismay, the suede could not be *washed* at home or *dry cleaned* at an ordinary place , *but had to be sent* to a specialist.

When the clauses of a compound sentence are long and are also subdivided by commas, a stronger mark of punctuation than a comma may be needed to separate the clauses from each other. For this purpose a semicolon is regularly used.

> For purposes of discussion, we will recognize two main varieties of English, Standard and Nonstandard ; and we will divide the first type into Formal, Informal, and Colloquial English.

32b

2. To separate elements in a series

Separate words, phrases, or clauses in a series by commas. The typical form of a series is *a, b,* and *c.* A series may contain more than three parallel elements, and any of the coordinating conjunctions may be used to connect the last two. If *all* the elements of a series are joined by coordinating conjunctions (*a and b and c*), no commas are necessary to separate them.

Series of adjectives

The shy devilfish blushes in *blue*, *red*, *green*, *or brown.*

Series of phrases

Water flooded *over the riverbed*, *over the culverts*, *and over the asphalt road.*

Series of predicates

The bear *jumped away from the garbage can*, *snarled at the camper*, *and raced up the tree.*

Series of nouns

Resistors, *transistors*, *capacitors*, *and connectors* are small electronic parts.

Series of independent clauses

Stone was hauled twelve miles, a casing was built as the hole deepened, and a well 109 feet deep was completed in Greensburg, Kansas.

The comma before the last item in a series is omitted by some writers, but its use is generally preferred because it can prevent misreading.

Misleading   The three congressional priorities are nuclear disarmament, the curtailment of agricultural trade and aid to underdeveloped countries.
[Without the comma before *and, agricultural trade* and *aid to underdeveloped countries* can be read as compound objects of *curtailment of,* and the reader reaches the end of the sentence still waiting for the third priority. No such misreading occurs if the comma is included.]

3. Uses with coordinate elements

Adjectives modifying the same noun should be separated by commas if they are coordinate in meaning. Coordinate adjectives are those that could be joined by *and* without distorting the meaning of a sentence.

32b

Bus lines provide *inexpensive*, *efficient* transportation.
[The adjectives are coordinate: transportation that is *inexpensive* and *efficient.*]

Sometimes, however, an adjective is so closely linked with the noun that it is thought of as part of the noun. Such an adjective is not coordinate with a preceding adjective.

> The Paynes bought a *spacious summer* cabin.
> [This does not mean *a cabin that is spacious and summer. Summer* indicates the kind of cabin; *spacious* describes the summer cabin.]

Note that numbers are not coordinate with other adjectives and are not separated by commas.

> They screened in *two large , airy* outdoor porches.
> [*Two* and *large* should not be separated by a comma. But since the two outdoor porches were *large* and *airy,* a comma is used to separate these two coordinate adjectives.]

Coordinate words or phrases that are sharply contrasted are separated by commas.

> He is *ignorant , not stupid.*

> Our aim is *to encourage question and debate , not criticism and argument.*

An idiomatic way of asking a question is to make a direct statement and add to it a coordinate elliptical question. Such a construction should be separated by a comma from the direct statement.

> You will come with us , *won't you?*

> He won't test us on last semester's units , *will he?*

Another idiomatic construction that requires a comma is the coordinate use of adjectives, as in *the more . . . , the more. . . .*

> *The faster* the bird , *the higher* the metabolism.

> *The more* a candidate meets voters , *the more* he may learn about their concerns.

Exercise 1

Insert the proper punctuation marks where they are required in the following sentences, and give a reason for your choice.

1. Seven legislators from the southern part of the state changed their votes and with their aid the bill was passed.
2. During many periods of history men's clothing has been no less extravagant in cut color and richness of fabric than women's and there have been times when men's clothes have been the gaudier.
3. By the end of the twenty-mile hike we were all fairly tired and some of us were suffering from sore feet as well.
4. Three of the editors argued that the article was biased and malicious and voted to reject it in spite of the distinguished name of the author.
5. The teller at the bank looked dubiously at the check I offered her and even though I knew the check was good I could feel a guilty look freezing on my face as her doubts increased.

32b

6. Painted surfaces should be washed with a detergent sanded lightly and covered with a thin coat of plastic varnish.
7. I painted the house a warm deep pearl gray.
8. Her latest novel was marred by pretentious writing the absence of solid characterization and a hackneyed plot.
9. I believe that a state lottery can be useful because it can provide revenue for education increase employment and relieve the tax burden.
10. I judge people by what they say and how they act not by their gender or race.

4. To set off nonrestrictive modifiers

A dependent clause, participial phrase, or appositive is nonrestrictive when it can be omitted without changing the main idea of the sentence. A **nonrestrictive modifier** gives additional information about the noun to which it refers. A **restrictive modifier,** on the other hand, restricts the meaning of the word to which it refers to one particular group or thing. If it is omitted, the main idea of the sentence is changed.

Nonrestrictive clauses and phrases

Note that *two commas* are required to set off a nonrestrictive modifier in the middle of a sentence; one comma is sufficient if the modifier is at the beginning or end of the sentence.

Nonrestrictive clause

My faculty advisor, *who had to sign the program card,* was hard to find.
[If the clause were omitted, some information would be lost, but the sentence would make the same point: that my advisor was hard to find.]

Restrictive clause

Faculty advisors *who are never in their office* make registration difficult.
[Omitting the clause here changes the sense completely. The purpose of the clause is to limit the statement to a certain kind of faculty advisor—those who are never in their offices.]

nonrestrictive clause
I found the letter under the door, *which had been locked.*

restrictive clause
The letter *that I found under the door* was a mystery.

nonrestrictive phrase
Uncle Sid's letter, *lying unclaimed in the dead letter office,* contained the missing document.

restrictive phrase
We have had many complaints about letters *undelivered because of careless addressing.*

32b

Notice how the meaning of a sentence may be altered by the addition or the omission of commas:

> The board sent questionnaires to all members, who are on Social Security.
> [Nonrestrictive clause. The sentence implies that all members are on Social Security.]

> The board sent questionnaires to all members who are on Social Security.
> [Restrictive clause. The questionnaire is sent only to some members, those on Social Security.]

Nonrestrictive appositives

Appositives are usually nonrestrictive and hence are set off by commas. If, however, an appositive puts a necessary limitation upon its noun, it is restrictive and no punctuation is necessary.

Nonrestrictive appositive

> Scientists working with cryogenics have produced temperatures within a thousandth of a degree of absolute zero, *approximately 459.7 below zero Fahrenheit.*

Restrictive appositive

> The noun *cryogenics* comes from a Greek word meaning "icy cold."

An appositive used to define a word is often introduced by the conjunction *or.* Such appositives are always set off by commas to distinguish them from the common construction in which *or* joins two coordinate nouns.

> The class found a fine specimen of pyrite, *or fool's gold.*

> We couldn't decide whether to plant *phlox or coral bells.*

An abbreviated title or degree (*K.C.B., USMC, M.D., Ph.D.*) is treated as an appositive when it follows a proper name.

> He was introduced as Robert Harrison, *L.L.D.*, and he added that he also held a Ph.D. from Cornell.

Exercise 2

Insert commas in the following sentences to set off nonrestrictive clauses and participial phrases. In doubtful cases, explain the difference in meaning produced by the insertion of commas.

1. King Leopold of Belgium who was Queen Victoria's uncle also gave her a great deal of advice.
2. Many people who have never been to the United States think of it as a country of wealth and luxury where everyone lives on the fat of the land.
3. Some years ago I lived in a section of town where almost everyone was a Republican.
4. With the advent of the jet engine which is more efficient at high than at low altitudes aircraft could attain greater heights.

32b

5. The astronauts who had been trained for any circumstance were calm when the launching was called off at the last minute.
6. The student hoping to get a "C" without too much work should stay out of Economics 152.
7. We will have to hire someone who can do a better job of keeping the place neat and orderly.
8. The packing plant where I worked all summer is on the Aleutian Islands.
9. She has made a special study of the native women who are monogamous.
10. The average American tired of last year's models and seeking something new is an easy prey for the designers who capitalize on herd psychology and the craving for novelty.

5. To set off parenthetic elements

Parenthetic is a general term describing explanatory words or phrases that are felt to be intrusive and subordinate. That is, they interrupt the normal sentence pattern to supply additional, supplementary information, and they are accordingly set off by commas or other punctuation marks. In the widest sense of the term, nonrestrictive modifiers are a kind of parenthetic element. Many other sentence elements may become parenthetic if they are removed from their regular place and inserted so that they interrupt the normal order of a sentence.

For example, adjectives normally are placed before the words they modify: *Two tired, hungry boys came into camp.* If the adjectives are inserted elsewhere in the sentence, they become parenthetic and should be set off: *Two boys, tired and hungry, came into camp.* Similarly, it is possible to rewrite a sentence like *I am certain that space science will bring some unexpected discoveries* so that one clause becomes parenthetic: *Space science, I am certain, will bring some unexpected discoveries.*

The minutes , *I regret to say* , need several additions.

The discovery that mammals can learn to breathe under water may , *in the opinion of some experts* , lead to a technique that will prevent drowning.

Transitional words

Transitional words and phrases, such as *however, moreover, indeed, consequently, of course, for example, on the other hand,* are usually set off by commas, especially when they serve to mark a contrast or the introduction of a new point. In short sentences where stress on the transitional word is not needed or desired, the commas are often omitted.

The beginning violinist needs patience. *For example* , six lines of music can have 214 bowing variations.

32b

The best beef should be bright red and be marbled with pure white fat. *However,* a customer may be fooled by tinted lighting, which, in fact, cheats the buyer.

The court ruled, *consequently,* that no damages could be collected.

Notice that *however* is sometimes used as a regular adverb, to modify a particular word rather than as a sentence modifier, and that when so used it is not set off by a comma.

However much he diets, he does not lose enough weight.
[Since *however* modifies *much*, it is not set off.]

Dates and addresses

Multiple elements of dates, addresses, and references are set off by commas. If only one element (day of month, year, city) appears, no punctuation is needed.

April 4 is her birthday.

New York is her native state.

Act IV moves toward the climax.

But if other elements are added, they are set off by commas.

April 4, 1963, is the date of her birth.

The return address was 15 South Main Street, Oxford, Ohio.

The quotation is from *King Lear,* II, ii, 2.

Direct address, interjections, yes and no

Nouns used as terms of direct address, interjections, and the words *yes* and *no* should be set off by commas.

Ms. Kuhn, would you like to be a teaching assistant?

This preposterous charge, *ladies and gentlemen,* reveals my opponent's ignorance.

Oh, *yes,* we have a more expensive rental.

Quotation expressions

Quotation expressions such as *he said* are set off by commas when used with a direct quotation.

"When I was in Africa," *he said,* "seeing an elephant was exciting."

Do not use a comma to set off an indirect quotation.

The jeweler said that he could reset the sapphire.

They told us that they had sent a wire.

32b

When the quotation contains two independent clauses and the quotation expression comes between them, a semicolon may be required to prevent a comma fault (see **31c**).

> "Please try*,*" *he said;* "you could win."
>
> "Please try*,*" *he said.* "You could win."
>
> "I'd like you to try*,*" *he said;* "I won't insist, though."

For other rules regarding the punctuation of direct quotations, see **32d**.

Absolute phrases

Absolute phrases should be set off by commas. An absolute phrase consists of a participle with a subject (and sometimes a complement) not part of the basic structure of the sentence but serving as a kind of sentence modifier. It usually tells when, why, or how something happened.

> *The gale having quieted,* highway workers began to clear fallen trees and signs from the roads.
>
> The marks on her transcript didn't annoy her, *grades representing only part of her education.*

Exercise 3

Insert commas where they are required to set off parenthetic elements or to follow conventional usage.

1. Money is not to be sure the only problem that people worry about.
2. Yes I have lived in Minnesota most of my life but I was born in Seattle Washington.
3. My uncle formerly one of the richest men in Woodstock promised to put me through college.
4. In the first place there is no evidence Mr. Jones that my client was driving a car on July 14 1985.
5. Teaching of course has certain disadvantages class size being what it is.
6. "From here" said Mr. Newman "you can see the car double-parked in the alley."
7. The study of Latin or of any other foreign language for that matter helps to clarify English grammar.
8. My cousins tired and wet returned from their fishing trip at sunset.
9. Stricter laws it is argued would be of no use without more machinery for their enforcement.
10. Portland Maine was not as I remember an unpleasant place for a boy to grow up in.

6. To set off introductory elements

32b

A dependent clause coming first in the sentence is usually set off by a comma. If a dependent clause follows the main clause, however, a comma is used only when the dependent clause is nonrestrictive.

If you see him, tell him to write me soon.
[Introductory adverbial clause, set off by a comma.]

Tell him to write me *as soon as he can.*
[Restrictive adverbial clause following main clause.]

Take a trip abroad now, *even if you have to borrow some money.*
[Nonrestrictive adverbial clause following main clause.]

An introductory verbal phrase (participial, gerund, or infinitive) is usually followed by a comma. A prepositional phrase of considerable length at the beginning of a sentence may be followed by a comma.

participial phrase

Suffering from disease, overcrowding, and poverty, the people of Manchester were prime victims of the early Industrial Revolution in England.

gerund phrase

After seeing the poverty and unfair treatment of the working-class people, Mrs. Gaskell wrote several protest novels.

infinitive phrase

To understand Hemingway's uneasy friendship with F. Scott Fitzgerald, one must know something of Hemingway's attitude toward Fitzgerald's wife, Zelda.

long prepositional phrase

Soon after his first acquaintance with Fitzgerald, Hemingway took an intense dislike to Zelda.

7. To prevent misreading

Use a commma to separate any sentence elements that might be incorrectly joined in reading and thus misunderstood. *This rule supersedes all others.*

Incorrect	Ever since he has devoted himself to athletics.
Correct	Ever since, he has devoted himself to athletics.
Incorrect	Inside the house was brightly lighted.
Correct	Inside, the house was brightly lighted.
Incorrect	Soon after the minister entered the chapel.
Correct	Soon after, the minister entered the chapel.
Incorrect	To elaborate the art of flower arranging begins with simplicity.
Correct	To elaborate, the art of flower arranging begins with simplicity.

8. Misuse of the comma

Modern practice is to use less rather than more punctuation in narrative and expository prose. A good working rule for the beginner is to use no commas except those required by the preceding conventions. Here are some examples

32b

of serious errors caused by excessive punctuation. In all the following sentences, the commas should be omitted.

Incorrect	His ability to solve the most complicated problems on the spur of the moment , never failed to impress the class. [The comma erroneously separates subject and predicate.]
Incorrect	The men who lived in the old wing of the dormitory , unanimously voted to approve the new rules. [If the clause is restrictive, no commas should be used; if the clause is nonrestrictive, two commas are required.]
Incorrect	During chapel the minister announced , that the choir would sing Handel's *Messiah* for Easter. [The comma erroneously separates an indirect quotation from the rest of the sentence.]
Incorrect	Gigi is so tall , that she may break the record for rebounds. [The comma erroneously splits an idiomatic construction, *so tall that*.]

Do not put a comma before the first member or after the last member of a series, unless the comma is required by some other rule.

Incorrect	For lunch I usually have , a sandwich, some fruit, and milk. [The comma after *have* separates the whole series from the rest of the sentence. It should be omitted.]
Incorrect	New Jersey, Rhode Island, and Massachusetts , were the most densely populated states in 1980. [The comma after *Massachusetts* erroneously separates the whole series from the rest of the sentence.]
Correct	New Jersey, Rhode Island, and Massachusetts , in that order , were the most densely populated states in 1980. [The comma after *Massachusetts* is required to set off the parenthetic phrase *in that order*.]

Exercise 4

Some of the following sentences omit necessary commas, while others contain unnecessary and misleading ones. Punctuate the sentences correctly and be prepared to justify each comma you use and the eliminations you make.

1. The person who used to speak precisely and clearly, may now mumble and run words together the way a favorite television star does.
2. Some parents feel there should be a limit to the amount of homework that students are assigned but I feel most teachers are quite reasonable about the amount given.
3. When people cheat, they cheat no one, but themselves.
4. This purity of spirit combined with the courage to stand up for what she believes, makes Hester the great character that she is.
5. Finally when Ike is fully initiated the chase begins.

32b

6. A certain coffee commercial is amusing because it uses puppets, and is different from other advertisements.
7. The skeptical writer proposes questions hoping for answers.
8. I could readily understand for instance, that primitive human beings who were ignorant and easily terrified, might develop a caste of medicine men.
9. The band, bunting and fireworks were planned but these were not enough to assure the parade's success.
10. It is soon evident, in the story, *Lucky Jim,* by Kingsley Amis, that Margaret is unstable, and that Dixon feels insecure and inferior.
11. He is apparently disgusted with his job, and the rest of his environment.
12. Their faces, like the faces of the rest of the villagers are placid and gentle.

32c The semicolon

The semicolon indicates a greater break in the sentence than the comma does, but it does not have the finality of a period. Its most important use is to separate two independent clauses not joined by a conjunction. As a device for creating compound sentences from shorter sentences, the semicolon may easily be overworked. If a conjunction expresses the relationship between two parts of a sentence, use the conjunction. The semicolon should be reserved for use when the relationship between two statements is so clear that it is unnecessary to state it explicitly.

1. To separate principal clauses

When the independent clauses of a compound sentence are not joined by a conjunction, a semicolon is required.

I do not say that these stories are untrue ; I only say that I do not believe them.

In India fourteen main languages are written ; several hundred dialectical variations are spoken.

The conjunctive adverbs (*so, therefore, however, hence, nevertheless, moreover, accordingly, besides, also, thus, still, otherwise,* and so on) are inadequate to join two independent clauses. A semicolon is required to separate two independent clauses not connected by a pure conjunction. Using a comma instead produces a comma splice (see **31c**).

Our plan was to sail from Naples to New York ; however, an emergency at home forced us to fly instead.

From the high board, the water looked amazingly far away ; besides, I was getting cold and tired of swimming.

The loan account book must be sent with each monthly payment ; otherwise, there may be disputes as to the amount still owing.

32c

If the clauses are short and closely parallel in form, commas are frequently used between them even if conjunctions are omitted.

> The picture dimmed, the sound faded, the TV failed.
>
> The curtains fluttered, the windows rattled, the doors slammed.

2. To separate clauses when commas are inadequate

Even when two independent clauses are joined by a coordinating conjunction, a semicolon may be used to separate the clauses if the clauses are long or are subdivided by commas.

> The Northwest Ordinance of 1787, drafted by Jefferson, is generally noted because it established government of territory north of Ohio and west of New York; *yet* one of its most important statutes was the allocation of land and support for public schools.
>
> In recognition of her services, the principal was given a farewell dinner, a record, and a scroll; *and* a new elementary school was named after her.

Use a semicolon to separate elements in a series when the elements contain internal commas. That is, when a comma is not a strong enough mark of separation to indicate the elements of a series unmistakably, a semicolon is preferable.

> **Incorrect** One day of orientation was led by Mr. Joseph, the chaplain, Mrs. Smith, a French teacher, and the Dean.
>
> **Correct** One day of orientation was led by Mr. Joseph, the chaplain; Mrs. Smith, a French teacher; and the Dean.
> [The punctuation of the corrected sentence indicates clearly how many people led the orientation.]
>
> **Correct** Bibliography may include Frank Kermode, *The Sense of an Ending*; Cynthia Ozick, *Art & Ardor*; Elaine Showalter, *A Literature of Their Own*; and Paul Zweig, *The Adventurer.*

Be sure that semicolons separate coordinate elements. Using a semicolon to separate an independent clause and a subordinate clause is an error similar to writing a sentence fragment, and just as serious.

> **Incorrect** Young people tend to reject parental authority; although they are searching for other adults as models.
>
> **Correct** Young people tend to reject parental authority, although they are searching for other adults as models.

Exercise 5

32c

Some of the following sentences contain semicolons that are unnecessary or incorrect, while other sentences lack needed semicolons. Correct the punctuation and be able to justify each semicolon you use or omit.

1. Joseph is reluctantly picked up by a passing stagecoach; and then only after one of the passengers notes that they could be held legally responsible if a naked stranger should die for lack of aid.

2. More understandable than any of her other criticisms are her remarks about the educational system, however, even these are not very specific.

3. Our technology has developed the telephone for the talebearer; the car for the speedster; and the elevator for children.

4. A novel dealing with the affectations of a past society may become dated, and one must consider this possibility when judging it, otherwise, the book will suffer undue criticism.

5. He was not admitted to the honor society; although he was a good athlete and a top student.

6. The second edition of the book, published in 1922, is relatively scarce and hard to find; but the third edition, published four years later, can be seen in almost any store selling old books.

7. Sometimes I get so interested in a book that I stay up until I finish it; regardless of whether I have classes the next morning or not.

8. Since air is dissolved by water at the surface only, the shape of an aquarium is important, too small an opening may cause an oxygen deficiency.

9. I might ask here; "What is the most important thing in life?"

10. The sculptor can work for more than a week on the same clay model; because clay can be kept soft and pliable for a long time.

Exercise 6

Explain the punctuation in the following sentences. To do so, you will need to distinguish among principal clauses, subordinate clauses, and phrases.

1. There are no set rules that actors must follow to become proficient in their art; however, there are certain principles regarding the use of mind, voice, and body that may help them.

2. The book covered the life of Lotta Crabtree from birth to death; it painted her as one of the most colorful figures of early California.

3. The unconscious sailor would then be taken to an outbound ship to be sold to the captain at a price ranging from $100 to $300, depending on how pressed the captain was for men; and he would regain consciousness somewhere on the Pacific Ocean, without the slightest idea of where he was or where he was going.

4. Among the colorful figures in the book are Johnny Highpockets, a simple-minded settler; Charley Tufts, formerly a professor at Yale; and the author of the book himself.

5. In most respects the hotel is admirably located; it is near the corner of Fifth Avenue and 52nd Street, within walking distance of convention headquarters.

6. On the postcard was a reproduction of a watercolor by John Piper; it showed the interior of Ingelsham Church.

7. My interview, which lasted over an hour, was successful; I got the job.

32c

32d Quotation marks

1. To enclose direct quotation

Use quotation marks to enclose a direct quotation, but not an indirect quotation. A direct quotation gives the exact words of a speaker. An indirect quotation is the writer's paraphrase of what someone said.

> **Indirect quotation** He said that he would call.
>
> **Direct quotation** He said, "I will call."

The expression *he said* is never included within the quotation marks. If the actual quotation is interrupted by such an expression, both halves must be enclosed by quotation marks.

> "I am interested," he said, "so let's talk it over."
>
> "It all began accidentally," Jackson said. "My remark was misunderstood."

2. To quote several sentences

If a quotation consists of several sentences, uninterrupted by a *he* or *she said* expression, use one set of marks to enclose the entire quotation. Do not enclose each separate sentence. If a quotation consists of several paragraphs, put quotation marks at the beginning of each paragraph and at the end of the last paragraph.

> Barbara replied, "Right now? But I haven't finished my paper for economics. Call me in a couple of hours."
>
> Poor Richard has a number of things to say about diet: "They that study much ought not to eat so much as those that work hard, their digestion being not so good.
>
> "If thou art dull and heavy after meat, it's a sign thou hast exceeded the due measure; for meat and drink ought to refresh the body and make it chearful, and not to dull and oppress it.
>
> "A sober diet makes a man die without pain; it maintains the senses in vigour; it mitigates the violence of the passions and affections."

3. Quotations within quotations

A quotation within a quotation is enclosed with single quotation marks. Be sure to conclude the original quotation with double marks.

> The lecture began, "As Proust said, 'Any mental activity is easy if it need not take reality into account.'"

32d

In the rare instance when a third set of marks must be included within a quoted passage, they become double:

In her edition of Flannery O'Connor's letters, Sally Fitzgerald writes: "Anything but dour, she never ceased to be amused, even in extremis. In a letter after her return from the hospital and surgery, in 1964, she wrote: 'One of my nurses was a dead ringer for Mrs. Turpin. . . . Her favorite grammatical construction was "it were." . . . I reckon she increased my pain about 100%.' "

4. To indicate implied speech

Quotation marks are frequently used for implied speech:

He tried to cry, "She is there, she is there," but he couldn't utter the words, only the sounds.

—Jan De Hartog

They are not customarily used for unspoken thoughts:

It was a momentary liberation from the pent-up anxious state I usually endured to be able to think: At least I'm not them! At least I'm not those heavy, serious, righteous people upstairs.

—Robert Lowry

5. Misuse in paraphrase

Use quotation marks around material directly quoted from another writer, but not around a paraphrase of an author's ideas.

John Selden pinpoints our attitude toward virtues when he defines humility: "Humility is a virtue all preach, none practice, and yet everybody is content to hear. The master thinks it good doctrine for his servant, the laity for the clergy, and the clergy for the laity."

John Selden describes humility as a virtue we all praise, but few practice. We expect to observe it in those who deal with us, while overlooking our own chances to be humble.

6. Longer quotations

When a borrowed quotation runs to several lines of print, it should be set off by indenting ten spaces and double-spacing. Quotation marks should not be used to set off such material, though they may be required within the quotation.

T. S. Eliot begins the essay "Tradition and the Individual Talent":

> In English writing we seldom speak of tradition,
> though we occasionally apply its name in de-
> ploring its absence. We cannot refer to "the
> tradition" or to "a tradition"; at most, we
> employ the adjective in saying that the poetry of

32d

So—and—so is "traditional" or even "too traditional." Seldom, perhaps, does the word appear
except in a phrase of censure. If otherwise, it
is vaguely approbative, with the implication,
as to the work approved, of some pleasing archae-
ological reconstruction.

7. Verse quotations

A quotation of more than one line of poetry should be set off by indenting and double-spacing, without quotation marks. Be sure to keep the line lengths exactly as they are in the original.

Blake characterizes this freshness of perception at the
beginning of "Auguries of Innocence":

> To see a World in a Grain of Sand
>
> And a Heaven in a Wild Flower,
>
> Hold Infinity in the palm of your hand
>
> And Eternity in a hour.

A quotation of one line of verse, or part of a line, should be enclosed in quotation marks and run in as part of your text.

Lytton disliked the false heroics of Henley's "My head is bloody but unbowed."

If parts of two lines of verse are run in to the text, indicate the line break by a slash (/):

Stark Young and Rex Stout both found book titles in Fitzgerald's "never grows so red / The rose as where some buried Caesar bled."

8. Punctuation with quotation marks

At the end of a quotation, a period or comma is placed inside the quotation mark; a semicolon or colon is placed outside the quotation mark.

"Quick," said my cousin, "hand me the flashlight."

The bride and groom in the film said, "I do"; the audience in the theatre cheered.

I have only one comment when you say, "All people are equal": I wish it were true.

32d

A question mark or exclamation mark goes inside the quotation mark if it applies to the quotation only, and outside the quotation mark if it applies to the whole sentence.

> My mother asked, "Did you arrive on time?"
>
> Did the invitation say "R.S.V.P."?
>
> He called irritably, "Move over!"
>
> Above all, don't let anyone hear you say, "I give up"!

9. To indicate titles

Use quotation marks for titles of articles, short stories, short poems, songs, chapters of books, lectures and speeches, and individual episodes of radio and television shows.

"Sharp Drop in Unemployment" (newspaper article)

"Doris Lessing's Heroines" (journal article)

"Young Goodman Brown" (short story)

"Jane Austen and the Dance" (lecture)

"Prelude to Tragedy" (episode of the television show *The Spanish Civil War*)

"Mending Wall" (poem)

"Summertime" (song)

"Fictions" (chapter)

Italics on the typewriter and in handwriting are represented by underlining. Italicize titles of books, plays, long poems, pamphlets, periodicals, films, radio and television programs, and major works of opera, dance, and music.

Crime and Punishment (book)

King Lear (play)

The Waste Land (long poem)

Advice for Literature Majors (pamphlet)

Washington Post (newspaper)

American Literature (journal)

Shane (film)

Concert America (radio show)

Dallas (television show)

Aida (opera)

Eight Jelly Rolls (dance)

Goldberg Variations (music)

Note that the titles of books of sacred scripture and the names of books of the Bible are neither underlined nor set in quotations.

Exodus   Vedas   Koran

Old Testament   Talmud   Upanishads

In reference to magazines or newspapers, the initial definite article is usually not treated as part of the title: the *New York Times,* the *San Francisco Chronicle.*

32d

10. Misuse for humorous emphasis or with slang

If occasionally you want to indicate that a word or phrase should be heavily stressed or deserves special attention, use italics, not quotation marks. Humor or irony should be indicated by the context. Using quotation marks to call attention to an ironic or humorous passage is like poking your listener in the ribs when you have reached the point of a joke. If you use slang at all, take full responsibility for it. Do not apologize for a phrase by putting it in quotation marks.

Exercise 7

Add punctuation marks and italics where they are needed.

1. The Dean replied that she knew very well that freshmen had trouble getting adjusted. But, she added, it doesn't usually take them eight months to find themselves.
2. I hope said Professor Turini that someone can identify a quotation for me. It's from the end of a sonnet, and all I can remember is like a lean knife between the ribs of Time.
3. I asked whether Professor Lawrence still began his first lecture by saying My name is Lawrence and I wish I were not here, as he always did when I was in college.
4. The program said that the musical Hello, Dolly is based on Thornton Wilder's play The Matchmaker.
5. Take a chair, said my tutor. He picked up my paper. Tell me honestly, he said. Is this the best you can do?
6. Madame Lenoir said, As my first number I will sing the song Der Leiermann, from Schubert's Winterreise.
7. When asked To what do you attribute your success? Henderson always answered Sleeping late in the morning.

32e Other punctuation marks: apostrophe, colon, dash, parentheses, brackets

1. The apostrophe

The chief uses of the apostrophe are to indicate the possessive case of nouns and indefinite pronouns, to mark the omission of letters in a contracted word or date, and to indicate the plural of letters or numerals.

Possessive case

Nouns and indefinite pronouns that do not already end in s form the possessive by adding an apostrophe and an s.

a child's toy   children's toys
one's dignity   Cole Porter's songs

32e

Plural nouns that end in s (*boys, girls*) form the possessive by adding an apostrophe only.

girls' hockey   the Ellises' orchard
boys' jackets   the Neilsons' garage

In joint possession, the last noun takes the possessive form.

Marshall and Ward's St. Paul branch

In individual possession each name should take the possessive form.

John's, Karl's, and Harold's separate claims

Singular nouns that end in s (*Thomas, kiss*) form the possessive by adding an apostrophe and an s if the s is to be pronounced as an extra syllable.

Thomas's poems   King James's reign   the kiss's effect

But if an extra syllable would be awkward to pronounce, the possessive is formed by adding the apostrophe only, omitting the second s.

Socrates' questions   Moses' life   Euripides' plays

The personal pronouns *never require an apostrophe*, even though the possessive case ends in s: *his, hers, its, ours, yours, theirs.*

Note also these preferred forms: *someone else's book; my sister-in-law's visit; nobody else's opinion.*

Contractions

Use an apostrophe to indicate omissions in contracted words and dates.

it is	it's	of the clock	o'clock
does not	doesn't	class of 1990	class of '90
have not	haven't	cannot	can't
is not	isn't	we are	we're

Plural of letters and numerals

The plural of letters and of numerals is formed by adding an apostrophe and an s. The plural of a word considered as a word may be formed in the same way.

Her *w*'s were like *m*'s, and her *6*'s like *G*'s.

His conversation is too full of *you know*'s punctuated by *well*'s.

2. The colon

The colon is a mark of punctuation used primarily to introduce a formal enumeration or list, a long quotation, or an explanatory statement.

32e

Consider these three viewpoints: political, economic, and social.

Tocqueville expresses one view: "In the United States we easily perceive how the legal profession is qualified by its attributes . . . to neutralize the vices inherent in popular government. . . ."

I remember which way to move the clock when changing from Daylight Saving Time to Standard Time by applying a simple rule: spring ahead, fall backward.

Note that a list introduced by a colon should be in apposition to a preceding word; that is, the sentence preceding the colon should be grammatically complete without the list.

Incorrect	We provide: fishing permit, rod, hooks, bait, lunch, boat, and oars.
Correct	We provide the following items: fishing permit, rod, hooks, bait, lunch, boat, and oars.
Correct	We provide the following: fishing permit, rod, hooks, bait, lunch, boat, and oars.
Correct	The following items are provided: fishing permit, rod, hooks, bait, lunch, boat, and oars.

The colon may be used between two principal clauses when the second clause explains or develops the first.

Intercollegiate athletics continues to be big business, but Robert Hutchins long ago pointed out a simple remedy: colleges should stop charging admission to football games.

A colon is used after a formal salutation in a business letter.

Dear Sir or Madam: Dear Mr. Harris: Ladies and Gentlemen:

A colon is used to separate hour and minutes in numerals indicating time.

The train leaves at 9:27 A.M., and arrives at Joplin at 8:15 P.M.

In bibliographical references, a colon is used between the place of publication and the name of the publisher.

New York: Oxford UP

Between the parts of a Biblical reference a colon may be used.

Proverbs 28:20

3. The dash

The dash, as its name suggests, is a dramatic mark. Like the comma and the parentheses, it separates elements within the sentence, but what the parentheses say quietly the dash exclaims. The dash is indicated on the type-

32e

writer by two hyphens with no spaces on either side. To signal a summary statement, the dash is more informal than the dignified colon—and more emphatic. Use the dash cautiously. Its flashy interruption can create suspense and energy in a sentence, but its frequent use often indicates a writer who has not learned how to punctuate with discrimination.

A dash is used, as a separator, to indicate that a sentence is broken off or to indicate a sharp turn of thought.

Tallulah Bankhead barged down the Nile last night as Cleopatra—and sank.

—John Mason Brown

The great tragedy of science—the slaying of a beautiful hypothesis by an ugly fact.

—T. H. Huxley

Dashes may be used to set off appositives or parenthetic elements when commas are insufficient.

Three pictures—a watercolor, an oil, and a silk screen—hung on the west wall.
[If commas were used to set off *a watercolor, an oil, and a silk screen* the sentence might be misunderstood to refer to six pictures. The dashes make it clear that only three pictures are meant.]

By the time the speech was over—it lasted almost two hours—I was dozing in my chair.
[Since the parenthetic element is an independent clause, commas would be insufficient to set it off clearly.]

When a sentence begins with a list of substantives, a dash is commonly used to separate the list from the summarizing statement which follows.

Relaxation, repose, growth within—these are necessities of life, not privileges.

So with Mr. Kipling's officers who turn their backs; and his Sowers who sow the Seed; and his Men who are alone with their Work; and the Flag—one blushes at all these capital letters as if one had been caught eavesdropping at some purely masculine orgy.

—Virginia Woolf

4. Parentheses

Parentheses, like dashes and commas, are used to enclose or set off parenthetic, explanatory, or supplementary material. Arbitrary rules indicating which marks to use cannot be laid down. Commas are most frequently used, and are usually sufficient, when the parenthetic material is very closely related in thought or structure to the rest of the sentence. If the parenthetic material is long or if it contains commas, dashes would customarily be used to set it off. Parentheses are most often used for explanatory or supplementary material of the sort which might be put in a footnote—useful information that is not

32e

essential. Parentheses are also used to enclose numbers that mark an enumeration within a sentence.

> The artist's concern (and especially, I should say, the novelist's) must be to save the particulars at all costs, even at the sacrifice of the perfection of the design.
>
> —Mary McCarthy

> His last story ("Success a la Steinberg") lacked imagination and any relevance to the cartoonist named in the title.

> In general, the war powers of the President cannot be precisely defined, but must remain somewhat vague and uncertain. (See Wilson's *Constitutional Government in the United States.*)

> The types of noncreative thinking listed by Robinson are (1) reverie, or daydreaming, (2) making minor decisions, (3) rationalizing, or justifying our prejudices.

5. Brackets

Brackets are used to enclose a word or words inserted in a quotation by the person quoting.

> "For the First Amendment does not speak equivocally. It prohibits any law 'abridging the freedom of speech, or of the press.' *It must be taken as a command of the broadest scope that explicit language, read in the context of a liberty-loving society, will allow.*" [Italics added.]

> "It is clear [the message read] that the Muscle Shoals development is but a small part of the potential public usefulness of the entire Tennessee River.

> "We know more about its state [the state of the language] in the later Middle Ages; and from the time of Shakespeare on, our information is quite complete."

The word *sic* (meaning *thus*) enclosed in brackets is sometimes inserted in a quotation after a misspelling or other error to indicate that the error occurs in the original.

> He sent this written confession: "She followed us into the kitchen, snatched a craving [sic] knife from the table, and came toward me with it."

If one parenthetical expression falls inside another, then brackets replace the inner parentheses. (Avoid this situation whenever possible; usually [as here] it is distracting.)

Exercise 8

Insert colons, dashes, parentheses, and brackets as they are needed in the following sentences.

1. Each of its large rooms there were no separate cells in this prison housed some twenty prisoners.
2. I took part in a number of activities in high school the rally committee, dramatics, *Ayer* staff the *Ayer* is our annual, and glee club.

32e

3. She joined the Quakers and became an occasional speaker the Quakers have no ordained ministers at their meetings in Philadelphia.
4. According to an inscription on the flyleaf, the book had been owned by Alburt sic Taylor.
5. The sect permits dancing but forbids some other seemingly innocent recreations card playing, for example, is banned as being the next thing to gambling.
6. According to the *Mason Report* Stearns testified as follows "I made his John Brown's acquaintance early in January 1857, in Boston."
7. The midnight programs at the Varsity Theater feature horror films, science-fiction thrillers, movies of strange monsters from the sea you know the kind of thing.

Exercise 9

Some of the following sentences contain incorrect or misleading punctuation, while others lack needed punctuation. Correct each sentence and be prepared to justify your changes.

1. The author mentions spontaneous and joyous effort, but what is a spontaneous joyous effort.
2. Lincoln born in 1809 in Kentucky, was brought up in a poor family in the woods.
3. It is the setting that is significant, without the setting there would be no story.
4. Now we reach the inevitable question, how do our liberally educated people make use of their knowledge when they enter the business world?
5. In our new house, the kitchen the bathroom and the utility rooms, will have plain wood floors.
6. Under the system just established a student from a family that cannot afford to send a child away to college, will have a chance for a scholarship, especially if he or she is interested in science or engineering.

Exercise 10

Punctuate the following paragraphs and be ready to give a reason for each mark used.

I could tell without turning who was coming. There wasnt a big flatfooted clop-clop like horses make on hard-pack but a kind of edgy clip-clip-clip. There was only one man around here would ride a mule at least on this kind of business. That was Bill Winder who drove the stage between Reno and Bridgers Wells. A mule is tough all right a good mule can work two horses into the ground and not know it. But theres something about a mule a man cant get fond of. Maybe its just the way a mule is just as you feel its the end with a man whos that way. But you cant make a mule part of the way you live like your horse is its like he had no insides no soul. Instead of a partner youve just got something else to work on along with the steers. Winder didnt like mules either but thats why he rode them. It was against his religion to get on a horse horses were for driving.

Its Winder Gil said and looked at Davies and grinned. The news gets around dont it.

I looked at Davies too in the glass but he wasnt showing anything just staring at his drink and minding his own thoughts.   —Walter Van Tilberg Clark

32e

33 *Spelling*

Orthography, or the art of correct spelling, is derived from two Greeks roots: *ortho* (right) and *graphy* (write). Spelling right, then, is writing straight. Since the time of Aristotle, correct spelling has distinguished the scholar from the dolt. Indeed, Lord Chesterton could write in the eighteenth century that one false spelling would fix ridicule on a gentleman for the rest of his life: "I know many of quality," he claims, "who never recovered from the ridicule of having spelled *wholesome* without the *w*." In the next century, such American rebels as Walt Whitman and Mark Twain could ridicule the English aristocratic passion for correctness. "Morbidity for nice spelling," Whitman scolded, "means . . . impotence in literature," and Twain pouted, "I don't see any use in spelling a word right, and never did. . . . We might as well make all our clothes alike and cook all dishes alike." No impotence in literature for Twain, who then wrote one of the greatest works in the language in which many of the words are (intentionally) misspelled.

In *The Adventures of Huckleberry Finn* Twain catches by means of misspellings the sound of Huck speaking a dialect that is not Standard English. Our language, which scholars began to standardize in the late seventeenth century, grows out of hundreds of dialects such as the one Huck spoke, and that variety of origins accounts for many of the peculiarities of English spelling. English is not an easy language to spell, and it is in the American spirit to chafe at the propriety of good spelling. Still, many people, especially college teachers, feel, like Aristotle, that good spelling is the result of study and memory, and that its presence on a piece of paper is a mark of intelligence and effort.

The first step in mastering orthography is to make a list of words you often misspell. Ask a friend to test you on the words listed in **33e**. Write down the words you miss. Add to this list all words that are misspelled on your themes, and study the list. Look carefully at the letters of each word, pronounce the word a syllable at a time, write the word repeatedly to fix the pattern in your mind. Invent mnemonic devices—pictures, jingles, associations—to help you remember particular spellings. If you have written the word "sent*an*ce" and it is circled on your paper, remember that a sentence is a f*en*ce built around an idea. If you have written "mispell," remember that in a spelling bee we mi*ss* a word when we "mi*ss*pell" it. Learn the common prefixes and suffixes, and analyze words to see how they are formed. For example:

disappoint = dis + appoint
dissatisfied = dis + satisfied
misspelling = mis + spell + ing
really = real + ly
unnecessary = un + necessary
undoubtedly = un + doubt + ed + ly
government = govern + ment
carefully = care + ful + ly
incidentally = incident + al + ly

See how many words in the list of Words Commonly Misspelled (pages 422–25) can be analyzed into a root word with prefixes or suffixes. If you find exceptions, look for an explanation in the Spelling Rules (pages 418–20).

When you have finished the final draft of a paper, proofread it carefully before you hand it in. Proofread for spelling errors separately if you have trouble with spelling. It is no excuse to say that you knew the correct spelling of a word but that your pen slipped. Misspellings because of typographical errors or general carelessness are still misspellings.

<u>33a</u> Trouble spots

Learn to look for trouble spots in words and concentrate on them. Common words are almost always misspelled in the same way. That is, a particular letter or combination of letters is the trouble spot, and if you can remember the correct spelling of the trouble spot, the rest of the word will take care of itself. *Receive,* like *deceive, perceive,* and *conceive,* is troublesome only because of the *ei* combination; if you can remember that it is *ei* after *c,* you will have mastered these words. To spell *beginning* correctly, all you need to remember is the double *n.*

Careful pronunciation may help you to avoid errors at trouble spots. In the following words, the letters in boldface are often omitted. Pronounce the words aloud, exaggerating the sound of the boldface letters:

accident**all**y	Feb**r**uary	liab**l**e
candi**d**ate	gener**all**y	lib**r**ary
ever**y**body	labo**r**atory	lit**e**rature
occasion**all**y	reco**g**nize	sur**p**rise
proba**b**ly	soph**o**more	tempe**r**ament
quan**t**ity	strict**l**y	usu**all**y

33a

Many people add letters incorrectly to the following words. Pronounce the words, making sure that no extra syllable creeps in at spots indicated by boldface type.

ath**l**etics	ent**r**ance	mischie**v**ous
disast**r**ous	height	remem**br**ance
drown**ed**	hind**r**ance	simil**ar**
e**lm**	light**n**ing	um**br**ella

Trouble spots in the following words are caused by a tendency to transpose the boldface letters. Careful pronunciation may help you to remember the proper order.

child**r**en	pe**r**form	preju**d**ice
hund**r**ed	pe**r**spiration	p**r**escription
irrele**v**ant	p**r**efer	trage**d**y

33b Similar words frequently confused

Learn the meaning and spelling of similar words. Many errors are caused by confusion of such words as *effect* and *affect*. It is useless to spell *principal* correctly if the word that belongs in your sentence is *principle*. The following list distinguishes briefly between words that are frequently confused.

accept	receive	alumna	a woman
except	aside from	alumnae	women
access	admittance	alumnus	a man
excess	greater amount	alumni	men
advice	noun	angel	celestial being
advise	verb	angle	corner
affect	to influence (verb)	ascent	climbing
effect	result (noun)	assent	agreement
effect	to bring about (verb)	berth	bed
		birth	being born
aisle	in church	boarder	one who boards
isle	island	border	edge
all ready	prepared	breath	noun
already	previously	breathe	verb
allusion	reference	capital	city
illusion	misconception	capitol	building
altar	shrine	choose	present
alter	change	chose	past

clothes	garments	loose	adjective
cloths	kinds of cloth	lose	verb
coarse	not fine	peace	not war
course	path, series	piece	a portion
complement	to complete	personal	adjective
compliment	to praise	personnel	noun
conscience	sense of right and wrong	principal	most important
		principle	basic doctrine
conscious	aware	quiet	still
corps	group	quite	entirely
corpse	dead body	respectfully	with respect
costume	dress	respectively	in the order named
custom	manner		
council	governmental group	shone	from shine
		shown	from show
counsel	advice	stationary	adjective
dairy	milk supply	stationery	noun
diary	daily record	than	comparison
decent	proper	then	at that time
descent	slope	their	possessive
desert	wasteland	there	in that place
dessert	food	they're	they are
device	noun	to	go to bed
devise	verb	too	too bad, me too
dual	twofold	two	2
duel	fight	weather	rain or shine
formally	in a formal manner	whether	which of two
		who's	who is
formerly	previously	whose	possessive
forth	forward	you're	you are
fourth	4th	your	possessive
ingenious	clever		
ingenuous	frank		
its	of it		
it's	it is		
later	subsequently		
latter	second of two		
lead	metal		
led	past tense of verb lead		

33b

33c Spelling rules

Learn the available spelling rules. Spelling rules apply to a relatively small number of words, and unfortunately almost all rules have exceptions. Nevertheless, some of the rules may help you to spell common words that cause you trouble, especially those words formed with suffixes.

It is as important to learn when a rule may be used as it is to understand the rule itself. Applied in the wrong places, rules will make your spelling worse, instead of better.

1. Final silent *e*

Drop a final silent *e* before suffixes beginning with a vowel (*-ing, -age, -able*). Keep a final silent *e* before suffixes beginning with a consonant (*-ful, -ly, -ness*).

hope + ing = hoping	hope + ful = hopeful
love + able = lovable	nine + teen = nineteen
stone + y = stony	arrange + ment = arrangement
guide + ance = guidance	late + ly = lately
plume + age = plumage	pale + ness = paleness
white + ish = whitish	white + wash = whitewash
write + ing = writing	sincere + ly = sincerely
dote + age = dotage	bale + ful = baleful

Learn the following exceptions:

dyeing	hoeing	judgment	awful
ninth	truly	duly	wholly

The *e* is retained in such words as the following in order to keep the soft sound of *c* and *g:*

noticeable	courageous
peaceable	outrageous

Exercise 1

Following the rule just given, write the correct spelling of each word indicated below.

use + ing	pale + ing
use + ful	manage + ment
argue + ment	write + ing
nine + ty	refuse + al
pale + ness	waste + ful
immediate + ly	hope + less
please + ure	absolute + ly
manage + able	sure + ly

33c

2. Doubling final consonant

When adding a suffix beginning with a vowel to words ending in one consonant preceded by one vowel (*red, redder*), notice where the word is accented. If it is accented on the last syllable or if it is a monosyllable, *double* the final consonant.

pre*fér* + ed = preferred   *béne*fit + ed = benefited
o*mít* + ing = omitting   *pró*fit + ing = profiting
oc*cúr* + ence = occurrence   *di*ffer + ence = difference
réd + er = redder   *trá*vel + er = traveler

Note that in some words the accent shifts when the suffix is added.

re*fér*red   *ré*ference
pre*fér*ring   *pré*ference

There are a few exceptions to this rule, such as *transferable* and *excellent;* and a good many words that should follow the rule have alternative spellings: either *worshiped* or *worshipped; traveling, traveler,* or *travelling, traveller.*

Exercise 2

Make as many combinations as you can of the following words and suffixes. Give your reason for doubling or not doubling the final consonant. Suffixes: *-able, -ible, -ary, -ery, -er, -est, -ance, -ence, -ess, -ed, -ish, -ing, -ly, -ful, -ment, -ness, -hood.*

occur	commit	defer	profit
happen	equal	sum	avoid
begin	ravel	stop	level
god	kidnap	clan	jewel
shrub	hazard	libel	
scrap	read	expel	
red	rid	rival	
equip	man	glad	

3. Words ending in *y*

If the *y* is preceded by a consonant, change the *y* to *i* before any suffix except *-ing*.

lady + es = ladies   lonely + ness = loneliness
try + ed = tried   accompany + es = accompanies
study + ing = studying

The *y* is usually retained if it is preceded by a vowel:

valleys   monkeys   displayed

Some Exceptions: laid, paid, said, ladylike

33c

Exercise 3

Add suffixes to the following words. State your reason for spelling the word as you do.

mercy	relay	hardy	bounty	medley
duty	study	wordy	jockey	galley
pulley	essay	fancy	modify	body

4. *ie* or *ei*

When *ie* or *ei* is used to spell the sound *ee*,
Put i before e
Except after c.

achi*e*ve	gri*e*ve	retri*e*ve	c*ei*ling
beli*e*f	ni*e*ce	shi*e*ld	conc*ei*t
beli*e*ve	pi*e*ce	shri*e*k	conc*ei*ve
bri*e*f	pi*e*rce	si*e*ge	dec*ei*t
chi*e*f	reli*e*f	thi*e*f	dec*ei*ve
fi*e*ld	reli*e*ve	wi*e*ld	perc*ei*ve
gri*e*f	repri*e*ve	yi*e*ld	rec*ei*ve

Some Exceptions: *ei*ther, l*ei*sure, n*ei*ther, s*ei*ze, w*ei*rd.

33d Hyphenation

A hyphen is used, under certain circumstances, to join the parts of compound words. Compounds are written as two separate words (*city hall*), as two words joined by a hyphen (*city-state*), or solid as one word (*townspeople*). In general, the hyphen is used in recently made compounds and compounds still in the process of becoming one word. Because usage varies considerably, no arbitrary rules can be laid down. When in doubt consult the latest edition of an unabridged dictionary. The following "rules" represent the usual current practice.

1. Compound adjectives

Words used as a single adjective *before* a noun are usually hyphenated.

fine-grained wood	three-quarter binding
strong-minded woman	matter-of-fact statement
far-sighted proposal	so-called savings
well-informed leader	old-fashioned attitude

33d

When these compound adjectives *follow* the noun, they usually do not require the hyphen.

> The *snow-covered* mountains lay ahead.

> The mountains are *snow covered.*

When the adverb ending in *-ly* is used with an adjective or a participle, the compound is not usually hyphenated.

> *highly praised* organization, *widely advertised* campaign

2. Prefixes

When a prefix still retains its original strength in the compound, use a hyphen. In most instances, however, the prefix has been absorbed into the word and should not be separated by a hyphen. Contrast the following pairs of words:

ex-president, excommunicate	pre-Christian, preconception
vice-president, viceroy	pro-British, procreation

Note that in some words a difference of meaning is indicated by the hyphen:

> She *recovered* her strength.

> She *re-covered* her sofa.

3. Compound numbers

A hyphen is used in compound numbers from twenty-one to ninety-nine.

Correct   twenty-six, sixty-three [*but* one hundred thirty]

4. Hyphen to prevent misreading

Use a hyphen if necessary to avoid ambiguity.

Ambiguous   A detail of *six foot soldiers* was on duty.

Clear   A detail of six *foot-soldiers* was on duty.

Clear   A detail of *six-foot* soldiers was on duty.

Exercise 4

Should the compounds in the following sentences be written solid, with a hyphen, or as two words? Consult a recent edition of a good dictionary, if necessary.

1. We need an eight foot rod.
2. All the creeks are bone dry.
3. She gave away one fourth of her income.
4. The United States is a world power.
5. Who was your go between?
6. He is extremely good looking.

33d

7. The younger son was a ne'er do well.
8. Let us sing the chorus all together.
9. They are building on a T shaped wing.
10. She is getting a badly needed rest.
11. Are you all ready?
12. The leak was in the sub basement.
13. He was anti British.
14. She does her work in a half hearted manner.
15. I don't like your chip on the shoulder attitude.
16. They always were old fashioned.
17. A high school course is required for admission.
18. I do not trust second hand information.
19. He is as pig headed a man as I ever knew.
20. She will not accept anything second rate.

33e Words commonly misspelled

The following list is composed of some ordinary words that are often misspelled. If you learn to spell correctly those which you usually misspell, and if you will look up in a dictionary words that are obviously difficult or unfamiliar, your spelling will improve remarkably.

Have a friend test you on these words—fifty at a time. Then concentrate on the ones you miss. To help you remember correct spellings, trouble spots are indicated by boldface type in most of the words.

ab**sence**	airp**lane**	ap**pro**priate
absor**p**tion	allo**t**ment	ar**c**tic
ab**s**urd	allo**tt**ed	argu**ment**
abund**a**nt	**all** right	arithmetic
academic	already	ar**r**angement
accidenta**lly**	altogether	arti**cle**
ac**comm**odate	always	ascend
accumulate	ama**teur**	as**so**ciation
accurate	among	ath**l**etic
achi**e**vement	analysis	attac**ked**
acquainted	an**nually**	attendance
acquire	apology	audience
across	appa**ratus**	available
addi**tionally**	ap**p**arent	a**wk**ward
add**ress**	appearance	bargain
adequately	appetite	basi**cally**
ag**g**ravate	appreciate	becom**ing**

beginning	coolly	especially
believe	copies	*etc.* (*et cetera*)
benefited	courteous	exaggerate
boundary	criticism	exceed
brilliant	dealt	excellent
Britain	deceive	exceptionally
business	decision	exercise
calendar	definitely	existence
candidate	descendant	exorbitant
career	describe	expense
category	description	experience
cemetery	desirable	explanation
certain	despair	familiar
challenge	desperate	fascinate
changeable	dictionary	feasible
changing	different	February
Christian	difficult	fictitious
column	dining room	finally
coming	disappear	foreign
commission	disappoint	forty
committee	disastrous	friend
comparatively	discipline	gauge
competent	disease	government
competition	dissatisfied	grammar
conceit	dissipate	guard
concentrate	divide	harass
condemn	doctor	hardening
confidence	dying	height
conqueror	effect	hindrance
conscientious	eighth	humorous
conscious	eliminate	hurriedly
consider	embarrass	hyprocrisy
consistent	emphasize	illiterate
contemporary	entirely	imagination
continuous	entrance	imitation
controlled	environment	immediately
convenience	equipped	incidentally

33e

incredibly
independent
indispensable
infinite
initiative
intelligence
interest
involve
irrelevant
irresistible
itself
jealousy
knowledge
laboratory
laid
led
leisure
library
license
literature
loneliness
lose
luxury
magazine
maintenance
manufacturer
marriage
mathematics
mattress
meant
medieval
merely
miniature
municipal
murmur
mysterious
necessary

neither
nineteen
noticeable
nowadays
nucleus
obstacle
occasionally
occurred
occurrence
omission
omitted
opinion
opportunity
optimism
origin
paid
pamphlet
parallel
paralyzed
parliament
particularly
partner
pastime
perform
perhaps
permanent
permissible
persistent
personnel
persuade
physical
pleasant
politician
possess
possible
practically
preceding

predominant
prejudice
preparation
prevalent
primitive
privilege
probably
procedure
proceed
profession
professor
prominent
pronunciation
prove
psychology
pursue
quizzes
really
receive
recognize
recommend
reference
referred
religious
reminisce
repetition
representative
rhythm
ridiculous
sacrifice
safety
scene
schedule
secretary
seize
sense
separate

sergeant	studying	truly
severely	succeed	typical
shining	suppress	tyranny
siege	surprise	undoubtedly
similar	susceptible	unnecessary
sincerely	syllable	until
soliloquy	sympathize	using
sophomore	temperament	usually
specimen	tendency	vengeance
speech	thorough	village
stopping	together	villain
strenuous	tragedy	weird
stretch	transferred	writing

Exercise 5

Write the infinitive, the present participle, and the past participle of each of the following verbs (e.g., *to stop, stopping, stopped*):

prefer	begin	acquit	equip
profit	hop	commit	recur
slam	differ	drag	confer

Exercise 6

Write the following words together with the adjectives ending in *-able* derived from them (e.g., *love, lovable*):

dispose	prove	console	imagine	measure
move	compare	blame	cure	

Exercise 7

Write the following words together with their derivatives ending in *-able* (e.g., *notice, noticeable*):

trace	change	charge	damage	manage
service	marriage	place	peace	

Exercise 8

Write the singular and the plural of the following nouns (e.g., *lady, ladies*):

baby	remedy	treaty	turkey
hobby	enemy	delay	decoy
democracy	poppy	alley	alloy
policy	diary	attorney	corduroy
tragedy	laundry	journey	convoy

33e

Exercise 9

Write the first and third persons present indicative, and the first person past, of the following verbs (e.g., *I cry, he cries, I cried*):

fancy	spy	vary	worry
qualify	reply	dry	pity
accompany	occupy	ferry	envy

Exercise 10

Study the following words, observing that in all of them the prefix is not *diss-* but *dis-:*

dis + advantage	dis + obedient
dis + agree	dis + orderly
dis + approve	dis + organize
dis + interested	dis + own

Exercise 11

Study the following words, observing that in all of them the prefix is not *u-* but *un-:*

un + natural	un + numbered
un + necessary	un + named
un + noticed	un + neighborly

Exercise 12

Study the following words, distinguishing between the prefixes *per-* and *pre-*. Keep in mind that *per-* means *through, throughout, by, for;* and that *pre-* means *before.*

perform	perhaps	precept
perception	perspective	precipitate
peremptory	perspiration	precise
perforce	precarious	precocious
perfunctory	precaution	prescription

Exercise 13

Study the following adjectives, observing that in all of them the suffix is not *-full,* but *-ful:*

peaceful	graceful	grateful	pitiful
dreadful	forceful	faithful	thankful
handful	shameful	healthful	plentiful

Exercise 14

Study the following words, observing that in all of them the ending is not *-us,* but *-ous:*

advantageous	specious	fastidious
gorgeous	precious	studious
courteous	vicious	religious
dubious	conscious	perilous

33e

Exercise 15

Study the following words, observing that in all of them the suffix -al precedes -ly:

accidentally	terrifically	exceptionally
apologetically	specifically	elementally
pathetically	emphatically	professionally
typically	finally	critically

Exercise 16

Study the following words, observing that the suffix is not -ess, but -ness:

clean + ness	plain + ness	stern + ness
drunken + ness	stubborn + ness	keen + ness
mean + ness	sudden + ness	green + ness

Exercise 17

Study the following words, observing that the suffix is not -able, but -ible:

accessible	horrible	legible
admissible	imperceptible	perceptible
audible	impossible	permissible
compatible	incompatible	plausible
contemptible	incredible	possible
convertible	indefensible	reprehensible
discernible	indelible	responsible
eligible	intelligible	sensible
feasible	invincible	susceptible
flexible	invisible	tangible
forcible	irresistible	terrible

Exercise 18

Study the following groups of words:

-ain	-ain	-ian	-ian
Britain	curtain	barbarian	guardian
captain	fountain	Christian	musician
certain	mountain	civilian	physician
chieftain	villain	collegian	politician

Exercise 19

Study the following groups of words:

-ede	-ede	-eed
accede	precede	exceed
antecede	recede	proceed
concede	secede	succeed

33e

Exercise 20

Fill the blanks with *principal* or *principle*. *Principle* is always a noun; *principal* is usually an adjective. *Principal* is also occasionally a noun: the *principal* of the school, both *principal* and *interest*.

1. The _____ will be due on the tenth of the month.
2. Her refusal was based on _____.
3. This is my _____ for going.
4. The _____ has asked that we hold our meeting tomorrow.
5. He did not even know the first _____ of the game.
6. Can you give the _____ parts of the verb?

Exercise 21

Fill the blanks with *affect* or *effect:*

1. I do not like his _____ ed manner.
2. An entrance was _____ ed by force.
3. The _____ upon her is noticeable.
4. The law will take _____ in July.
5. It will be an _____ ive remedy.
6. The hot weather will _____ the crops.
7. There was no serious after _____.
8. She _____ ed ignorance of the whole matter.

Exercise 22

Fill the blanks with *passed* or *past*. *Passed* is the past tense or past participle of the verb *pass; past* can be an adjective, noun, adverb, or preposition.

1. We _____ your house.
2. She went _____ me.
3. They whistled as they _____ by.
4. He is a man with a _____.
5. My cousin is a _____ master at the art of lying.
6. That vocalist is _____ her prime.
7. Many years _____ before he returned.
8. It is long _____ bedtime.

Exercise 23

Fill the blanks with:

1. *Its* (pronoun in the possessive case) or *it's* (contraction of *it is*).
   a. _____ raining.
   b. The cat has had _____ supper.
   c. The clock is in _____ old place again.
   d. _____ now six years since the accident.
   e. I think that _____ too late to go.

2. *Your* (pronoun in the possessive case) or *you're* (contraction of *you are*).

    a. _____ mistaken; it is _____ fault.

    b. _____ position is assured.

    c. _____ to go tomorrow.

    d. I hope that _____ taking _____ vacation in July.

3. *There* (adverb or interjection), or *their* (pronoun in the possessive case), or *they're* (contraction of *they are*).

    a. It is _____ turn.

    b. _____ ready to go.

    c. _____, that is over with.

    d. _____ car was stolen.

    e. _____ back from _____ trip.

4. *Whose* (pronoun in the possessive case) or *who's* (contraction of *who is*).

    a. _____ turn is it?

    b. There is the woman _____ running for mayor.

    c. _____ responsible for this?

    d. _____ book is this?

    e. He is one _____ word can be trusted.

    f. Bring me a copy of _____ *Who*.

    g. _____ ready to go?

Exercise 24

Circle the italicized words that are spelled correctly in each of the following sentences. Consult section **33b** if necessary.

1. Everyone is going *accept, except* me.
2. People came to her every day for *advice, advise,* and she was always ready to *advice, advise* them.
3. At so high an altitude it was hard to *breath, breathe.*
4. His *breath, breathe* came in short gasps.
5. One of the sights of Washington, D.C., is the *Capital, Capitol.*
6. Albany is the *capital, capitol* of New York.
7. Before dinner I had time to change my *clothes, cloths.*
8. The tickets were sent with the *complements, compliments* of the manager.
9. The country was as dry and dreary as a *desert, dessert.*
10. The shack in which we *formally, formerly* lived is still standing.
11. It's *later, latter* than you think.
12. The winners were *lead, led* up onto the stage.
13. Button the money in your pocket so you won't *lose, loose* it.

33e

34 *Mechanics*

The appearance of a paper, like the appearance of a person, indicates regard for self and for the world at large. Accurate typing, a clean page, observance of editing conventions—all of these suggest a writer's confidence and authority. Wise writers use any available means—including care with mechanics—to win the favor and attention of their readers.

34a Manuscript

Unless your instructor specifies otherwise, you should prepare your essays on standard 8½ x 11 white paper. Typed papers—which are preferable—should be double-spaced on unruled white bond. If your instructor permits handwritten papers, use wide-ruled paper, write legibly in black or dark blue ink, and skip lines. An instructor or an editor grows weary with a manuscript that has to be puzzled out one word at a time. Give your thoughts and sentences a fair chance by presenting them neatly on the page.

If a reading of your final draft shows the need for minor corrections, make them unmistakably clear. It is not necessary to recopy an entire page for the sake of one or two small insertions or alterations, but recopying is called for if the number of corrections would make the page difficult to read or messy in appearance. Words to be inserted should be written above the line, and their proper positon should be indicated by a caret (∧) placed below the line. Inserted words should not be enclosed in parentheses or brackets unless these marks are required by the sense of the sentence. Cancel words by drawing a neat line through them, not by enclosing them in parentheses or brackets.

Below are some additional widely accepted conventions for preparing your manuscript:

1. Type or write on one side of the sheet only.

2. Leave a margin of one inch on the top, bottom, and sides of typed papers, slightly more for handwritten essays.

3. On four double-spaced lines in the upper left corner of the first page, give your name, your instructor's name, the course number, and the date.

34a

Double-space again (or skip another line) and center your title. Do not use quotation marks or underline your title unless it includes words that require such punctuation (see **34e**). Capitalize all words in the title except articles, short conjunctions, and short prepositions. Quadruple-space after your title and begin the first line of your essay.

4. Indent paragraphs five spaces when you type. In hand-written manuscripts, indent about an inch.

5. Number all pages with arabic numbers in the upper right corner, one-half inch from the top of the page.

When you reproduce quotations in your text, observe the following conventions. (For an extended discussion of the correct use of quotations, see **21c**.)

1. A quotation of only a few words should be incorporated into your sentences:

> In Childhood and Society, Erik Erikson notes
> that the young adult, "emerging from the search
> for and insistence on identity," has become
> "ready for intimacy."

2. A quotation of more than three or four lines of prose, or more than two lines of verse, should be set off from the main text without quotation marks by indenting. Introduce the quotation with a colon in most cases. Begin prose quotations on a new line and indent the entire quotation ten spaces from the left margin; center poetry on the page. In both cases, double-space the quotation itself.

3. A quotation of poetry should be divided into lines exactly as the original is divided. If an entire line of verse does not fit on one line of the page, the words left over should be indented on the next line:

> Allons! the inducements shall be greater,
> We will sail pathless and wild seas,
> We will go where winds blow, waves dash, and the
> Yankee clipper speeds by under full sail.
>
> —Walt Whitman

4. When quoting dialogue from a story, novel, or play, be sure that the paragraphing and punctuation of the quotation are exactly as in the original.

34a

"Are you better, Minet—Chéri?"

"Yes. I can't think what came over me."

The grey eyes, gradually reassured, dwelt
on mine.

"I think I know what it was. A smart little
rap on the knuckles from Above."

I remained pale and troubled and my mother
misunderstood:

"There, there now. There's nothing so ter—
rible as all that in the birth of a child, nothing
terrible at all. It's much more beautiful in real
life. The suffering is so quickly forgotten,
you'll see! The proof that all women forget is
that it is only men——and what business was it of
Zola's, anyway?——who write stories about it."

—Colette

Note that British writers commonly use a single quotation mark (') where
American convention requires double quotation marks (").

34b Capital letters

The general principle governing capitalization is that proper nouns are
capitalized and common nouns are not. A proper noun is the name of a particular
person, place, or thing:

Richard Wright	Alaska	the Capitol
Virginia Woolf	New Orleans	Colorado River

A common noun is a more general term that can be used as a name for a number
of persons, places, or things:

author	state	building
woman	city	river

Note that the same word may be used as both a proper and a common noun.

34b

Of all the *peaks* in the Rocky Mountains, *Pike's Peak* is the mountain I would most
like to climb.

Our beginning *history* class studied legislative procedure and the part our representatives play in it. When I took *History 27* our class visited the Legislative Committee hearing in which the Representative from Ohio expressed his views on the Alliance for Progress.

Abbreviations are capitalized when the words they stand for would be capitalized: USN, ROTC, NBC.

1. Proper nouns

Capitalize proper nouns and adjectives derived from them. Proper nouns include the following:

1. Days of the week, months, and holidays:

   Sunday   October   Thanksgiving

2. Organizations such as political parties, governmental bodies and departments, societies, institutions, clubs, churches, and corporations:

   Socialist Party   Boston Public Library
   U.S. Senate   Optimists' Club
   Department of the Interior   Greek Orthodox Church
   American Cancer Society   Raytheon Company

3. Members of organizations:

   Republicans   Buddhists
   Lions   Girl Scouts

4. Historical events and periods:

   Battle of Hastings   Baroque Era
   Medieval Age   Synod of Whitby

5. Geographic areas:

   Latin America   the Midwest
   the Far East   Sahara

6. Names of races and languages:

   Japanese   Caucasian
   Urdu   Hebrew

7. Many words of religious significance:

   the Lord   the Bible
   the Son of God   the Book of Mormon
   Allah   Koran

34b

8. Names of members of the family when used in place of proper names:

I received a letter from Mother today.

9. In biological nomenclature, the names of genera but not of species:

Homo sapiens   *Equus caballus*

Salmo irideus   *Aquila heliaca*

10. Stars, constellations, and planets, but not the earth, sun, or moon unless used as astronomical names:

Sirius   Taurus

Arcturus   Jupiter

2. Titles

Capitalize titles of persons when they precede proper names. When used without proper names, titles of officers of high rank should be capitalized; other titles should not.

Senator Marsh   Professor Stein   Admiral Byrd   Aunt Elsa

Both the Governor and the Attorney General endorsed the candidacy of our representative.

The postmaster of our town appealed to the Postmaster General.

Capitalize the first word and the important words of the titles of books, plays, articles, musical compositions, pictures, and other literary or artistic works. The unimportant words are the articles *a, an,* and *the;* short conjunctions; and short prepositions.

I, Claudius   *Summer in Williamsburg*   *Friar Felix at Large*

Childhood and Society   *Measure for Measure*   Beethoven's *Third Symphony*

Brancusi's "Bird in Space"   Bruce Springsteen's "Born in the U.S.A."

Capitalize the first word and any titles of the person addressed in the salutation of a letter.

Dear Sir: Dear President Stark: Dear Ms. Loebel:

In the complimentary close, capitalize the first word only.

Yours sincerely,   Sincerely yours,

3. Sentences and quotations

Capitalize the first word of every sentence and of every direct quotation. Note that a capital is not used for the part of a quotation that follows an interpolated expression like "he said" unless that part is a new sentence.

34b

"Mow the lawn diagonally," said Mrs. Grant, "and go over it twice."

"Mow the lawn twice diagonally," said Mrs. Grant. "It will be even smoother if the second mowing crosses over the first one."

Mrs. Grant said, "Mow the lawn twice."

Following a colon, the first word of a series of short questions or sentences may be capitalized.

The first-aid questions were dull but important: What are the first signs of shock in an accident victim? should he be kept warm? should he eat? should he drink?

Capitalize the first word of every line of poetry except when the poem itself does not use a capital.

I'll walk where my own nature would be leading:
   It vexes me to choose another guide:
Where the grey flocks in ferny glens are feeding;
   Where the wild wind blows on the mountain-side.

—Emily Brontë

last night i heard
a pseudobird;
or possibly
the usual bird
heard pseudome.

—Ebenezer Peabody

Exercise 1

What words in the following sentences should be capitalized? Why?

1. A canary-colored buick convertible was driving north on fountain avenue.
2. Although many of the natives can speak spanish, they prefer their own indian dialect.
3. A novel experiment in american education was announced on monday by the yale school of law and the harvard school of business administration.
4. "I'm going out to the country club," said chris; "want to come along?"
5. Although technically a veteran, he had served in the coast guard for only two weeks toward the end of the second world war.
6. the douglas fir, often sold under the name oregon pine, is neither a fir nor a pine.
7. He makes these regional divisions: the east, the old south, the middle west, and the far west.
8. When I left high school I intended to major in english literature, but in college I became interested in science.
9. Buddhists, christians, jews, and moslems attended the conference, which was held at ankara, the capital of turkey.
10. Both the rotarians and the lions meet in the private dining room of the piedmont inn.

34b

34c Numbers

In general, treat all numbers in a particular context similarly; in the interest of consistency, do not use words for some and figures for others. The following additional guidelines for writing numbers are widely accepted.

1. Numbers from one to ten and round numbers that can be expressed in one or two words are usually written out.

   three people in line

   seven hundred reserved seats

   five thousand tickets

   All numbers that begin a sentence are spelled out, even though they would ordinarily be represented by figures.

   Four hundred sixty dollars was too much.

2. For ordinary usage, figures are appropriate for the day of the month, the year, and street numbers.

   June *23, 1985*   *123* Spring Street

3. Figures are used for long numbers, page and chapter numbers, time expressed by A.M. and P.M., and exact percentages, decimals, and technical numbers.

   1,275 gallons   chapter *14,* page *372*

   from *11* A.M. to *2* P.M.   *7.31* inches

   8.5 percent   *38th* parallel

4. After a dollar sign ($) figures are always used.

   My share of the job paid *$177.90,* but I had *$27.50* in expenses.

   If a number is short and followed by *dollars* or *cents,* it may be spelled out.

   I paid *twelve dollars* for the book.

34d Abbreviations

Minimize the use of abbreviations in ordinary expository prose. Spell out first names, the words in addresses (*Street, Avenue, New Jersey*), the days and months of the year, units of measurement (*ounces, pounds, feet, hour, gallon*). Volume, chapter, and page should be spelled out in references in the text, but abbreviated in parenthetical citations and bibliographies.

34d

Eliott Brodie of 372 West 27th *Avenue,* Kenosha, moved on *December* 16, 1970.
The quotation is on *page* 267 of the *third edition.*

For further information on proper terms for addressing dignitaries, consult the appropriate section in the latest Webster unabridged dictionary ("Forms of Address," *pp.* 51a–54a).

The following conventions are generally observed:

1. A few standard abbreviations are in general use in all kinds of writing: *i.e.* (that is), *e.g.* (for example), *etc.* (and so forth), *vs.* (versus), A.D., B.C., A.M., P.M., (or *a.m., p.m.*), Washington, *D.C.* Names of some organizations and of many government agencies are commonly represented by their initials: *CIA, GOP, NATO, CAA, NAACP.* Dictionaries vary in their preferences for using periods with these abbreviations.

   Some abbreviations require periods (*Ph.D., N.B., Feb., oz.*), but others are regularly written without periods (*FBI, Na, ERA*). The correct form of standard abbreviations can be found in your dictionary, usually in regular alphabetical order, sometimes in a separate appendix.

2. Civil, religious, and military titles are spelled out except the following ones:
   a. Preceding names: *Mr., Messrs., Ms., Mrs., Dr., St.* (for *Saint*). (*The*) *Rev.* and (*The*) *Hon.* are used only when the surname is preceded by a first name: *Rev. Henry Mitchell* (or *Mr. Mitchell* or *Father Mitchell*), not *Rev. Mitchell.*
   b. Following names: *Esq., M.D., Sr., Jr., Ph.D., M.A., LL.D.* Do not duplicate a title before and after a name.

   Incorrect   *Dr.* Rinard Z. Hart, *M.D.*

   Correct   *Dr.* Rinard Z. Hart, or Rinard Z. Hart, *M.D.*

   For the correct forms of titles used in addressing officials of church and state, consult an unabridged dictionary.

3. In technical writing, directions, recipes, and the like, terms of measurement are often abbreviated when used with figures.

   Correct   32°*F;* 1,500 *rpm;* 25 *mph;* ½ *tsp.* salt and 2 *tbs.* sugar; 12 *ft.* 9 *in.;* 5 *cc;* 2 *lb.* 4 *oz.*

   Abbreviations such as *Co., Inc., Bros.,* should be used only when business organizations use them in their official titles. The ampersand (&) is used only when the company uses the symbol in its letterhead and signature.

   Incorrect   D. C. Heath & Co., D. C. Heath and Co.

   Correct   D. C. Heath and Company

34d

Correct any errors in abbreviations in the following sentences.

1. Dr. Geo. C. Fryer lives on Sandy Blvd. near Walnut St.
2. I have worked for the Shell Oil Co. since Oct., '57.
3. We expected to go to N.Y. for Xmas.
4. The Acme Corp. ships mail-order goods C.O.D.
5. I was in Wash., D.C., on Aug. 10, 1975.
6. Mt. Whitney, which is 14,495 ft. high, is located in SE California.
7. The drive to Lexington, Ky., took us 3 hrs., 17 min.
8. A temperature of 32°F is equivalent to zero on the cent. scale.
9. He bought three fl. oz. of aromatic spirits of amm.
10. Turn back to the 1st page of Ch. 3 and read pp. 18–22.

34e Italics

Italics are used for certain titles, unnaturalized foreign words, scientific names, names of ships and aircraft, and words considered *as* words. To italicize a word in a manuscript, draw one straight line below it, or use the underlining key on the keyboard: `King Lear.`

1. In the titles of books, monographs, musical works, and such separate publications, italicize all words. (Do not italicize the author's name.) In the titles of newspapers, magazines, and periodicals, only the distinctive words are italicized. The article *The* in newspaper titles is usually not italicized, but printed in regular (roman) type. (Note that *The* is italicized in the preceding sentence since it refers to the word itself, used as the subject of *is*.)

The Blithedale Romance

Edmund Wilson's *The Shock of Recognition*

Of Stars and Men

Dictionary of Foreign Terms

The *Atlantic Monthly*

Christian Science Monitor

The *Southern Review*

The *New York Times*

Titles of parts of published works and articles in magazines are enclosed in quotation marks.

The assignment is "Despondency" from William Wordsworth's long narrative poem, *The Excursion.*

I always read filler material in the *New Yorker* entitled "Letters We Never Finished Reading."

She hoped to publish her story entitled "Nobody Lives Here" in a magazine like *Harper's*.

2. Italicize foreign words that have not yet become accepted in the English language. If you are not certain whether a foreign word has become naturalized, consult a dictionary. Be sure to consult the Explanatory Notes to see how foreign words are indicated. Scientific names for plants and animals are italicized.

> The dancer unties a knot with her feet in the Mexican *reboza*.
>
> The technical name of Steller's jay is *Cyanocitta stelleri*.

3. Italicize the names of ships and aircrafts, but *not* the names of the companies that own them.

> The liner *S.S. Constitution* sails for Africa tomorrow.
>
> He went to Hawaii on a Matson liner and returned on one of United's *Royal Hawaiian* flights.

4. When words, letters, or figures are spoken of as such, they are usually italicized.

> The misuse of *cool* and *real* is a common fault.
>
> The letter *e* and the figure *2* on my typewriter are worn.

Exercise 3

Correct in the following sentences any errors in abbreviations, numbers, capitals, and italics.

1. He made a survey of Athletics in the Universities and Colleges in the U.S.
2. When grandmother was a girl, she lived in Lincoln, Nebr.
3. She always adds a P.S. to her letters.
4. He was traveling in the East last Winter.
5. I spent fifty cents for a pattern, $6.80 for my material, and a dollar and ten cents for trimming; so you see that my dress will cost only $8.40.
6. 1985 brought us good fortune.
7. "You will surely decide to go," he said, "For you will never have such a chance as this again."
8. After each war we resolve "That these dead shall not have died in vain."
9. Our country entered the second world war in nineteen hundred and forty-one.
10. The use of the word like as a conjunction is a very common error.
11. I've had several good history teachers, but my history 141 professor, Doctor Charney, is the best professor I have met.
12. Roosevelt was elected president for a 2nd term by an Overwhelming Majority.
13. They discussed the eighteenth amendment and the methods of repealing an amendment to the constitution.
14. The president of the United States rose to greet the president of our university.
15. Queen Elizabeth 1 tried to preserve the status quo.

34e

<u>34f</u> Syllabication

Dividing a word at the end of a line is mainly a printer's problem. In manuscripts it is not necessary to keep the right-hand margin absolutely even, so it is seldom necessary to divide a word at the end of a line. If such a division is essential, observe the following principles, and mark the division with a hyphen (-).

1. Divide words only *between* syllables—that is, between the normal sound divisions of a word. When in doubt as to where the division between syllables comes, consult a dictionary. One-syllable words, such as *though* or *strength,* cannot be divided. Syllables of one letter should not be divided from the rest of the word. Nor should a division be made between two letters that indicate a single sound. For example, never divide *th* as in *brother, sh* as in *fashion, ck* as in *Kentucky, oa* as in *reproaching, ai* as in *maintain.* Such combinations of letters may be divided only if they indicate two distinct sounds: *post-haste, dis-hon-or, co-au-thor.*

| **Incorrect** | li-mit, sinec-ure, burg-lar-ize, ver-y, a-dult, co-ord-in-a-tion |
| **Correct** | lim-it, sine-cure, bur-glar-ize, very, adult, co-or-di-na-tion |

2. A division comes at the point where a prefix or suffix joins the root word, if pronunciation permits.

   be-half, sub-way, anti-dote, con-vene, de-tract

   lik-able (or like-able), like-ly, place-ment, Flem-ish, en-force-ment, tall-er, tall-est, fall-en

Exceptions because of pronunciation

   prel-ate, pred-e-cessor, res-ti-tu-tion, bus-tling, prej-u-dice, twink-ling, jog-gled

3. When two consonants come between vowels (me*mb*er), the division is between the consonants if pronunciation permits (*mem-ber*). If the consonant is doubled before a suffix, the second consonant goes with the suffix (*plan-ning*).

   remem-ber, pas-sage, fas-ten, disman-tle, symmet-rical (*but* symme-try), prompt-er (*but* promp-ti-tude), impor-tant, clas-sic, rum-mage, as-sur-ance, oc-cident, at-tend, nar-ration, of-fi-cial-ly, com-pen-di-um, fit-ting

   BUT NOTE: knowl-edge

4. The division comes after a vowel if pronunciation permits.

   modi-fier, oscilla-tor, ora-torical, devi-ate

Glossary of Usage

This Glossary discusses only more commonly misused words. In recommending that you observe rules of usage, we are not suggesting that you abandon your natural speech for what may to your taste seem stilted. But remember that written language is selective. The choice of whether or not to observe standards of usage is yours, but the choice should be an informed and prudent one. A good college dictionary will often help you distinguish among levels of usage.

a, an Indefinite articles. *A* is used before words beginning with a consonant sound, *an* before words beginning with a vowel sound. Before words beginning with *h,* use *an* when the *h* is silent, as in *hour,* but *a* when the *h* is pronounced, as in *history.*

accept, except Different verbs which sound alike. *Accept* means "to receive," *except* "to leave out."

I **accepted** the diploma.

When assigning jobs, the dean **excepted** students who had already worked on a project.

adapt, adopt To *adapt* is to change or modify to suit a new need, purpose, or condition.

Human beings can **adapt** to many environments.

The movie was **adapted** from a novel.

To *adopt* something is to make it one's own, to choose it.

The couple **adopted** a child.

Our club **adopted** "Opportunity knocks" as its motto.

adverse, averse Often confused, but important to distinguish. *Adverse* means "antagonistic" or "unfavorable."

Adverse weather forced postponement of the regatta.

Averse means "opposed to"; only sentient beings can be *averse.*

She was **averse** to sailing under such conditions.

441

advice, advise   *Advice* is a noun, *advise* a verb.

> He gave me some good **advice**.

> I **advise** you to listen carefully.

affect, effect   Words close in sound and therefore often confused. *Affect* as a verb means "to influence." *Effect* as a verb means "to bring about."

> Smoking **affects** the heart.

> How can we **effect** a change in the law?

> As a noun, *effect* means "result."

> One **effect** of her treatment was a bad case of hives.

aggravate   Means "to intensify" or "to make worse."

> The shock **aggravated** his misery.

> Colloquially, it means "to annoy," "irritate," "arouse the anger of."

ain't   A nonstandard contraction of *am not, is not* or *are not.* Not to be used in most writing.

all ready, already   Not synonyms. *All ready* refers to a state of readiness.

> The twirlers were **all ready** for the half-time show.

> *Already* means "by or before the present time."

> Has the game **already** started?

all right   Unlike the pairs of words in the preceding and following entries, *all right* stands alone. There is no word *alright,* although many people, misled by the existence of *altogether* and *already,* assume that there is.

all together, altogether   *All together* refers to a group with no missing elements.

> If we can get our members **all together,** we can begin the meeting.

> *Altogether* means "completely."

> You are **altogether** mistaken about that.

allude, refer   To *allude* is to make an indirect reference.

> Did her letter **allude** to Sam's difficulties?

> To *refer* is to call attention specifically to something.

> The instructor **referred** us to Baudelaire's translations of Poe.

allusion, illusion, delusion   An *allusion* is a brief, indirect reference.

> Anyone who speaks of "cabbages and kings" is making an **allusion** to *Alice in Wonderland.*

An *illusion* is a deceptive impression.

He enjoyed the **illusion** of luxury created by his imitation Oriental rugs.

A *delusion* is a mistaken belief, implying self-deception and often a disordered state of mind.

She fell prey to the **delusion** that she was surrounded by enemy agents.

a lot, alot   The only correct spelling is *a lot*.

among, between   *Among* always refers to more than two.

He lived **among** a tribe of cannibals.

Between is used to refer to two objects or to more than two objects considered individually.

The scenery is spectacular **between** Portland and Seattle.

The governors signed the agreement **between** all three states.

amoral, immoral   Anything *amoral* is outside morality, not to be judged by moral standards.

The behavior of animals and the orbits of the planets are equally **amoral**.

Anything *immoral* is in direct violation of some moral standard.

Plagiarism is generally considered to be an **immoral** act.

amount, number   *Amount* is used as a general indicator of quantity; *number* refers only to what can be counted.

An immense **amount** of food was prepared for the picnic, but only a small **number** of people came.

an   See **a**.

ante, anti   As a prefix, *ante* means "before": *ante*date, *ante*cedent. *Anti* means "against": *anti*war, *anti*knock. Do not confuse these prefixes.

anxious, eager   *Anxious* refers to worry about the future.

He was **anxious** about the outcome of his exam.

Eager indicates hopeful excitement.

She was **eager** to meet her relatives from Ohio.

anyone, any one   *Anyone* is an indefinite pronoun and means "any individual at all." *Any one* designates a particular person or thing.

Anyone could see the obvious error.

Any one of us could have pointed out the error.

Everyone, every one, and *someone, some one* follow this pattern.

Everyone enjoyed the Olympics, and **every one** of the events was well-attended.

Someone should do the job. **Some one** person will have to be responsible.

Also see **everybody, every body.**

apt   See **liable.**

as   Dialectal when used in place of *that* or *who.*

I don't know **that** (not **as**) we can go.

There are some **who** (not **as**) trust him.

Because and *since* are clearer than *as* for introducing clauses showing causal relationship.

Because (or **since**) I was late, I missed the opening curtain.

at about   Prefer *about* in writing; *at about* is overworked and redundant.

Preferred in writing   It happened **about** three o'clock.

awhile, a while   *Awhile* is an adverb.

I'm tired so I'll sit **awhile.**

A while consists of a particle and a noun, often used as the object of a preposition.

I'm tired so I'll sit for **a while.**

bad, badly   Formal usage employs *bad* as an adjective with linking verbs like *feel* and *look.*

I feel **bad** (not **badly**) because of my headache.

Badly is an adverb used with most verbs.

I served **badly** during the tennis match because of my headache.

barely   See **hardly.**

between   See **among.**

but   Often used colloquially in such idioms as "I can't help but think." In writing "I can't help thinking" is preferred. If the nonstandard expression "I don't know but what he wants it" leads to confusion (does he or doesn't he?), it should be avoided in speech, too.

can, may   In formal speech and in writing, *can* is used to indicate ability, *may* to indicate permission.

If you **can** open that box, you **may** have whatever is in it.

In informal questions, *can* is often used even though permission is meant.

Can I try it next? Why **can't** I?

censor, censure To *censor* something (such as a book, letter, or film) is to evaluate it on the basis of certain arbitrary standards to determine whether it may be made public.

All announcements for the bulletin board are **censored** by the department secretary.

Censor is often used as the equivalent of "delete."

References in the report to secret activities have been **censored**.

Censure means "to find fault with," "to criticize as blameworthy."

Several officers were **censured** for their participation in the affair.

compare to, compare with, contrast with *Compare to* is used to show similarities between different kinds of things.

Sir James Jeans **compared** the universe **to** a corrugated soap bubble.

Compare with means to examine in order to note either similarities or differences.

Compare this example **with** the preceding one.

Contrast with is used to show differences only.

Contrast the life of a student today **with** that of a student in the middle ages.

complementary, complimentary *Complementary* means "serving to fill out" or "to complete."

His tenor and her soprano are **complementary**.

Complimentary means "freely given" or "giving praise."

Members of the audience were quite **complimentary** about the couple's recital.

concur in, concur with *Concur in* refers to agreement with a principle or policy.

She **concurred in** their judgment that the manager should be given a raise.

Concur with refers to agreement with a person.

She **concurred with** him in his decision to give the manager a raise.

conscious, conscience *Conscious* is an adjective meaning "aware of."

She was **conscious** of the others in the room.

Conscience is a noun meaning "the sense of moral goodness or badness."

Her **conscience** told her to leave.

gl

contact The use of *contact* as a verb meaning "to get in touch with" has gained wide acceptance, but a more exact term such as *ask, consult, inform, meet, see, telephone,* or *write* is generally preferable.

continual, continuous The first is widely used to indicate an action that is repeated frequently, the second to indicate uninterrupted action.

We heard the **continual** whimpering of the dog.

The dog kept a **continuous** vigil beside the body of his dead master.

contrast with See **compare to.**

data, criteria, phenomena Latin plural, not singular forms, and so used in formal writing. But the use of *data* (rather than *datum*) with a singular form is widespread.

These **data** have been taken from the last Census Report.

Criteria and *phenomena* are always plural. The singular forms are *criterion* and *phenomenon.*

Scientists encountered a **phenomenon** that could not be evaluated under existing **criteria.**

delusion See **allusion.**

different from, different than *Different from* is always acceptable usage.

College is **different from** what I had expected.

Different than is not acceptable in formal writing.

dilemma, problem A *dilemma* is a choice between two equally distasteful alternatives.

We faced the **dilemma** of paying the fine or spending three days in jail.

A *problem* is wider in meaning, referring to a difficulty or a question that must be solved.

The United States must soon resolve the **problem** of guaranteeing an energy supply for the 1990s.

disinterested, uninterested *Disinterested* means "unbiased," "impartial." *Uninterested* means "without any interest in," or "lacking interest."

Although we were **uninterested** in her general topic, we had to admire her **disinterested** treatment of its controversial aspects.

don't A contraction of *do not.* Not to be used in formal writing with a subject in the third person singular.

| Nonstandard | He **don't** know. |
| Standard | He **doesn't** know. |

due to   In writing, *due to* should not be used adverbially to mean *because of.*

| Colloquial | I made many mistakes **due to** carelessness. |
| Preferred in writing | I made many mistakes **because of** carelessness. |

Due to is an adjective and usually follows the verb *to be.*

His illness was **due to** exhaustion.

each other, one another   When two individuals are involved in a reciprocal relationship, *each other* is used.

My sister and I respected **each other.**

When more than two individuals are mutually related, *one another* is appropriate.

The sheep rubbed against **one another** in the chill.

eager   See **anxious.**

effect   See **affect.**

either, neither   As subjects, both words are singular. When referring to more than two, use *none* rather than *neither.*

Either (Neither) red or (nor) pink **is** appropriate.

I asked Leahy, Mahoney, and another Irishman, but **none** of them **was** willing.

eminent, imminent   *Eminent* means "prominent," "well known."

She was an **eminent** judge.

Imminent means "impending," "menacing," "about to occur."

The jury's verdict is **imminent.**

enthused   Either as a verb (he *enthused*) or adjective (he was *enthused*), the word is strictly colloquial. In writing, use "showed enthusiasm" or "was enthusiastic."

equally as good   A confusion of two phrases: *equally good* and *just as good.* Use either of the two phrases in place of *equally as good.*

Their TV set cost much more than ours, but ours is **equally good.**

Our TV set is **just as good** as theirs.

-ess   Feminine ending acceptable in such traditional words as *waitress, actress, hostess.* But many persons object to *poetess, authoress, sculptress* as patronizing and demeaning. Unless an *-ess* word has a long history and you are sure there are no objections to its use, it is best to avoid it.

etc.   Avoid the vague use of *etc.*; use it only to prevent useless repetition or informally to represent terms entirely obvious from the context.

Vague	The judge was honorable, upright, dependable, **etc.**
Preferred	The judge was honorable, upright, **and** dependable.
Standard	Use even numbers like four, eight, ten, **etc.**

Avoid *and etc.*, which is redundant.

everybody, every body   *Everybody* is an indefinite pronoun.

Everybody is welcome.

Every body consists of a noun modified by "every."

We could see every lake and **every body** of land as we flew north.

Somebody and *some body* are similar to *everybody, every body.*

Somebody did this inaccurate sketch.

The drawing should be redone to give it some shading and **some body.**

Be careful of "every" in other contexts.

Every day that I waited seemed longer.

Everyday events soon become habitual.

everyone, every one   See **anyone.**

except   See **accept.**

expect   Colloquial when used to mean "suppose," "presume": I *expect* it's time for us to go.

Preferred	I **suppose** it's time for us to go.

factor   Means "something that contributes to a result."

Industry and perseverance were **factors** in her success.

Avoid using *factor* to mean vaguely any thing, item, or event.

Vague	Ambition was a **factor** that contributed to the downfall of Macbeth. [Since *factor* includes the notion of "contributing to," such usage is redundant as well as vague and wordy.]
Preferred	Ambition contributed to the downfall of Macbeth.

farther, further   In careful usage *farther* indicates distance; *further* indicates degree and may also mean "additional." Both are used as adjectives and as adverbs: *a mile farther, further disintegration, further details.*

faze, phase   *Faze* is a colloquial verb meaning "to perturb," "to disconcert." *Phase* as a noun means "stage of development" (a passing *phase*); as a verb it means "to carry out in stages." Be wary of *phase in* and *phase out*, which have the ring of jargon.

fewer, less   *Fewer* refers to number, *less* to amount. Use *fewer* in speaking of things that can be counted and *less* for amounts that are measured.

Fewer persons enrolled in medical schools this year than last.

Less studying was required to pass chemistry than we had anticipated.

flaunt, flout   Commonly misspelled, mispronounced, and, therefore, confused. *Flaunt* means "to exhibit arrogantly," "show off."

He **flaunted** his photographic memory in class.

Flout means "to reject with contempt."

They **flouted** the tradition of wearing gowns at graduation by showing up in bluejeans.

former, latter   Preferably used to designate one of two persons or things. For designating one of three or more, write *first* or *last*.

further   See **farther.**

get, got, gotten   *Get to* (*go*), *get away with*, *get back at*, *get with* (something), and *got to* (for *must*) are acceptable in colloquial usage but should be avoided in writing. Either *got* or *gotten* is acceptable as the past participle of *get*.

good   An adjective. Should not be used in formal writing as an adverb meaning "well."

Colloquial	She plays tennis **good.**
Standard	She plays tennis **well.**
	She plays a **good** game of tennis.

had of   Nonstandard when used for *had*.

Nonstandard	If he **had of** tried, he would have succeeded.
Standard	If he **had** tried, he would have succeeded.

had ought   Nonstandard as a past tense of *ought*. The tense of this verb is indicated by the infinitive that follows.

He **ought to go**; she **ought to have gone.**

hanged, hung   When *hang* means "to suspend," *hung* is its past tense.

The guard **hung** a black flag from the prison to signal the execution.

When *hang* means "to execute," *hanged* is the correct past tense.

After the flag was **hung,** the prisoner was **hanged.**

hardly, barely, scarcely Since these words convey the idea of negation, they should not be used with another negative.

| Nonstandard | We **couldn't hardly** see in the darkness.
We **hadn't barely** finished. |
| Standard | We **could hardly** see.
We **had barely** finished. |

hopefully Although widely used in speech to mean "it is to be hoped," or "I hope" (*Hopefully,* a check will arrive tomorrow), the adverb *hopefully* is used in writing to mean "in a hopeful manner."

They spoke **hopefully** of world peace.

illusion See **allusion.**

imminent See **eminent.**

immoral See **amoral.**

imply, infer *Imply* means "to suggest" or "hint"; *infer* means "to reach a conclusion from facts or premises."

His tone **implied** contempt; I **inferred** from his voice that he did not like me.

incredible, incredulous Both are adjectives or, more rarely, nouns, but *incredible* means "unbelievable," "unlikely," while *incredulous* means "skeptical," "unbelieving."

The ad made **incredible** claims for the product, but I remained **incredulous.**

inside of Omit the superfluous *of* when this is used as a preposition.

I'll meet you **inside** the station.

See **outside of.**

insupportable, unsupportable Often confused, but not synonymous. *Insupportable* means "unable to be endured."

The noise of the bulldozers during the lecture was **insupportable.**

Unsupportable means "not capable of support."

The building program, though imaginative, is financially **unsupportable.**

inter, intra As a prefix *inter* means "between" or "among": *international, intermarry; intra* means "within" or "inside of": *intramuscular, intramural.*

irony See **sarcasm.**

irregardless A nonstandard combination of *irrespective* and *regardless.*

Regardless (or **irrespective**) of the minority opinion, we included the platform in the campaign.

is when, is where   Avoid using these as parts of a definition.

"Smog is polluted air" (rather than "Smog **is when** the air is polluted").

"Literacy is the ability to read and write" (rather than "Literacy **is where** a person can read and write").

its, it's   Often confused. *Its* is the possessive form of *it*.

My suitcase has lost one of **its** handles.

It's is the contracted form of *it is* or *it has*.

It's a good day for sailing.

It's been a month since I mailed the check.

kind, sort   Colloquial when used with a plural modifier and verb: *These* kind (or *sort*) of books *are* trash.

> **Standard**   **This sort** of book **is** trash.
> **These kinds** of books **are** classics

In questions, the number of the verb depends on the noun that follows *kind* (or *sort*).

What kind of **book is** this?

What kind of **books are** these?

kind of, sort of   Colloquial when used to mean "rather."

> **Colloquial**   I thought the lecture was **kind of** dull.
> **Standard**   I thought the lecture was **rather** dull.

later, latter   *Later* designates time; *latter* designates the second of two items, choices, or objects.

I'll see you **later** in the day.

The pound had a young poodle and a young terrier. I chose the **latter**.

Also see **former**.

latest, last   *Latest* means "most recent"; *last* means "final."

I doubt that their **latest** contract proposal represents their **last** offer.

lay, lie   Often confused. *Lay* is a transitive verb meaning "to put" or "place" something. It always takes an object. Its principal parts are *lay, laid, laid*. *Lie* is intransitive; that is, it does not take an object, and means "to recline" or "to remain." Its principal parts are *lie, lay, lain*. When in doubt, try substituting the verb *place*. If it fits the context, use some form of *lay*.

> **Present tense**   I **lie** down every afternoon.
> Every morning I **lay** the paper by his plate.

Past tense	I **lay** down yesterday after dinner.
	I **laid** the paper by his plate two hours ago.
Perfect tense	I **have lain** here for several hours.
	I **have laid** the paper by his plate many times.

lend See **loan.**

less See **fewer.**

let's Contraction of *let us.* In writing, it should be used only where *let us* can be used.

| Colloquial | **Let's don't** leave yet. **Let's us** go. |
| Standard | **Let's not** leave yet. **Let's** go. |

liable, likely, apt In careful writing, the words are not interchangeable. *Likely* is used to indicate a mere probability.

They are **likely** to be chosen.

Liable is used when the probability is unpleasant.

We are **liable** to get a parking ticket.

Apt implies a natural tendency or ability.

She is **apt** to win the musical competition.

lie See **lay.**

like The use of *like* to introduce a clause is widespread in informal English, especially that used by advertising agencies. In edited writing, *as, as if,* and *as though* are preferred.

Colloquial	This rose smells sweet, **like** a flower should.
Standard	This rose smells sweet, **as** a flower should.
	This perfume smells **like** roses.

literally Means "precisely," "without any figurative sense," "strictly." It is often inaccurately used as an intensive, to emphasize a figure of speech: I was *literally* floating on air. This makes sense only if one is capable of levitation. Use the word *literally* with caution in writing.

loan, lend Traditionally, *lend* is a verb, *loan* a noun, but *loan* is also used as a verb, especially in business contexts.

The company **loaned** us money for the down payment.

loose, lose *Loose* is usually an adjective meaning "unfixed," "unattached." *Lose* is a verb meaning "to misplace," "forget."

The screws are **loose** and the door wobbles.

Don't **lose** patience and don't **lose** your temper.

may   See **can.**

moral, morale   As an adjective or noun, *moral* refers to ethical conduct or values. As noun, *morale* refers to a prevailing mood or level of confidence.

gl

> She is a **moral** person.
>
> He always looks for the **moral** of the novel.
>
> His last three failures have hurt his **morale.**

most   As a noun or adjective, *most* means "more than half."

> **Most** of us plan to go to the dance.
>
> **Most** people admire her paintings.

> As an adverb, *most* means "very."

> His playing was **most** impressive.

> *Most* is colloquial when used to mean "almost," "nearly."

| Colloquial | **Most** everyone was invited. |
| Preferred in writing | **Almost** everyone was invited. |

much   See **very.**

myself   Correctly used as a reflexive: I cut *myself,* sang to *myself,* give *myself* credit. Colloquial when used as an evasive substitute for *I* or *me.*

Colloquial	My brother and **myself** prefer coffee.
	She spoke to my brother and **myself.**
Preferred in writing	My brother and **I** prefer coffee.
	She spoke to my brother and **me.**

neither   See **either.**

notorious   Means "of bad repute"; as, a *notorious* gambler. Not to be used for "famous," "celebrated," or "noted."

number   See **amount.**

of   *Could of, may of, might of, must of, should of,* and *would of* are slurred pronunciations for *could have, may have, might have, must have, should have,* and *would have;* they are nonstandard in writing.

off of   A colloquial usage in which *of* is superfluous.

| Colloquial | Keep **off of** the grass. |
| Preferred in writing | Keep **off** the grass. |

one another   See **each other.**

outside of   Correct as noun: He painted the *outside of* the house. Colloquial as a preposition: He was waiting *outside of* the house. Omit the *of* in writing. Colloquial as a substitute for *except for, aside from.*

over with   *With* is superfluous.

The regatta is **over** (not **over with**).

part, portion   A *part* is any piece of a whole; a *portion* is that part specifically allotted to some person, cause, or use.

We planted beans in one **part** of our garden.

She left a **portion** of her estate to charity.

party   Colloquial when used to mean "person," as in "The *party* who telephoned left no message." Write *person*.

percent   In formal writing use *percent,* or *per cent,* only after a numeral—either the spelled-out word (six) or the numerical symbol (6). The sign (%) is used only in strictly commercial writing. The word *percentage,* meaning "a part or proportion of a whole," is used when the exact amount is not indicated.

A large **percentage** were Chinese.

Thirty-one **percent** were Chinese.

phase   See **faze.**

phenomena   See **data.**

portion   See **part.**

principal, principle   As a noun, a *principal* is the head or leading figure in an institution, an event, or a play.

The **principals** in the negotiations were Henry Kissinger and Le Duc Tho, who later shared the Nobel Peace Prize.

Used as an adjective, *principal* refers to a leading feature or element in a group.

The **principal** types of telescopes are the refracting and the reflecting, or Newtonian, telescope.

A *principle* is a rule.

The main **principle** in skiing is to keep on one's feet.

problem   See **dilemma.**

raise, rise   Often confused. Remember that *raise* means to "cause something to rise." Therefore *raise* must always have an object. Remember the principal parts of each verb:

Standard		
I rise	I rose	I have risen
I raise	I raised	I have raised
(something)	(something)	(something)

gl

Standard   I **rise** at six o'clock every morning.
I **raise** flowers for sale.
I **rose** at six o'clock.
I **raised** flowers for sale.
I **have risen** at six o'clock for years.
I **have raised** flowers for years.

real   Colloquial when used for "very." Write *very* hot (not *real* hot).

reason is because, reason why   Both of these expressions are wordy. Eliminate *is because,* or *why,* or *the reason is.*

> **Wordy**   The **reason** we came **is because** we knew you needed help.
>
> **Concise**   We came **because** we knew you needed help.

refer   See **allude.**

regarding, in regard to, with regard to, in relation to, in terms of   These windy phrases are usually dispensable. Replace them with concrete terms.

> **Wordy**   **With regard to** grades, she was very good.
>
> **Concise**   She **got** very good grades.

sarcasm, irony   *Sarcasm* is not interchangeable with *irony. Saracastic* remarks, like *ironic* remarks, convey a message obliquely, but sarcasm contains the notion of ridicule, of an intention on the part of the writer to wound. Only persons can be *sarcastic,* while both persons and events can be *ironic.*

The sergeant inquired **sarcastically** whether any of us could tell time; it was **ironic** that his watch turned out to be ten minutes fast.

scarcely   See **hardly.**

sensual, sensuous   Both words refer to impressions made upon the senses. Their connotations, however, are widely different. *Sensual* often carries unfavorable connotations. It is frequently applied to the gratification of appetite and lust.

Sensual delights are often considered inferior to spiritual pleasures.

Sensuous, on the other hand, is used literally or approvingly of an appeal to the senses (the *sensuous* delight of a swim on a hot day), and can even refer to such abstract appeals as those found in poetry.

Milton's **sensuous** imagery calls upon sight, touch, and even smell to form the reader's impression of Eden.

gl

set, sit *Set* is a transitive verb meaning "to put" or "place" something. It should be distinguished from *sit,* an intransitive verb.

Present tense	I **sit** in the chair.
	I **set** the book on the chair.
Past tense	I **sat** on the chair.
	I **set** the book on the table.
Perfect tense	I **have sat** in the chair.
	I **have set** the book on the table.

shall, will The distinction between these words is rapidly fading. Most writers now use *will* throughout. *Shall* may still be used for emphasis (He *shall* be heard); since it is less common than *will,* it has a formal tone.

should, would *Should* substitutes for "ought to" (He *should* go on a diet); *would* for "wanted to" (He could do it if he *would*). *Should* indicates probability (I *should* be finished in an hour); *would* indicates custom (He *would* always call when he got home).

so, such Avoid using *so* and *such* as vague intensifiers: I am *so* glad; I had *such* a good time.

I was **so** glad to find that print **that** I bought copies for all my friends.

some Colloquial when used as an adverb meaning "somewhat" (I am *some* better today) or when used as an intensifying adjective (That was *some* dinner).

Preferred in writing	I am **a little** (or **somewhat**) better today.
	That was **an excellent** dinner.

somebody, some body See **everybody.**

someone, some one See **anyone.**

sort of See **kind of.**

such See **so.**

sure Colloquial when used for "certainly," "surely," as in "He *sure* can play poker."

that, which *That* is largely used to introduce restrictive clauses, which limit or define the antecedent's meaning and are not set off by commas.

The law **that** gave women the right to vote was passed in 1920.

Which is used to introduce nonrestrictive clauses, which do not limit or define the meaning of the antecedent. Nonrestrictive clauses are always set off by commas.

The 19th Amendment, **which** gave women the right to vote, was passed in 1920. [The amendment is already identified by number; the clause "which gave women the right to vote" merely gives additional information.]

Often the antecedent will be identified in a preceding sentence, in which case the clause is still nonrestrictive.

The 19th Amendment gave women the right to vote. This amendment, **which** passed in 1920, marked the entry of women into party politics.

their, there   Often confused. *Their* is the possessive form of *they.*

Their time will come.

There refers to place.

Put the book **there.**

this here, these here, that there, those there   Nonstandard. Say *this, these, that,* or *those.*

to, too, two   Sometimes confused. *To* is a preposition.

We went **to** the late show.

Too is an adverb meaning "more than enough" or "also."

He has made the same mistake **too** many times.

She **too** shares this feeling.

Two is an adjective or a noun designating number.

Two people were early.

We found only **two** of the people who had been there.

toward, towards   Interchangeable. *Toward* is more common in America, *towards* in Britain.

transpire   In formal writing, where the word properly belongs, it means "to become known." It is colloquial in the sense of "happen," or "come to pass."

try and   Often used for "try to," but should be avoided in writing.

I must **try to** (not **try and**) find a job.

uninterested   See **disinterested.**

unique   Adverbs such as *rather, more, most, very* are colloquial when used to modify *unique.* Since the word means "being the only one of its kind," no thing can be more (or less) unique than another.

This copy of the book is **unique.**

This copy of the book is **very rare.**

unsupportable   See **insupportable.**

up   Do not add a superfluous *up* to verbs: We opened *up* the box and divided the money *up.* Write: We opened the box and divided the money.

gl

very, much (with past participles) A past participle that is felt to be a part of a verb form, rather than an adjective, should not be immediately preceded by *very* but by *much, greatly,* or some other intensive. A past participle that can be used as an adjective may be preceded by *very.*

Colloquial	He was **very** admired by other students.
	He was **very** influenced by the teacher.
Preferred in writing	He was **very much** admired by other students.
	He was **greatly** influenced by the teacher.
	He was a **very** tired boy.

wait on Colloquial for *wait for.*

ways Colloquial in such expressions as *a little ways*. In writing, the singular is preferred: *a little way.*

where . . . to, where . . . at Colloquialisms whose prepositions are redundant or dialectal.

| Colloquial | **Where** are you going **to**? **Where** is he **at**? |
| Preferred in writing | **Where** are you going? **Where** is he? |

which, who Do not use *which* to refer to persons. Save it for objects or things. Use *who* to refer to a person or persons.

This is the book **which** I will give Eileen, **who** should enjoy it.

Also see **that.**

who, whom (For the choice between these forms, see **28b.**)

will See **shall.**

wise Commerical jargon when attached to nouns in such combinations as *taxwise, languagewise, timewise, moneywise.* To be avoided in serious writing.

would See **should.**

would have Colloquial when used in *if* clauses instead of *had.*

| Colloquial | If he **would have stood** by us, we might have won. |
| Preferred in writing | If he **had stood** by us, we might have won. |

write-up Colloquial for a description, an account, as in "a write-up in the newspaper."

you was Use *you were* in writing. *You was* is nonstandard.

your, you're Often confused. *Your* is the possessive of *you.*

Your train is late.

You're is a contraction of *you are.*

If **you're** ready, we can leave.

Grammatical Terms

absolute construction, absolute phrase An absolute phrase consists of a participle with a subject (and sometimes a complement) grammatically unconnected with the rest of the sentence but usually telling when, why, or how something happened.

The floodwaters having receded, people began returning to their homes.

I hated to leave home, **circumstances being as they were.**

abstract language Words expressing general ideas, states, or conditions: *generosity, love, goals.* See **concrete language.**

active voice See **voice.**

adjective A part of speech used to describe or limit the meaning of a substantive. There are the following kinds:

Descriptive	a **true** friend, a **poor** man
Limiting	**an** apple, **the** woman, **two** boys

Notice that many kinds of pronouns regularly perform the function of an adjective.

Possessive	**my** book, **his** sister, **your** house
Demonstrative	**this** chair, **these** papers
Interrogative	**hose** hat? **which** one?
Indefinite	**any** card, **each** boy, **some** candy

adjective clause See **clause.**

adverb A part of speech used to modify a verb, an adjective, or another adverb. An adverb answers the questions: *Where? When? How? Why?* or *To what extent?*

He bowed **politely.**
["Politely" modifies the verb "bowed."]

A **very** old woman came in.
["Very" modifies the adjective "old."]

He was **too** much absorbed to listen.
["Too" modifies the adverb "much."]

Substantives may be used adverbially:

He walked **two miles.**
["Two miles" modifies the verb "walked."]

He walked **two miles** farther.
["Two miles" modifies the adverb "farther."]

adverb clause   See **clause.**

agreement   The correspondence in number and person between the subject and verb in a sentence and the correspondence in number, person, gender, and case between a pronoun and its antecedent (see Chapter **27**).

antecedent   A word, phrase, or clause to which a pronoun refers.

I saw the **house** long before I reached **it.**
["House" is the antecedent of "it."]

This is a **problem which** cannot be solved without calculus.
["Problem" is the antecedent of "which."]

appositive   A substantive attached to another substantive and denoting the same person or thing. A substantive is said to be **in apposition** with the substantive to which it is attached.

Alice, my **cousin,** was enjoying her favorite sport—**sailing.**
["Cousin" is in apposition with "Alice"; "sailing" is in apposition with "sport."]

article   The word *the* is called the **definite article;** the word *a* or *an* is called the **indefinite article.** In function, articles can be classed with adjectives.

auxiliary   When the verbs *be, have, do, shall, will, may, can, must,* and *ought* assist in forming the voices, modes, and tenses of other verbs, they are **auxiliaries.**

A message **was** given to me.

He **should have** known better.

He **has been** gone a week.

cardinal number   Any of the numbers *one, two, three, four,* etc., denoting quantity, in distinction from *first, second, third,* etc., which are **ordinal numbers** and show sequence. Cardinal and ordinal numbers can function as adjectives or as nouns.

case   The inflection of a noun (*girls', friend's*) or pronoun (*she, her, hers*) to show its relationship to other words. In English, pronouns are classified into three cases (see Chapter **28**).

Nominative (or subjective)   **I** spoke; **they** listened; **she** dozed.
[The inflected pronouns function as subject.]

Objective	John tossed **me** the ball.
	I collided with two other players and knocked **them** down.
	[The inflected pronouns function as indirect object, and object of the verb.]
Possessive (or genitive)	**His** score and **mine** were identical.
	Our scores were higher than **theirs**.
	They wondered **whose** grade was the highest.
	[The inflected pronouns show possession or a similar relationship.]

gr

In modern times, English nouns are inflected only to indicate the genitive case: *Jerry's* money and *Sarah's* money was invested at their *parents'* advice; this allayed the *relatives'* fears about the *boy's* future and the *girl's* education.

clause   A group of words containing a subject and predicate (see Chapter **9**). Clauses that can stand alone as complete sentences are **independent (principal** or **main)** clauses. Clauses that are not by themselves complete in meaning are **dependent (subordinate)** clauses. Subordinate clauses are used as nouns, adjectives, or adverbs. They are usually introduced by subordinating conjunctions or relative pronouns.

We heard him **when he came in.**
["We heard him" is the main clause; "when he came in" is the subordinate clause.]

That she will be late is certain.
[Subordinate clause used as a noun.]

The woman **who spoke to us** is our sheriff.
[Subordinate clause used as an adjective.]

He will come in **when he is ready.**
[Subordinate clause used as an adverb.]

Clauses that play the same part in a sentence, whether they are main or subordinate, are called **coordinate clauses.**

The bell rang and **everyone stood up.**
[Coordinate main clauses.]

He left **because he did not like the work** and **because the pay was low.**
[Coordinate subordinate clauses.]

collective noun   A noun that is singular in form (*class, crowd, orchestra*) but that denotes a group of members.

colloquial language   Language appropriate to speech but not to formal writing, unless a relaxed and casual tone is intended.

comma splice   A sentence error in which two independent clauses are joined by a comma with no coordinating conjunction.

> **Comma splice**   The car was an ancient model, it made the trip successfully.
>
> **Revised**   The car was an ancient model, **but** it made the trip successfully.

See Chapter **31**.

gr

comparison   Inflection of an adjective or adverb to indicate an increasing degree of quality, quantity, or manner.

> **Positive degree**   Our house is **cold.**
>
> **Comparative degree**   Their house is **colder.**
>
> **Superlative degree**   Their house is the **coldest** in town.

When adjectives have one or two syllables, the comparative degree is usually formed by adding *-er* to the positive; and the superlative degree is usually formed by adding *-est* to the positive. To form the comparative degree of adverbs and of adjectives with more than two syllables, place *more* before the positive form; the superlative degree is usually formed by placing *most* before the positive. Some adjectives have irregular comparison: e.g., *good, better, best; bad, worse, worst.* See Chapter **29**.

complement   Traditionally, a word or phrase added to a verb to complete the sense of the statement. It may be the direct object of a transitive verb, an indirect object, or a predicate noun or adjective. See Chapter **9**.

> **Direct object**   A big wave swamped our **boat.**
>
> **Indirect object**   I paid **him** the money.
>
> **Predicate noun**   Our destination was **Corsica.**
>   The referee called Sanchez the **winner.**
>
> **Predicate adjective**   The waves were **enormous.**
>   A limber branch made the tree-house **shaky.**

complex sentence   See Chapter **9**.

compound sentence   See Chapter **9**.

concrete language   Words describing specific things, perceptible by the senses: *smooth, bitter, yellow, creaky, shrill.* See **abstract language.**

conjugation   The inflected forms of a verb which show person, number, tense, voice, and mood. The following is a simplified conjugation of the indicative mood of the verb *see:*

	Active voice	Passive voice

Present tense

		Active voice	Passive voice
singular	1.	I see	I am seen
	2.	you see	you are seen
	3.	he (she, it) sees	he is seen
plural	1.	we see	we are seen
	2.	you see	you are seen
	3.	they see	they are seen

Past tense

singular	1.	I saw	I was seen
	2.	you saw	you were seen
	3.	he saw	he was seen
plural	1.	we saw	we were seen
	2.	you saw	you were seen
	3.	they saw	they were seen

Future tense

singular	1.	I will see	I will be seen
	2.	you will see	you will be seen
	3.	he will see	he will be seen
plural	1.	we will see	we will be seen
	2.	you will see	you will be seen
	3.	they will see	they will be seen

Perfect tense

singular	1.	I have seen	I have been seen, etc.
	2.	you have seen	
	3.	he has seen	
plural	1.	we have seen	
	2.	you have seen	
	3.	they have seen	

Past perfect tense

singular	1.	I had seen	I had been seen, etc.
	2.	you had seen	
	3.	he had seen	
plural	1.	we had seen	
	2.	you had seen	
	3.	they had seen	

Future perfect tense

1.	I will have seen, etc.	I will have been seen, etc.

gr

gr

conjunction A part of speech used to connect words, phrases, and clauses. There are the following kinds:

> **Coordinating** Pure, or simple, conjunctions: **and, or, nor, but, for, so, yet.** Correlatives: **either . . . or, neither . . . nor, both . . . and, not only . . . but [also].**
>
> **Subordinating** Conjunctions introducing noun clauses, adjective clauses, or adverb clauses: **that, when, where, while, whence, because, so that, although, since, as, after, if, until,** etc.

Coordinating conjunctions (see Chapter **9**) connect sentence elements that are logically and grammatically equal; i.e., they may connect two subjects or two verbs or two clauses, etc. Subordinating conjunctions (see Chapter **8**) connect subordinate (or dependent) clauses with their principal (or independent) clauses.

conjunctive adverb An introductory adverb, or sentence modifier, that indicates the relationship between principal clauses: *however, moreover, therefore, nevertheless, also, hence, consequently, then, furthermore,* etc. Between independent clauses a conjunctive adverb must be preceded by a semicolon or by a coordinating conjunction. See Chapter **31**.

connotation The associations, suggestions, feelings that a word brings to mind as opposed to its literal, dictionary meaning. For example, both *baby* and *infant* denote, or mean literally, a small child, but *baby* connotes coddling, affection, and tender protection. See **denotation.**

coordinate Sentence elements that are parallel in grammatical construction are coordinate. In the sentence *He and she talked lengthily and earnestly, and at last agreed, he* and *she* are coordinate; *talked* and *agreed* are coordinate; *lengthily* and *earnestly* are coordinate.

dangling modifier A word or phrase that does not modify another word or phrase or that cannot be easily linked to the sentence.

> **Dangling** *Dashing out the door,* the mat caused me to stumble.
>
> **Revised** Dashing out the door, *I* stumbled on the mat.

See Chapter **14** and **absolute construction.**

declension See **inflection.**

demonstrative See **adjective** and **pronoun.**

denotation The literal or dictionary definition of a word. See **connotation.**

diction Choice of words, especially as those words affect the tone of the writer's voice, depending on their formality or informality, the range of which is suggested below:

highly formal ⟶ highly informal

residence	home	house	pad
affluent	wealthy	rich	loaded
obtuse	ignorant	stupid	dumb

direct address   A grammatical construction in which the speaker or writer addresses a second person directly.

> **Mary,** wait for me.
>
> **Friends, Romans, countrymen,** lend me your ears.

direct object   See **object** and Chapter **9**.

double negative   A nonstandard form consisting of two negatives.

> **Double negative**   He **doesn't** have **no** place to go.

elliptical expression   An expression that is grammatically incomplete, but the meaning of which is clear because the omitted words are implied.

> **Elliptical**   **If possible,** bring your drawings along.
>
> **Complete**   **If it is possible,** bring your drawings along.
>
> **Elliptical**   To me he gave his watch; **to Mary,** [he gave] **his favorite painting.**

euphemism   The substitution of an "inoffensive," often trite and sentimental expression for one considered to be unpleasant or indelicate: *in an interesting condition* or *in the family way* are old-fashioned euphemisms for *pregnant.* See Chapter **15**.

finite verb   A verb that makes an assertion and can serve as a predicate, as distinguished from infinitives, participles, and gerunds.

> **Finite verb**   The alarm **rang** and I **got** up.
>
> **Verbal**   The **ringing** alarm awoke me and I hurried **to get** up.

gender   In grammar, the division of nouns (*actor, actress*) and pronouns (*he, she, it*) into sexual categories: masculine, feminine, and neuter.

genitive   See **case.**

gerund   A verb form ending in *-ing* and used as a noun. It should be distinguished from the present participle, which also ends in *-ing* but is used as an adjective. See **participle.**

> **Subject of verb**   **Fishing** is tiresome.
>
> **Object of verb**   I hate **fishing.**
>
> **Object of preposition**   I have a dislike of **fishing.**
>
> **Predicate noun**   The sport I like least is **fishing.**

Like a noun, the gerund may be modified by an adjective. In the sentence *They were tired of his long-winded preaching, his* and *long-winded* modify the gerund *preaching.* A noun or pronoun preceding a gerund is normally in the possessive case—e.g., *his* preaching. Since a gerund is a verb form, it may take an object and be modified by an adverb.

He disapproved of our **taking luggage** with us.
["Luggage" is the object of the gerund "taking."]

Our success depends upon his **acting promptly.**
["Promptly" is an adverb modifying the gerund "acting."]

idiom An expression whose meaning cannot be determined from the literal meaning of the individual words, but which as a whole is understood and used by speakers of a particular language or region.

She **was taken in** by the practical jokes.

Every now and then, I **have a mind** to **tell her off.**

He is, **after all,** my brother, and I have to **stick up for him.**

He was **out of his head** for a while, but he finally **pulled himself together.**

imperative See **mood.**

indicative See **mood.**

indirect object See **object** and Chapter **9.**

infinitive That form of the verb usually preceded by *to. To* is called the **sign of the infinitive.** Since it is a verb form, the infinitive can have a subject, can take an object or a predicate complement, and can be modified by an adverb.

They wanted **me to go.**
["Me" is the subject of "to go."]

They asked **to meet him.**
["Him" is the object of "to meet."]

We hope **to hear soon.**
["Soon" is the adverbial modifier of "to hear."]

The infinitive may be used as a noun (*To meet her* is a pleasure. He wanted *to buy my car*), or as an adjective or adverb (He gave me a book *to read.* He waited *to see you.* We are happy *to help*).

inflection A change in the form of a word to show a change in meaning or use. Nouns may be inflected to show number (*man, men*) and the genitive case (*dog, dog's*). Pronouns may be inflected to show case (*he, him*), person (*I, you*), number (*I, we*), and gender (*his, hers*). Verbs are inflected to show person (I *go,* he *goes*), number (she *is,* they *are*), tense (he *is,* he *was*), voice

(I *received* your letter, your letter *was received*), and mood (if this *be* treason). Adjectives and adverbs are inflected to show relative degree (*strong, stronger, strongest*). The inflection of substantives is called **declension;** that of verbs, **conjugation;** that of adjectives and adverbs, **comparison.**

intensive pronoun   When the pronouns *myself, himself, yourself,* etc., are used in apposition, they are called **intensives** because they serve to emphasize the substantives that they are used with; e.g., *I myself will do it. I saw the bishop himself.* When one of these words is used as the object of a verb and designates the same person or thing as the subject of that verb, it is called a **reflexive pronoun;** e.g., *I hurt myself. They benefit themselves.*

interjection   An exclamation that has no grammatical relation with the rest of the sentence; e.g., *oh, alas, please.*

intransitive   See **verb.**

irregular verb   A verb which does not form its past tense by adding *-ed* or *-t: sing, sang, sung; drink, drank, drunk.* Such a verb is sometimes called a **strong verb.** See Chapter **30** for a table of irregular verbs.

jargon   The specialized, technical language of a profession, class, group, or discipline that is usually obscure to the general public.

linking verb   A verb like *to be, to seem, to appear, to become, to feel,* or *to look,* which acts mainly as a connecting link between the subject and the predicate noun or predicate adjective.

misplaced modifier   A modifier that is awkwardly placed—usually too far from the term it modifies—so that its relation to rest of the sentence is confusing.

> **Misplaced**   I sped across the river which was frozen **on skates.**
>
> **Revised**   I sped **on skates** across the river which was frozen.

See Chapter **14.**

mixed construction   The fusion within a sentence of two parts that do not fit together grammatically or semantically.

> **Mixed**   Because she was early is the reason she found a seat.
>
> **Revised**   Because she was early she found a seat.

modifier   A word or group of words that functions as an adjective or an adverb to limit, define, or qualify another word or group of words. In the sentence "I dislike these sour oranges," *sour* describes *oranges* and *these* limits them to a nearby group. They are adjectival modifiers. In the sentence "She sang for half an hour" the phrase *for half an hour,* which tells how long she sang, is an adverbial modifier.

mood Inflection of a verb to indicate whether it is intended to make a statement or command or to express a condition contrary to fact.

The **indicative mood** is used to state a fact or to ask a question.

The wind is blowing.

Is it raining?

The **imperative mood** is used to express a command or a request.

Do it immediately.

Please answer the telephone.

The **subjunctive mood** is used to express a wish, a doubt, a concession, a condition contrary to fact (see Chapter **30**). In speech and in all but "edited" writing, the subjunctive mood has largely been replaced by the indicative.

Wish　I wish that I **were** able to help you.

Condition contrary to fact　If she **were** older, she would understand.

nominative See **case**.

nonrestrictive modifier A dependent clause or phrase that adds information without limiting the meaning of the word it modifies. See Chapter **32**.

noun A part of speech: a noun names a person, place, thing, or abstraction. There are the following kinds:

A **common noun** refers to any member of a group or class of things, or to abstract qualities; e.g., *man, village, book, courage*. Common nouns are not usually capitalized.

A **proper noun** or **proper name** is the name of a particular person, place, thing, or event; e.g., *Jane Austen, Chicago, Domesday Book, Revolutionary War*. Proper nouns are capitalized.

A **collective noun** is the name of a group or class considered as a unit; e.g., *flock, class, group, crowd, gang, team*.

Nouns may also function as modifiers; e.g., *town hall*. Such constructions are sometimes called **compound nouns**.

noun clause See **clause**.

number Inflection of verbs, nouns, and pronouns to indicate singular or plural.

object The **direct object** (see Chapter **9**) of a verb names the person or thing that completes the assertion made by a transitive verb. It answers the question *what* or *whom*.

Father dried the **dishes** and broke a **plate**.

I trusted **him** and followed his **advice**.

The **indirect object** (see Chapter **9**) of a verb is the person or thing to which something is given or for which something is done. The indirect object can usually be made the object of the preposition *for* or *to*.

I built my **wife** a shelf. = I built a shelf **for my wife.**

I wrote **him** a letter. = I wrote a letter **to him.**

objective (accusative)   See **case** and Chapter **28.**

objective complement   Either a noun or an adjective that completes the predicate by telling something about the direct object.

noun

They call him a **fool.**

adj.

I like my coffee **hot.**

ordinal number   See **cardinal number.**

parallelism   The stylistic device of putting equal ideas into equivalent structures in a sentence.

She wants **fame, prestige,** and **power.**
[The boldface words are equally weighted as objects of the verb "wants."]

That she must work hard, that many obstacles stand in her way, that few encourage her endeavors—these facts do not affect her pluck one bit.
[Clause is balanced against clause to create parallel structure.]

participle   A verb form used as an adjective. The present participle ends in *-ing*; e.g., *eating, running.* The past participle ends in *-ed, -d, -t, -en, -n* or is formed by vowel change; e.g., *stopped, told, slept, fallen, known, sung.*

Since a participle is a verbal adjective, it has the characteristics of both a verb and an adjective. Like an adjective, it modifies a substantive.

The **inquiring** reporter stopped him.

Encouraged by his help, she continued her work.

Having just **returned** from my vacation, I had not heard the news.

Like a verb the participle may take a direct or an indirect object and may be modified by an adverb:

Wishing us success, he drove away.
["Us" is an indirect object, "success" a direct object, of the participle "wishing."]

Stumbling awkwardly, he came into the room.
["Awkwardly" is an adverb modifying the participle "stumbling."]

gr

parts of speech   The classification of words according to the special function that they perform in a sentence: *nouns, pronouns, verbs, adjectives, adverbs, prepositions, interjections,* and *conjunctions.*

passive voice   See **voice** and Chapter **14.**

person   Inflection of verbs and personal pronouns to indicate the speaker **(first person),** the person spoken to **(second person),** and the person spoken of **(third person).**

First person   I am, we are; I go, we go.

Second person   you are; you go.

Third person   she is, they are; he goes, they go.

phrase   A phrase is a group of words without a subject and predicate, and used as a single part of speech—as a *substantive, verb, adjective,* or *adverb.* See Chapter **9.**

predicate   A group of words that makes a statement about, or asks a question about, the subject of the sentence (see Chapter **9**). Thus in the sentence *Jim drove the car,* "drove the car" is the predicate, because it tells what the subject *Jim* did. The predicate always contains a finite verb; e.g., *drove, had driven.*

The **simple predicate** is the verb alone. The **complete predicate** is the verb and its modifiers and complements.

Jim drove the car into the garage.
["Drove" is the simple predicate. "Drove the car into the garage" is the complete predicate.]

predicate adjective, predicate noun   See **complement.**

prefix   Letters added before a word's base to form a new word: *pre-, re-, com-.* See **suffix.**

preposition   A part of speech that shows the relationship between a substantive and another word in the sentence; e.g., *in, on, into, to, toward, from, for, against, of, between, with, without, before, behind, under, over, above, among, at, by, around, about, through.* The word that completes the meaning of the preposition is called the **object of the preposition.** In English many words may be used as either prepositions or adverbs, their classification depending on their function in the sentence. If they are followed by a substantive which, with them, forms a phrase, they are prepositions (see Chapter **9**); if by themselves they modify a verb, they are adverbs.

He stood **behind** the chair. [Preposition]

The money is **in** the bank. [Preposition]

They came **in** while we were there. [Adverb]

principal clause   See **clause.**

principal parts   In English, the three forms of a verb from which all other forms are derived. They are (1) the present infinitive, (2) the past tense, and (3) the past participle: *send, sent, sent; choose, chose, chosen; swim, swam, swum.* All present and future tense forms, including the present participle, are derived from the first principal part: I *send,* he *sends,* we *will send.* The second principal part is used for the simple past tense: he *sent,* I *chose,* you *swam.* Compound past tenses and the forms of the passive voice employ the third principal part: he *has chosen,* they *had swum,* the package *was sent,* or *may be sent, is being sent, will be sent,* etc.

gr

In learning a foreign language or in correcting unconventional English, one must know the principal parts of the irregular verbs (see Chapter **30**). The verb *to be* is too irregular to be reduced to three principal parts.

pronoun   A part of speech, a word used to refer to a noun already used (or implied). Pronouns may be classified as follows:

Personal	**I, you, he, she, it,** and their inflectional forms I listened to **her.**
Demonstrative	**this, that, these, those** **This** is my favorite book.
Interrogative	**who, which, what** **Who** can answer this question?
Relative	**who, which, that,** and compounds like **whoever** This is the house **that** Jack built.
Indefinite	**any, anyone, some, someone, no one, nobody, each, everybody, either,** etc. **Someone** has my pen.
Reflexive	**myself, yourself,** etc. I hurt **myself.**
Intensive	**myself, yourself,** etc. He **himself** is to blame.
Reciprocal	**each other, one another** John and Mary looked at **each other.**

regular verb   A verb that forms its past tenses by adding *-ed* or *-t: start, started; dream, dreamed* or *dreamt.* Also called a **weak verb.**

relative pronoun   A pronoun (*who, which,* or *that*) used with a double function: to take the place of a noun and to connect clauses as does a subordinating conjunction (see Chapter **28**).

restrictive modifier A dependent clause or phrase intended to define or limit the word it modifies (see Chapter **32**).

restrictive

The students **who come regularly to class** do better work and earn

restrictive

higher marks than the students **who attend only periodically.**

gr

run-on sentence A sentence error in which two independent clauses are joined without any punctuation or conjunction. Also called a **fused sentence.**

Run-on The car stalled at the corner it was out of gas.

Revised The car stalled at the corner. It was out of gas.

See Chapter **31**.

sentence An independent utterance, usually including a subject and predicate, that can stand by itself and is set off by capitalization of its beginning and a period or other terminal punctuation at the end. A sentence may range in length from one word (*Why?*) or short phrases (*What an absurd idea!*) to a main clause (*I saw him sitting on the fence*). See Chapter **9**.

From the point of view of structure, sentences are classified as **simple, compound, complex,** or **compound-complex.** See Chapter **9**.

From the point of view of meaning or function, sentences may be classified as follows:

1. A **declarative sentence** asserts something about a subject.

   The man felt ill and called the doctor.

2. An **interrogative sentence** asks a question.

   When is she coming?

3. An **imperative sentence** expresses a command.

   Call him again.

4. An **exclamatory sentence** expresses strong feeling.

   What a fool he was!

   For further discussion, see Chapters **9** and **10**; see also Chapter **31**, especially for the discussion of so-called "incomplete" forms.

sentence fragment Dependent clauses or phrases which are punctuated as sentences but which should be joined to an independent clause or made into one.

Fragment   I accepted jury duty. **Being as I was free.**

Revised   I accepted jury duty **since I was free.**

See Chapter **31**.

subject   The part of the sentence or clause naming the person or thing about which something is said. The subject of a sentence is usually a noun or pronoun, but it may be a verbal, or phrase, or a noun clause. See Chapter **9**.

Noun   Beyond the ridge lay a high **plateau.**

Verbal   Nowadays **flying** is both safe and cheap.

Phrase   **"To fear the worst** oft cures the worse."

Clause   **That she will be promoted** is certain.

The simple subject is a substantive, usually a noun or pronoun. The **complete subject** is the simple subject and its modifiers.

The young trees that we planted last year have grown tall.
["Trees" is the simple subject. "The young trees that we planted last year" is the complete subject.]

subjunctive   See **mood** and Chapter **30**.

subordination   Making one element of a sentence grammatically dependent on another in order to show the relationship of ideas.

When the party was over, I left.
[The subordinate clause with "when" limits the time of the action.]

See Chapter **9**.

substantive   Any word or group of words used as a noun. It may be a noun, a pronoun, a clause, an infinitive, or a gerund.

suffix   Letters added at the end of a word's base to form a new word: *-tion, -ship, -ing*. See **prefix**.

syntax   The way in which words are put together to make phrases, clauses, and sentences.

tense   Different forms of a verb that indicate distinctions in time. In English there are six tenses: the present tense, the past tense, the future tense, the perfect (present perfect) tense, the past perfect tense, and the future perfect tense. See **conjugation** for examples.

verb   A part of speech whose function is to assert that the subject exists, acts, or has certain characteristics. (The man who *is* on my left *wrote* the book; he *is* very difficult to talk to.) The verb may be a word or a group of words, but in either case its form changes to indicate time, person, mood. (He *was saying* that I *am* too young but *should have* a chance next year.)

A **transitive verb** is a verb that requires a direct object (noun or other substantive) to complete its meaning.

He **shut** the **door.**
["Door" completes the statement by telling what was shut.]

They **greeted her.**

An **intransitive verb** is a verb that does not require a direct object.

After a heated argument, he **left.**

The child **sat** near the fire.

A **linking verb** acts mainly as a connecting link between the subject and the predicate noun or predicate adjective.

That **is** correct.

He **seems** sleepy.

She **felt** warm.

verbals Forms of a verb (*stealing, stolen, to steal*) used as nouns, adjectives, or adverbs. See **gerund, participle, infinitive,** and Chapter **9.**

voice Inflection of a verb to indicate the relation of the subject to the action expressed by the verb. A verb is in the **active voice** when its subject is the doer of the action. A verb is in the **passive voice** when its subject is acted upon.

Active voice I **rang** the bell.
[The subject "I" did the act of "ringing."]

Passive voice The bell **was rung** by me.
[The subject "bell" was acted upon by "me."]

weak verb See **regular verb.**

word order The ordering of words in a sentence, a major determinant of meaning in English.

Peter broke up with Mary.

Mary broke up with Peter.

I saved the lifeguard.

I was saved by the lifeguard.

gr

Index